Volume 35 in the Series

Major Problems in Neurology
PROFESSOR CP WARLOW, BA, MB, BChir, MD, FRCP
PROFESSOR J VAN GIJN, MD, FRCPE
Consulting Editors

OTHER MONOGRAPHS IN THE SERIES

NEUROLOGY OF THE INFLAMMATORY CONNECTIVE TISSUE DISEASES

FRANS G.I. JENNEKENS
Professor of Neuromyology
Department of Neurology
University of Utrecht

LOUIS KATER
Professor of Clinical Immunopathology
Department of Internal Medicine, Division of Rheumatology
and Clinical Immunology
University of Utrecht

 W.B. Saunders Company

London · Edinburgh · Philadelphia · New York · Sydney · Toronto

WB SAUNDERS
An imprint of Harcourt Brace and Company Limited

© Harcourt Brace and Company Ltd 1999

First published 1999

ISBN 0–7020–22314

British Library Cataloguing in Publication Data
A catalogue record for this book is available from the British Library

Library of Congress Cataloguing in Publication Data
A catalog record for this book is available from the Library of Congress

Note
Medical knowledge is constantly changing. As new information becomes available, changes in treatment, procedures, equipment and the use of drugs become necessary. The editors/authors/contributors and the publishers have, as far as it is possible, taken care to ensure that the information given in this text is accurate and up-to-date. However, readers are strongly advised to confirm that the information, especially with regard to drug usuage, complies with the latest legislation and standards of practice.

Typeset by Phoenix Photosetting, Chatham, Kent
Printed and bound in China

The
Publisher's
policy is to use
**papaer manufactured
from sustainable forests**

Contents

Acknowledgements

This book covers a large part of the field of neurology, a small part of psychiatry and a considerable number of immune-mediated internal medicine diseases. Overlooking such a wide field carries the risk of incompleteness, superficialness, and worst of all mistakes. Fortunately, friends and colleagues appeared prepared to read critically previous versions of chapters and parts of chapters. Without their advice this would have been just another book. Their names and fields of expertise are: Dr. Harold Baart de la Faille, dermatology; Prof. Hans Bijlsma, rheumatology; Dr. Ron Derksen, clinical immunology; Dr. Gert W. van Dijk, neurology; Dr. Frits Gmelig Meyling, immunology; Prof. Jan van Gijn, neurology; Prof. Cees Kallenberg, clinical immunology; Dr. Aike Kruize, rheumatology; Prof. Jan Robbertze, psychiatry; Dr. Annet van Royen-Kerkhof, paediatric immunology; Dr. Charles Vecht, neurology; and Prof. Marianne de Visser, neuromuscular disorders.

Especially, we thank Dr. Lino Ramos for his hours of wit and expertise and for providing most of the radiology figures.

Our partners, Mrs. Debby Kater-Schipper and Dr. Aagje Jennekens-Schinkel, greatly stimulated us in this undertaking: without them this book would not have been written.

FRANS GI JENNEKENS AND LOUIS KATER

Foreword

Inflammatory connective tissue diseases confuse neurologists because, not only do they rather rarely cause or present with neurological complications, but most neurologists are unlikely to know much about their underlying pathology and biology. On the other hand, rheumatologists for whom these diseases are their stock in trade, may find the neurological syndromes difficult to sort out and understand. Also, when it comes to treatment, everyone is handicapped by the serious lack of good evidence from randomised controlled trials. Any account of the neurology of inflammatory connective tissue diseases must therefore be written by a neurologist and a rheumatologist who have a clear view of the difficulties. This is precisely what Frans Jennekens and Louis Kater have combined to do in a way which first explains the "neurology" to the non-neurologist and others and secondly the mysteries of the autoantibodies and treatments to the neurologist. They then take us through the clinical features, diagnosis and treatment of the various disorders with a welcome tendency to be over-rather than under-inclusive. This is certainly the sort of book I will reach for the next time I ask myself about a patient "is it multiple sclerosis or systemic lupus?", or when I need to know how to treat a patient with the antiphospholipid antibody syndrome. Even if the authors don't always tell me precisely what I need to know (because no-one knows), they at least tell me what is known and, as importantly, what is not known, and point me towards the appropriate references. I hope that my rheumatological friends and colleagues, and others involved with the care of patients with these disorders, will find this book just as useful.

CHARLES WARLOW
Edinburgh

1

Introduction

Inflammatory connective tissue diseases (ICTDs) are a group of diseases of the musculoskeletal system and allied disorders that that are all considered to be immunologically mediated. The main representatives of this group are rheumatoid arthritis (RA), systemic lupus erythematosus (SLE), Sjögren's syndrome, scleroderma, dermatomyositis and polymyositis, and the vasculitides. Other diseases – from the neurological point of view less prominent, but not necessarily less serious – in this group are juvenile chronic arthritis, adult Still's disease, acute rheumatic fever, polymyalgia rheumatica and relapsing polychondritis. Though clinically there is a marked overlap between these diseases, the difference in immunopathology is nevertheless considerable. With rheumatic fever as the only exception, the aetiology has not been identified yet, despite much research and many theories.

What then – apart from clinical characteristics – do the ICTDs have in common? They have all immunological abnormalities: inflammatory reactions, auto-antibodies and immune complexes. In contrast to the antibodies in diseases such as Lambert-Eaton myasthenic syndrome (LEMS) and myasthenia gravis (MG), the auto-antibodies in the inflammatory connective tissue diseases are usually not organ specific and seem to act merely as epiphenomena. The antinuclear antibodies (ANAs) are probably the best example. They most likely reflect a disturbance in the immune regulation: for instance, a loss of immune suppressor activity of the T-cell system, which in turn may be caused by immunogenetic, hormonal and environmental factors. The occurrence of auto-antibodies like ANAs and rheumatoid factor (RF) in healthy individuals in low titre (*e.g.*, in the elderly) is generally taken to express a decreased suppressor activity. Significant elevated titres may be associated with diseases and may serve as diagnostic tools, if they are at least specific for one or several of the ICTDs or subgroups thereof.

Strong indications exist for a pathogenetic role of genetic factors, as for instance the immune response gene make-up (HLA system) and genetic deficiencies of the complement system. However, none of the ICTDs show clear inheritance patterns.

Recently, the conception that many clinical features are mediated through vasculitis, spreading the diseases throughout the body, was challenged by the dis-

1

covery of antiphospholipid antibodies and their association with disease manifestations (see Chap. 8, the Hughes' syndrome). What generally was considered to be inflammation-mediated, is at least in some cases due to vasculopathy and to arterial and venous thrombotic events. The ongoing gradual conceptual shift from vasculitis to vasculopathy as causative mechanism, for the internal as well as for neurological manifestations of the ICTDs, has contributed to the growing uncertainty about the best method of treatment. At present, only a few of the available guidelines for drug treatment of the ICTDs are based on results of intervention studies. Choices for treatment policies often have to be made on insecure grounds. Added to the already existing dilemmas is that at least some neurological manifestations may be due primarily to an abnormality in coagulation instead of vasculitis.

In this book, the neurological manifestations are described against the general background of the respective diseases. Aetiology, pathogenesis and laboratory features are discussed as far as necessary for understanding clinical characteristics and for decisions on treatment. Chapter 2 is written primarily as an update for those readers who are not busy daily with keeping abreast of the developments in the neurological field. It deals with the neurological syndromes in the ICTDs and gives the foundation to which subsequent chapters refer. Chapters 3 and 4 are short, clinically oriented overviews, which respectively discuss antibodies relevant for diagnosis and treatment and immuno-therapy. Chapters 5 and 6 concentrate on the inflammatory disorders of two systems, the vascular and the skeletal muscle system. The neurological aspects of the other ICTDs are described in Chapters 7–12. The antiphospholipid syndrome is given the name Hughes' syndrome, according to Drs. Khamashta and Petri's proposal. For practical reasons, Chapters 9 and 12 deal with several more or less closely related disorders.

2

Update on Neurological Syndromes Featuring Inflammatory Connective Tissue Diseases

CHAPTER AIM

The mutual relationship of the inflammatory connective tissue diseases (ICTDs) is expressed in shared clinical and laboratory features. Neurological manifestations are frequent in the ICTDs, and together cover a large part of the field of neurology. To prevent undue repetition in succeeding chapters, the present chapter is used as an update, as far as deemed relevant, on some of these neurological manifestations. The first part of this chapter is devoted to syndromes of the central nervous system (CNS), the second to those of the peripheral nervous system (PNS) and the third to disturbances of the neuromuscular junctions. Table 2.1 summarizes the syndromes that will be discussed. For skeletal muscle syndromes, the reader is referred to Chapter 6 and for neuro-vasculitic syndromes to Chapter 5.

THE CENTRAL NERVOUS SYSTEM (CNS)

INTRODUCTION

The CNS is an incredibly complicated structure. It contains approximately 10^{10} post-mitotic neurones and the wiring required to connect these neurones, which consists of axons and dendrites in the grey substance and short and long fibre tracts in the white substance. In between neurones and nerve fibres are the astrocytes, subserving metabolic and supportive functions, and the oligodendroglia cells, which form the myelin sheaths of the nerve fibres. In addition, there are microglia cells, which are the macrophages of the CNS. Each neuronal cell body is covered by synapses (Fig. 2.1). Tens of neurotransmitters and hundreds of different receptors are found in the brain.

The endothelium of the CNS vessels constitutes a barrier between the blood and the CNS tissue to which the endothelial extracellular matrix and the perivascular

Table 2.1 The main neurological syndromes featuring inflammatory connective tissue diseases

	Vasc	Myos	SLE	Hugh	RA	JCA	RF	Scler	Sjö	MCT	PMR	RP
Coma	+	−	+	+	−	+/−	−	−	−	−	−	−
Delirium, OBS	+	−	+	+	+	−	−	−	−	+	−	+
Dementia	+	−	+	+	−	−	−	−	+/−	−	−	+/−
Psychosis	−	−	+	−	−	−	−	−	−	+/−	−	−
Epilepsia	+	−	+	+	+	−	−	+	+	+	−	+/−
Infarct	+	−	+	+	−	−	−	−	+	+/−	−	−
CVT	+	−	+	+	−	−	−	−	+	−	−	−
Intr haemorr	+	−	+	−	−	−	−	−	+	+/−	−	−
White matt d	+	−	+	+/−	−	−	−	−	+	−	−	+
Optic neurit	+	−	+	+	+/−	−	−	−	+	+/−	−	+
Transv myel	+	−	+	+	−	−	−	+/−	+	+	−	−
Chorea	−	−	+	+	−	−	+	−	−	−	−	−
Mening synd	+	−	+	−	+	+/−	−	−	+	+	−	+
Trig neurop	+	−	+	−	+	−	−	+	+	+	−	−
Spin ganglion	+/−	−	−	−	−	−	−	−	+	−	−	−
Infl neurop	−	−	+	−	−	−	−	−	+	+	−	−
MG	−	−	+	−	+	−	−	+	+	−	−	−
LEMS	−	−	+	−	−	−	−	−	−	−	−	+
Acq neuromy	−	−	+	−	−	+	−	−	−	−	−	−

Horizontal abbreviations: Vasc, vasculitis; Myos, myositis; SLE, systemic lupus erythematosus; Hugh, Hughes' syndrome or antiphospholipid syndrome; RA, rheumatoid arthritis; JCA, juvenile chronic arthritis; RF, rheumatic fever; Scler, scleroderma; Sjö, Sjögren's syndrome; MCT, mixed connective tissue disease; PMR, polymyalgia rheumatica; RP, relapsing polychondritis.

Vertical abbreviations: OBS, organic brain syndrome; CVT, cerebral venous thrombosis; Intr haemorr, intracranial haemorrhage; White matt d, white matter disease; Optic neurit, optic neuritis; Transv myel, transverse myelitis; Mening Synd, meningeal syndrome; Tig neurop, tigeminal neuropathy; Spin ganglion, spinal ganglinitis; Infl neurop, inflammatory neuropathy; MG, myasthenia gravis; LEMS, Lambert-Eaton myasthenic syndrome; Acq neuromy, acquired neuromyotonia.

glia limitans contribute. This barrier protects the CNS tissue from the entrance of some specific dyes and other substances, as shown in experimental investigations (Reese and Karnowsky, 1967; Cserr and Knopf, 1992). The barrier is, however, easily permeable to hydrophilic compounds and has a number of carrier-mediated transport systems. Activated T-cells can also enter the CNS (Ludowyk *et al.*, 1992). Under pathological conditions, the barrier may cease to function, thus providing a free entrance to cells and substances into the CNS compartment.

DIFFUSE AND FOCAL DYSFUNCTION AND LESIONS

Lesions of the CNS may be diffuse, affecting one or several elements of the nervous tissue to varying degrees, or they may be focal. Diffuse lesions often only affect part of the CNS and a specific neuronal population or a specific structure in the CNS. In some disorders, for instance, only Purkinje cells are affected. Amyotrophic lateral sclerosis (ALS) causes widespread degeneration throughout the CNS, predominantly of the motor neurones. The preferential susceptibility of some specific neurones may be due to antibodies against specific proteins, *e.g.* anti-Yo antibodies

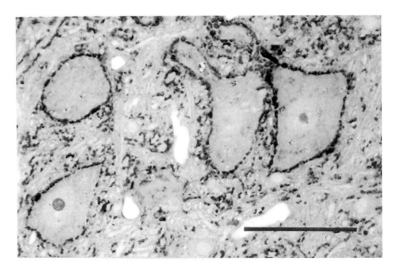

Figure 2.1 Synapses (black dots) on cell bodies of four lower motor neurones in facial nucleus of rat. Synapses are stained immunohistochemically by antisynaptophysin antibodies. Synaptophysin is an integral membrane glycoprotein of presynaptic vesicles. Synapses are also present in the neuropil, *e.g.* between axons and dendrites. Bar: 50 μm. (Courtesy of Dr. Herman JLM Ulenkate.)

against Purkinje cells in paraneoplastic disorders (Smith *et al.*, 1988; see Lai, 1997), or to a gene mutation leading to a disorder in protein synthesis, as in familial amyotrophic lateral sclerosis (Rosen *et al.*, 1993). The clinical features of these diffuse diseases depend on the population of neurones or synapses involved. Cerebellar ataxia is a clinical feature in disorders of Purkinje cells and a pyramidal syndrome and muscle weakness are features in familial ALS. Diffuse lesions may also result from a disorder of a structure subserving neuronal functioning, as for instance widespread small vessel disease in SLE (see Chapter 7, *Encephalopathy due to Small Vessel Disease*).

Focal lesions concern damage at a specific site and are usually due to a space occupying or traumatic lesion, or to a vascular accident. All cells present at that site are at risk. The clinical features depend on the role of the neurones at that site or the fibre tract that is interrupted.

Diffuse dysfunction can result from an evanescent abnormal condition (*e.g.*, intoxications), a widespread diffuse lesion (*e.g.*, due to hypoxia or trauma), or a local lesion (*e.g.*, in the brainstem that disturbs arousal of the cortical neurones, or which acts, as epileptic focus for secondary generalized seizures).

COMA AND DELIRIUM

Two aspects of consciousness that should be distinguished are arousal and content (Plum and Posner, 1982). Arousal is stirred up by elements in the reticular formation of the brainstem, extending from pons to diencephalon. Consciousness is the whole of cognitive and affective functions. The brainstem system arouses the cortex of the hemispheres and is, along with the cortex, responsible for self-awareness and conscious behaviour. Coma is due to widespread cortical lesions, to a local lesion of the reticular formation in the brainstem, or to both. The stages between full consciousness and coma are best assessed with the Glasgow Coma Scale (Table 2.2) (Jennett and Teasdale, 1977). The pupillary reactions deserve special attention for differential diagnostic reasons. They are commonly lost in coma due to traumatic brain injury or to space occupying lesions, since the nuclei controlling pupillary motility and the brainstem structures governing the arousal system are close to each other. The nuclei and nerves regulating pupil width are, on the other hand, not easily influenced by metabolic substances. Coma is therefore likely to be metabolic when pupillary motility is preserved.

Organic brain syndrome refers to a condition that resembles delirium but has not yet fully developed into a delirium. Consciousness of individuals in a delirium is disturbed, and this contributes to or is responsible for a state of disorientation and for mistaken interpretations of perceptions, in particular visual perceptions. Patients in this condition are agitated, restless and fearful (see Chapter 7, *criteria of delirium*). The pathogenetic mechanism underlying delirium has not been clarified yet. It is not known whether it is always due to diffuse dysfunction or, in some cases, to a diffuse or local lesion.

COGNITIVE DISORDERS AND DEMENTIA

Several specific cognitive domains are distinguished, *e.g.* memory disorders, aphasia, apraxia, agnosia, and disorders of executive functions among others. Impairment of cognition may be generalized, affecting all cognitive domains, or specific. According to the Diagnostic and Statistical Manual of Mental Disorders 1994 (DSM-IV), the designation dementia is applicable when there are multiple cognitive deficits, including memory deficit, sufficiently severe to cause impairment

Table 2.2 The Glasgow Coma Scale

Eye-opening (E)	Spontaneous	4	
	To speech	3	
	To pain	2	
	Nil	1	
Motor response (M)	Obeys	6	
	Localizes	5	
	Withdraws	4	
	Abnormal flexion	3	
	Extensor response	2	
	Nil	1	
Verbal response (V)	Oriented	5	
	Confused conversation	4	
	Inappropriate words	3	
	Incomprehensible words	2	
	Nil	1	
Coma Score	E+M+V	Minimal 3	
		Maximum 15	

From Jennet and Teasdale (1977), with permission.

in occupational or social functioning. It has been suggested that subcortical (white matter) dementia which is characterized by slowed information processing, apathy, depression or euphoria, memory retrieval failure, and impaired reasoning skills, should be distinguished from cortical dementia in which the instruments of cognition (*e.g.*, language) are also affected (Jennekens-Schinkel *et al.*, 1990). Disorders of specific cognitive domains are due to localized brain lesions.

A thorough investigation of cognition requires assessment of problem solving, memory, learning, conceptional reasoning, language, constructional skills, attention, reaction times and motor speed (Table 2.3). These investigations require expertise and at least twice as much time as, for instance, magnetic resonance imaging (MRI) of the brain, and are therefore not always adequately performed. The Mini Mental State Examination (MMSE) is a short list of queries that is often used to screen for dementia. Its advantage is that it requires little time and no expertise. Its drawback is that it is inaccurate and insensitive. The Screening Examination For Cognitive Impairment (SEFCI) and the Cambridge Cognitive Examination

Table 2.3 Comprehensive assessment of cognition. Example of a choice of tests.

Test name	Test purpose	Time required
Standard progressive matrices (Raven)	Tests accuracy of discrimination and evaluation of logical relations in visual display	25 min.
*WAIS vocabulary test	To test general mental ability; to demonstrate effects of dominant hemisphere disease	15 min.
Wechsler memory scale	Traditional clinical memory battery	10 min.
Cube imitation test	Non-verbal immediate memory test	3 min.
Wisconsin card sorting test	Test of abstract reasoning and shifting of mental set	10 min.
California verbal learning test	Assessment of immediate free recall and delayed recall	20 min.
Pattern learning	Recall and recognition of dot patterns	5 min.
Colour word test	To test occurrence of perceptual interference	3 min.
Naming to confrontation	Description and analysis of errors	5 min.
Word generation according to lexical rules	Number of correct words; perseveration in four trials	5 min.
Hundred words reading test	Test of rapid and accurate reading	1 min.
Writing to dictation	Analysis of errors	2 min.
Figure copying	Test of constructional skill	2 min.

For description of tests see Lezak (1995).
*WAIS, Wechsler Adult Intelligence Scale.

(CAMCOG) have been put forward as alternatives (Beatty *et al.*, 1995; Kwa *et al.*, 1996). Disorders of cognition occur in SLE, Hughes' syndrome (antiphospholipid syndrome), perhaps in Sjögren's syndrome and in a number of the vasculitides (see Table 2.1)

PSYCHOSIS

Psychotic conditions are characterized by disorders of thought and perception. Patients complain about delusions and hallucinations and may demonstrate a series of changes in language and behaviour. Consciousness is entirely undisturbed. The prototype of all psychoses is schizophrenia (Sedvall and Farde, 1995; Ross and Pearlson, 1996). The present insights into the changes underlying psychotic behaviour are due in part to the study of the cellular pharmacology of drugs that provoke psychotic reactions. One of these drugs, phencyclidine, has attracted considerable scientific interest because it induces schizophrenia-like symptoms and worsens symptoms of schizophrenic patients (Javitt and Zukin, 1991; Gorelick and Balster, 1995; Olney and Farber, 1995).

Phencyclidine (PCP), also known as 'angel dust', is a synthetic arylcyclohexyl-amine and was initially developed as a general anaesthetic. Following anaesthesia with PCP, a high percentage of the individuals treated with it, proved to be psychotic for periods of up to 72 hours, and occasional subjects even for 7–10 days. PCP concentrations in serum associated with these psychotic reactions were up to 100 ng/ml (0.4 µmol). The molecular target of PCP, which is responsible for the psychotic reaction, should have the affinity to bind PCP that is present in such concentrations. PCP is lipid soluble and crosses the blood-brain barrier without any difficulty. A brain receptor with the required affinity was discovered in 1979 and appeared to be a site located in the ion channel of the N-methyl-D-aspartate (NMDA) receptor. PCP appeared to inhibit non-competitively glutamatergic neurotransmission and to cause NMDA receptor hypofunction. This conclusion was supported by studies of cloned NMDA receptor sub-units that were shown to be PCP sensitive ion channels. Other NMDA antagonists were demonstrated to induce, in appropriate dosages, phencyclidine-like psychotic reactions. The evidence is therefore in favour of the notion that NMDA receptor hypofunction is psychotogenic.

The relevant point here is that psychotic reactions appear to be related, at least in some conditions, to abnormal interaction between neurones and to imbalance between different neuronal circuits. These disorders come into being at the synaptic level, which explains why they cannot be visualized easily or related to structural damage. Antibody binding may well cause channel-blocking and channel-hypofunction and may conceivably induce psychotic episodes. Psychosis as described here is not a feature of vascular brain lesions. Entirely reversible psychotic reactions occur in patients with SLE and may be induced by treatment with corticosteroids. The DSM-IV criteria for a psychotic condition due to a general medical condition are described in chapter 7. Treatment of psychosis is described there also.

EPILEPSY

Approximately 40 different epileptic syndromes have been described in humans. Primary generalized seizures with widespread changes occurring simultaneously over the whole cortex are to be distinguished from seizures with focal onset (Dreifuss and Henriksen, 1992).

Primary generalized epilepsy

The behavioural manifestations of primary generalized epilepsy are absences, myoclonic- and tonic-clonic fits and atonia. Absences are believed to be related to disturbances in thalamocortical rhythms. Some thalamic relay neurones have axons that are widely ramifying and can fire in bursts that entail the whole cortex. Studies in animal models of primary convulsive epilepsy point to regulatory roles of brainstem neurones, or more specifically neurones in the inferior- and superior-colliculus and the substantia nigra (Dichter, 1994; Hosford, 1995).

Management. The drug of first choice for treatment of convulsive primary generalized epilepsy is either carbamazepine or valproic acid.

Partial epilepsy

Every cortical area has its local circuit with inhibitory and excitatory connections. Input into this local circuit from neurones in other regions is also either inhibitory or excitatory. Ion channels, neurotransmitters and neurotransmitter receptors all play a role in these circuits. Events that disturb the balance between excitation and inhibition may cause a seizure. Spreading of simultaneous discharges of a local group of neurones is usually prevented by 'surround inhibition.' However, in some circumstances, nearby neurones also start to discharge and seizure activity may then propagate over the whole hemisphere or the whole cortex, thus causing a secondary generalized tonic-clonic seizure (Dichter, 1994; McNamara, 1994; Hosford, 1995).

Now the question is how a focal lesion may cause focal discharges of nearby neurones and partial epilepsy. Experimental investigations have shown that repeated focal application of subliminal electrical stimulations may eventually induce partial epilepsy and secondary generalized convulsions. The repeated stimulations apparently cause a local increase of sensitivity. Similarly, focal lesions, such as neoplasms or vascular anomalies, also may induce focal hyperexcitability with some spreading to synaptically related nearby neurones.

Several ICTDs are associated with epilepsy, usually partial epilepsy or secondary generalized epilepsy, more often than explainable by chance (Aarli, 1993). Among these are vasculitis, SLE, and Hughes' syndrome, as will be discussed in Chapters 5, 7 and 8.

Management. Drugs of first choice for partial epilepsy or secondary generalized epilepsy are carbamazepine or phenytoine in that order.

Status epilepticus in older children and adults

The nature of the mechanisms that generally abort isolated seizures and fail in status epilepticus is insufficiently known. Lowenstein and Alldredge (1998) proposed the following as a working definition for status epilepticus: continuous seizures lasting at least 5 minutes or two or more discrete seizures with incomplete recovery of consciousness in between. Status epilepticus of patients with CNS diseases of recent onset, like vascular disorders and infections, are relatively difficult to control. The status epilepticus of patients with ICTDs belongs to this category.

Management. Care for a patient in a status epilepticus involves a few general measures and drug therapy. The algorithms proposed by Lowenstein and Alldredge for management of status epilepticus include:

 – that the airway be kept free and 100% oxygen given to compensate for the periods of apnoe in between seizures;
 – that high fever in patients with CNS injury be prevented as it is unfavourable for the nervous tissue (see management of ischaemic stroke);
 – that lorazepam be the drug of first choice (0.1 mg/kg at 2 mg/min) because it is as equally fast acting and effective as diazepam and has a longer antiseizure effect. The adverse effects on respiration (depression), blood pressure (hypotension), and consciousness (impairment of consciousness) are also similar as of diazepam;
 – that phenytoin be added if lorazepam is not sufficient to stop seizures. The recommended dose is 20 mg/kg intravenously at a maximum rate of 50 mg/min. Up to 50% of patients receiving phenytoin at this dose and rate develop hypotension and 2% bradycardia and ectopic beats.

For out of hospital treatment, Lowenstein and Alldredge advocate either rectal administration of diazepam fluid or gel (0.5 mg/kg, maximum 20 mg) or intramuscular administration of midazolam (0.15 to 0.3 mg/kg). These two forms of therapy usually terminate seizures within 10 to 15 minutes.

INFARCTS AND ISCHAEMIC STROKES

It may be that effective treatment of ischaemic strokes with either neuro-protectiva or thrombolytica will be available in the very near future. First, we shall discuss the effects of oxygen shortage on nerve cells and then we will describe the actual situation concerning diagnosis and treatment of ischaemic stroke.

How do nerve cells die?
Commonly, nerve cells die by necrosis or apoptosis, as do cells in other organs (Wyllie and Duvall, 1992) (Table 2.4). In the process leading to necrosis, a reversible

Table 2.4 Features of necrosis and apoptosis

	Necrosis	*Apoptosis*
Cytological aspect	Swelling	Shrinkage
Cell membrane	From an early stage permeable for vital stains	Initially not permeable
Cell nucleus	Swelling and fading	Coarse chromatin granules
When occurring	In pathological conditions, groups of cells	May be physiological, programmed, single cells
Biochemistry	Energy supply fails and protein synthesis stops	Dependent on energy supply and protein synthesis
Histological reaction	Inflammatory, glial cell proliferation	Phagocytosis

Data from James (1994) and Bär (1996).

and an irreversible phase can be distinguished. The reversible part is morphologically characterized by swelling of the cytoplasm and the cisterns of the smooth endoplasmatic reticulum and by loss of ribosomes from the rough endoplasmatic reticulum. The cell membrane starts bulging at places where the cytoskeleton is weakened and blebs develop. These blebs may tie off from the cell. After the 'point of no return' has passed, floccular densities appear in swollen mitochondria. The cell membrane becomes permeable, Ca^{++} and Na^+ ions enter into the cells and proteins leak out. The cell nucleus fades away (karyolysis) or disintegrates (karyorrhexis).

Characteristic for the nervous system is a process labelled *excitotoxic cell death*, which means that nerve cells may become necrotic and die by abnormal interaction between neurones. Excitotoxity as the basis for neuronal cell disease and death was hypothesized in the second half of the seventies by Olney, and it is now accepted as an important mechanism underlying various acute and chronic diseases (Olney, 1978; Lipton and Rosenberg, 1994; Doble, 1995). In brief, amino acids serve in many CNS synapses as neurotransmitters. Glutamic acid is the main excitatory transmitter in the CNS and acts at approximately 30% of all CNS synapses. Receptors of two of the three excitatory amino acid receptor classes are ligand-gated cation channels. Various subtypes of these receptors are expressed by cells in different cell populations. When substrates for energy metabolism are no longer available to neurones, due to anoxia or vascular occlusion, energy production decreases and then stops, making maintenance of the membrane potential no longer feasible. The membrane becomes depolarized and Na^+ and Ca^{++} ions enter into the cells by voltage-gated ion channels (Fig. 2.2). Sodium entry is followed by the entry of water, by osmotic swelling and cell lysis. Entry of Ca^{++} ions impedes the functional capacity of mitochondria and stimulates many enzymes, including Ca-dependent proteases. It also stimulates release of vesicles containing neurotransmitters, many of which contain the transmitter glutamic acid. What follows is an excessive rise of extracellular glutamic acid, entry of Na^+ and Ca^{++} by excitatory receptor ion channels in nearby neurones, spreading of depolarization to nearby neurones, Ca overload of these neurones, etc. This *glutamergic loop* amplifies and spreads tissue necrosis (Doble, 1995).

Cells can initiate and regulate their own death (apoptosis). *Apoptosis* is an essential feature in orderly development, allowing the organism to dispose neatly of cells in excess. Once the process of apoptosis has started, it takes probably an hour or less before the cell is cleared away, and it does not create any reaction in its environment, as does necrosis. The morphological definition of apoptosis includes (1) cell shrinkage, (2) condensation of chromatin and nuclear fragmentation, (3) development of blebs and break away of cell fragments (apoptotic bodies), and (4) phagocytosis by nearby cells or macrophages (Fig. 2.3). Apoptosis is controlled by pro- and inhibitory genes, one of these being the inhibitory gene *bcl-2*. How its gene product, *bcl-2*, inhibits the apoptotic process is not yet fully known (Bär, 1996).

Recovery after damage of neurones

Neurones in the human brain are probably all postmitotic and dead neurones will therefore not be replaced by new neurones. The tasks that had been fulfilled by these now dead neurones can be taken over, however, by other neurones. Image analysis in laboratory animals and in humans has shown that this is more than a theoretical option (Mano *et al.*, 1995). Not all damaged neuronal cell bodies necessarily die. Some may recover when the cause of the damage is removed.

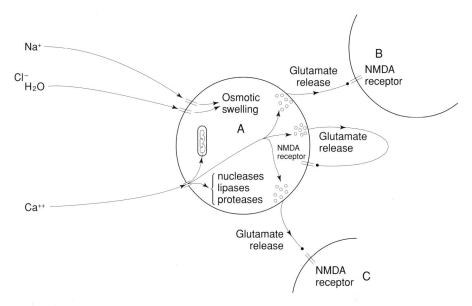

Figure 2.2 Consequences of anoxia-induced depolarization of a nerve cell. Due to anoxia, the membrane of nerve cell A is depolarized and voltage-gated ion channels in the cell membrane open, allowing for excess influx of Na^+ and Ca^{++}. The influx of sodium ions has excess influx of Cl^- and H_2O, and osmotic swelling of the cell and cell lysis as consequences. The influx of Ca^{++} stimulates proteases, nucleases and lipases and leads to breakdown of cell elements. Excess accumulation of Ca^{++} in mitochondria causes damage to ATP-synthesis by the mitochondria. Excessive uptake of Ca^{++} ions leads also to excessive stimulation of transmitter release, in this example the excitotoxic aminoacid glutamate. Dramatic amounts of the neurotransmitter glutamate may arrive in the intercellular spaces and cause prolonged opening of glutamate responsive receptors of the releasing cell A itself and nearby cells B and C, with subsequent excess entrance of ions Na^+ and Ca^{++} and imminent cell death.

Recovery from damage is expressed clinically by a variable degree of return of function within a matter of weeks or months.

Infarcts
Cerebral infarcts consist of a central region where neurones, glial cells and other cells are dead. This central area is surrounded by a border-zone, called the *penumbra*, where ischaemia is partial and some cells are still viable (Pulsinelli, 1992) (Fig. 2.4). Some cells die by necrosis and others by apoptosis. In general, insults that are not severe enough to produce necrosis but approach the necrosis threshold may induce apoptosis (Bredesen, 1995). Agents that block apoptosis seem to reduce the size of the infarct (Linnik *et al.*, 1993). In transgenic mice that overexpress the product of the death suppressor gene *bcl-2* (see *How do nerve cells die*), the volume of experimental infarcts is about 50% that of infarcts in control animals (Martinou *et al.*, 1994). Inhibition of *bcl-2* gene expression in rats exacerbates neuronal death after ischaemia (Chen *et al.*, 1996). Reperfusion of the ischaemic region is not favourable per se. The damage induced by ischaemia to the walls of small vessels carries the risk of oedema and haemorrhage.

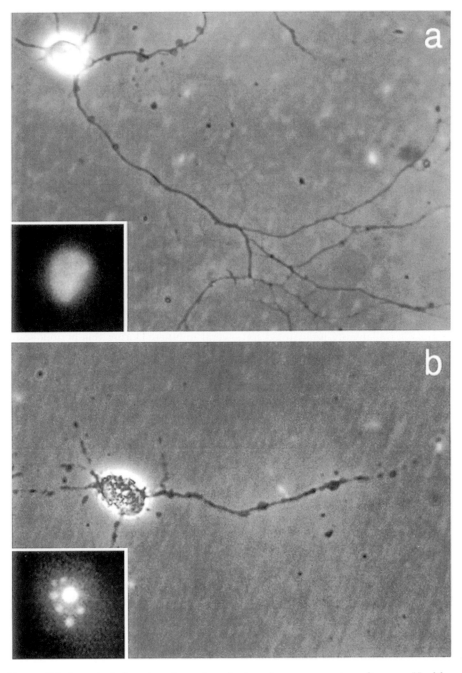

Figure 2.3 Apoptosis in rat embryonic spinal motor neurones in culture. *a*. Healthy phase-bright motor neurone with a normal kidney-shaped nucleus (insert). *b*. Apoptosis of motor neurone induced by free radical treatment. The nucleus is fragmented (insert). (Courtesy of Dr. Evert CA Kaal.)

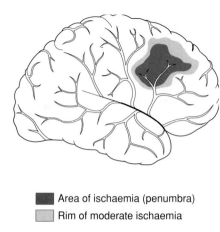

■ Area of ischaemia (penumbra)
▨ Rim of moderate ischaemia

Figure 2.4 Penumbra: infarct (black) is surrounded by a zone of damaged, threatened cells (hatched).

What exactly happens when the bloodflow in an artery is impeded depends on the degree and duration of hypoxia/ischaemia. When endarterectomy is performed for carotid stenosis, the circulation in the common, internal, and external carotid arteries is unilaterally interrupted for several minutes. During this period, some patients develop neurological deficit in the contralateral limbs that almost invariably disappears within hours after onset of reperfusion. The neurological deficit in transient ischaemic attacks (TIAs) disappears within minutes or hours and is probably caused by transient vessel occlusion in most cases. These examples indicate that there is a certain time interval before interruption of blood flow in a vessel leads to the loss of neurological function, thus offering a 'window for therapeutic opportunities'. How wide this window is, is not easy to establish (Zivin, 1998). It depends in part on the degree of collateral circulation and is different for different neuronal cell types. In acute ischaemic stroke, thrombolytic therapy with recombinant tissue plasminogen activator (rt-PA) may be beneficial when administered within 3 hours after onset (NINDS, 1995).

Ischaemic stroke in inflammatory connective tissue diseases
The main causes of ischaemic stroke in the ICTDs are vasculitis (see Chapter 5) or vasculopathy (*e.g.*, in SLE, see Chapter 7), abnormalities of coagulation (Hughes' syndrome, see Chapter 8), and cardiac emboli (valve disorders, myocardial infarcts or myocarditis in SLE, Churg–Strauss syndrome, and other vasculitides). The clinical manifestations depend on the size and localization of the infarcts. Onset is acute or subacute. Nausea and vomiting are rare, and up to 20% of patients have headache. Loss of consciousness is a feature of infarcts in the reticular formation of the brainstem. Multiple infarcts of the brain may cause dementia.

Diagnosis and management. Ischaemic stroke is diagnosed on the basis of clinical evidence and by computed tomography (CT) scanning to exclude intracerebral haemorrhage (Gilman, 1998a). Infarcts become visible on CT scans one to two days after onset. For detection of small infarcts magnetic resonance imaging (MRI) is superior.

Treatment includes (1) measures to prevent progression of ischaemic damage, (2) prevention of complications, and (3) attempts to foster reperfusion. The first point includes measures aimed at normalization of serum glucose levels if abnormal, of body temperature, and of oxygen saturation in the blood. Plasma glucose levels above 8 mmol/L have been shown to predict poorer outcome (Weir *et al.*, 1997). Though the effect of active control of glucose levels has not been clarified yet, it seems sensible to strive for normalization. Body temperature is raised in up to 25% of patients with acute stroke, and this has been shown to increase the risk of progressive neurological deterioration (Castillo *et al.*, 1997; Ginsberg and Busto, 1998; de Keyser, 1998). It is advised to keep body temperature in the range of 36.6–37°C within the first several days after acute stroke (Ginsberg and Busto, 1998). In case of abnormal respiration (Cheyne-Stokes), oxygen saturation should be determined and corrected if insufficient. In general, hypertension in the acute phase is left uncorrected because no benefit has been shown from lowering of blood pressure and because hypertension may decrease marginal perfusion in the penumbra (Powers, 1993). Prevention of complications includes the control of aspiration and pneumonia and the prevention of urine retention. rt-PA has been licensed in the USA for thrombolytic treatment of ischaemic stroke in carefully selected persons within the first 3 hours of onset (NINDS, 1995; Adams *et al.*, 1996). This decision has been disputed because it is based on the outcome of a single trial, the results of other thrombolytic trials show considerable variation, and not all cases of ischaemic stroke are due to vessel occlusion (Caplan *et al.*, 1997). In a systematic review of the available data, Wardlaw *et al.* (1997) conclude that additional investigations are needed. The American Heart Association (AHA) guidelines for application of thrombolytic therapy recommend administration of intravenous rt-PA to selected persons within 3 h of onset of stroke (0.9 mg/kg, maximum 90 mg; 10% as bolus followed by an infusion of the remaining 90% in 60 min), when the diagnosis has been established by physicians with expertise in stroke diagnosis and in reading CT scans of the brain (Adams *et al.*, 1996) (Box 2.1). Given the other recommendations by the AHA, as enumerated in Box 2.1, it appears that patients with ICTDs and ischaemic stroke are not excluded from this kind of treatment beforehand. Due to the risk of bleeding associated with administration of rt-PA and to the management of bleeding complications, patients admitted for this form of therapy should be treated in an intensive care unit according to a detailed protocol (Adams *et al.*, 1996).

At present only acetyl salicylic acid is available for secondary prevention of ischaemic stroke. A daily dose of 30–100 mg reduces the relative risk of recurrence of an ischaemic cerebral event by 13% (The Dutch TIA study group, 1994).

CEREBRAL VENOUS THROMBOSIS (CVT)

For an extensive review of all aspects of *cerebral venous thrombosis* the reader is referred to Bousser and Ross Russell (1997). The incidence and prevalence of CVT are not known exactly, due in part to under-diagnosis of the condition. However, CVT is surprisingly frequent in Behçet's disease (see Chapter 5), is not very exceptional in SLE (Chapter 7) and has been described in Wegener's granulomatosis (see Chapter 5), Hughes syndrome (Chapter 8), and Sjögren's syndrome (Chapter 11).

Box 2.1 Who should be excluded from treatment with thrombolytic therapy in case of ischaemic stroke? Recommendations by the American Heart Association.

- those who use oral anticoagulants or have a prothrombin time greater than 15 s
- those who have used heparin in the previous 48 h and have a prolonged partial thromboplastin time
- those who have a platelet count less than 100.000/mm^3
- those who have had another stroke or a serious head injury in the previous 3 months
- those who have had major surgery in the past 14 days
- those who have pre-treatment systolic blood pressure greater than 185 mm Hg or diastolic blood pressure greater than 110 mm Hg
- those whose neurological signs improve rapidly
- those whose neurological signs are mild
- those who have had prior intracranial haemorrhage
- those who have a blood glucose level < 50 mg/dl or > 400 mg/dl
- those who have had a seizure at the onset of stroke
- those who have had gastrointestinal or urinary bleeding within the preceding 21 days
- those who have had a recent heart infarct
- caution is required before giving rt-PA to persons with severe ischaemic stroke
- there is no experience with persons younger than 18 years
- the risks and potential benefits should be discussed with the patient and her/his family

---

Modified from Adams *et al.* (1996), with permission.

Clinical features

Cerebral blood is drained by a system of deep and superficial veins and guided to the venous sinuses in the dura mater. From there, the blood flows to the internal jugular veins and pterygoid plexus back to the heart. Obstruction in one of the main parts of this system (primarily the sinus sagittalis superior) leads to increase of intracranial venous and cerebrospinal fluid (CSF) pressure with headache, papilloedema and VIth cranial nerve palsy as clinical signs. Insufficient venous drainage may cause cerebral oedema, cerebral haemorrhages, unilateral or bilateral venous infarcts, depressed consciousness, seizures, focal motor and sensory deficit, agnosia, and other clinical manifestations (Fig. 2.5). If a smaller vein is obstructed and collateral circulation is insufficient, local blood flow may be seriously impeded, causing a venous infarct and haemorrhage, but the intracranial pressure will not be raised. The clinical manifestations are thus very variable and not very specific. Alternation of neurological signs, in the left and right side of the body, was previously thought to be both characteristic for CVT and frequent, but the latter is unfortunately not true.

Headache is the most frequent symptom and is present in approximately 80% of patients, and in up to 40% it is the only symptom. It can be acute in onset, but also chronic and is in some, but not in all, cases accompanied by papilloedema.

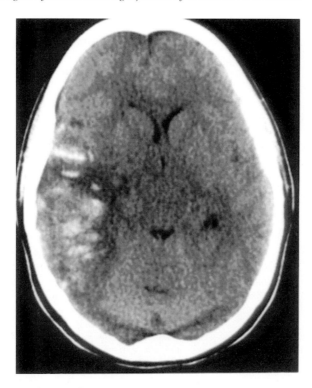

Figure 2.5 Haemorrhagic infarct in right temporal lobe due to thrombosis of right sinus sigmoideus. CT scan. See also Figs. 2.6, 2.7 and 2.8. (Courtesy of Dr. Lino Ramos.)

Periorbital oedema, redness of the face, proptosis, optic neuropathy and ophthalmoplegia are features of cavernous sinus thrombosis. Transverse sinus thrombosis can be the cause of isolated, single or multiple cranial nerve palsies, particular of nerves VIII, VII and VI (Kuehnen *et al.*, 1998). According to Bousser and Ross Russel (1997), some patients with thrombosis of an unpaired sinus (sagittalis superior or straight sinus) present with an encephalopathic syndrome without localizing signs. Thrombosis in the vena jugularis can cause lung emboli.

Diagnosis and management. To diagnose CVT, awareness of the condition and its clinical features are required. CVT can best be visualized by MRI and MR angiography (Figs. 2.6 and 2.7). In a minority of patients, CT shows the so-called empty delta sign after enhancement. It is due to opafication of the walls of the sinus sagittalis superior and the contrast with the low density of the thrombus in the lumen (Fig. 2.8).

Most authors agree that the treatment of choice is with heparin in all cases, regardless whether there is evidence of haemorrhage at imaging of the brain. Heparin is given by continuous intravenous infusion or subcutaneous injections. The dose should be adjusted to double the initial activated partial thromboplastin time (PTT). Heparin treatment is continued until the patient improves or at least until symptoms stabilize, and is then replaced by warfarin, adjusted to obtain an international normalized ratio (INR) between 2 and 3. Duration of treatment is 3

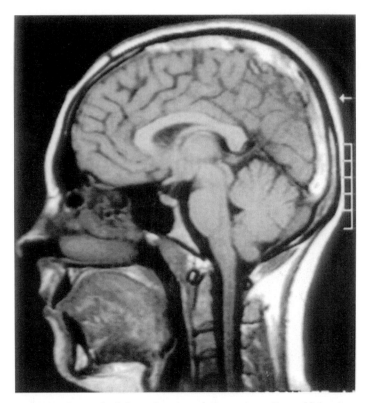

Figure 2.6 Increased signal of thrombus in subacute stage (1 week) in sinus sagittalis superior. MRI, T1-Wi image, sagittal projection. See also Figures 2.5, 2.7 and 2.8. (Courtesy of Dr. Lino Ramos.)

months when there is at least no extra risk of recurrence of thrombosis, but it is prolonged when risk continues to be present as in SLE and Behçet's disease (Bousser and Ross Russell, 1997). In a recently closed, and not yet published, double-blind placebo-controlled Dutch-British study, one group of patients received low molecular weight heparin in high therapeutic doses for 3 weeks and warfarin for 3 months (Stam, 1997).

INTRACRANIAL HAEMORRHAGE

The main risk factors for intracranial haemorrhage in patients with ICTDs are hypertension, vasculitis, a history of vasculitis and treatment with anticoagulants (*e.g.*, in Hughes' syndrome). Vasculitis weakens vessel walls and may induce aneurysmatic widenings. At the time that vasculitis is active, or months to years after vasculitis has recovered, one of these aneurysmata may succumb to the pressure of the blood and break open (see Chapter 5, *Polyarteritis nodosa*). High intensity anticoagluant therapy (international normalized ratio ≥ 3) has proven to carry the risk of bleeding, and some of these bleedings may occur intracranial (SPIRIT, 1997).

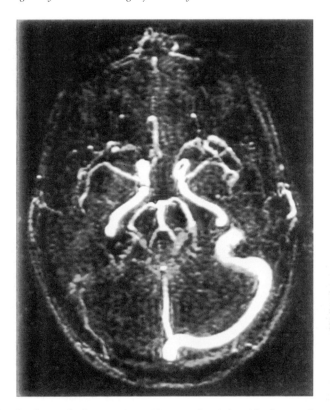

Figure 2.7 Lack of signal of sinus sigmoideus at the right side due to absence of flow. Phase-contrast MR-angiogram, 2 dimensional axial slice. See also Figures 2.5, 2.6 and 2.8. (Courtesy of Dr. Lino Ramos.)

Clinical features

Frequent symptoms at onset of intracerebral haemorrhage are headache, vomiting, seizures and lowering of consciousness (Feldmann, 1991; Caplan, 1992). This last symptom is due to rupture of a haematoma into the ventricles, obstruction hydrocephalus, or pressure on the brain stem (directly, or more often indirectly by an expanding haematoma or by oedema around the haematoma). The development of other signs depends on the localization of the haematoma.

A vasculitis-induced aneurysm occasionally ruptures directly into the subarachnoid space. In principle, the clinical manifestations do not differ from those due to bleeding of a circle of Willis aneurysm. They comprise sudden headache, depressed consciousness or coma, often but not always neck stiffness, and in some cases local symptoms dependent on the localization of the aneurysm. Some patients develop preretinal haemorrhages during the sudden increase of the intracranial pressure.

Chronic unilateral or bilateral subdural haematoma may develop in persons treated with anticoagulants and may cause depressed consciousness, psychiatric behaviour, hemiparesis and other focal neurological disorders.

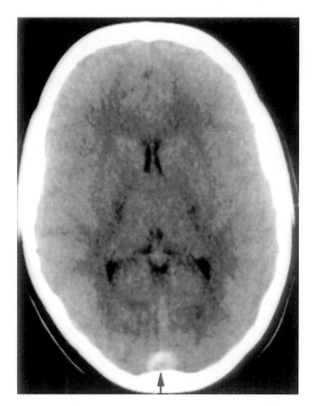

Figure 2.8 Empty delta sign on enhanced CT scan, due to thrombosis of sinus sagittalis superior (arrow). There is enhancement of the walls of the sinus sagittalis, contrasting markedly with the central hypodensity, due to filling defect of the sinus. Cerebral venous thrombosis is a potential manifestation of Behçet's disease, SLE, Hughes' syndrome, and (seldom) Sjögren's syndrome. See also Figures 2.5, 2.6 and 2.7. (Courtesy of Dr. Lino Ramos.)

Diagnosis and management. Diagnosis is based on the clinical picture and on CT scanning, preferably within 24 h after onset (Gilman, 1998a). In patients suspected of subarachnoid haemorrhage without evidence of bleeding on a CT, lumbar puncture to detect a bleeding or remnants of a bleeding should be performed at least 12 h after onset in order to be able to detect blood breakdown products.

When intracranial haemorrhage occurs in a patient treated with anticoagulants, immediate correction of coagulability is required. Intracerebral bleeding is often associated with transient hypertension for which treatment is not required. Though surgical intervention for intracerebral haematoma is disputed, most authors agree that surgical drainage is justifiable in patients with large haematomata in relatively good condition. Drainage of the CSF may be necessary in case of obstruction of the CSF circulation and hydrocephalus. The prognosis of intracerebral haematoma is often unfavourable: mortality at 6 months after onset is approximately 45% (Lampl *et al.*, 1995).

Though aneurysmatic widenings due to vasculitis are often not single and not suited for surgical intervention, imaging to detect the cause of the haemorrhage should be performed as in all other cases of subarachnoid haemorrhage, if only because classical isolated circle of Willis aneurysms can also occur in patients with ICTDs. MR angiography or CT angiography may be sufficient to detect aneurysms larger than 3 mm. For smaller aneurysms conventional angiography is needed (Gilman, 1998a).

The main complications in classical subarachnoid haemorrhage are: rebleeding, which in some cases is provoked by seizures; vasospasm-induced ischaemia; hyponatraemia due to renal sodium loss; and obstruction hydrocephalus. Although there is no sufficient information on the incidence of these complications in vasculitis-induced aneurysmatic bleeding, there is no reason why they should not occur similarly as those in classical subarachnoid haemorrhage. Guidelines for prevention or treatment of subarachnoid haemorrhage complications have been given by the Stroke Council of the AHA (Mayberg et al., 1994). The chance of rebleeding will not diminish by treatment of subarachnoid haemorrhage associated hypertension. Prophylactic administration of anticonvulsants is advisable to reduce the risk of seizures. Prescription of the calcium blocker nimodipine is indicated to prevent vasospasm related ischaemic lesions (oral nimodipine 60 mg every four h. Intravenous administration is more expensive and should be reserved for patients who cannot take nimodipine orally) (Feigin et al., 1998). In case of hyponatriaemia, volume contraction should be prevented and may necessitate intravenous administration of isotonic solutions. Hydrocephalus is treated first by lumbar punctures, and if this has no sustained effect then by ventriculostomy (Mayberg et al., 1994).

Drainage may be necessary of an anticoagulant-induced chronic subdural haematoma.

WHITE MATTER LESIONS

Axonal degeneration, demyelination and the effect of anoxia
When an axon (nerve fibre) is lesioned, the part distal from the lesion degenerates and disappears. How long it takes before degeneration actually starts is not known exactly, but it is probably approximately one day (Griffin and Hoffman, 1993; Griffin et al., 1995). After many months axonal remnants are still demonstrable, and myelin debris is not fully cleared away even after a year. Proximal of the lesion, axon and cell body undergo a series of changes but often survive. Axons may survive when only the myelin sheaths (or oligodendrocytes including the myelin sheaths) are affected by immune mediated, viral, toxic or metabolic processes, or by compression (Ludwin, 1995).

Nerve fibres in the CNS are dependent on aerobic metabolism for normal function and integrity. Following anoxia for 8–10 min, nerve fibres in the optic tracts of rats are not able to conduct anymore. After one hour of anoxia, partial recovery of conduction is still possible, however (Stys et al., 1995). Three to 6 h after death, axonal transport is still feasible in some nerve fibres in the human brain (Dai et al., 1998).

Recovery of nerve fibres in the CNS
In principle, lesioned (interrupted) nerve fibres in the CNS have the power to regenerate, but their growth is hampered by growth-inhibiting substances in oligodendrocytes (Bähr and Bonhoeffer, 1994; McKerracher et al., 1995). The capacity of CNS

axons to regenerate, when in a suitable environment, has been demonstrated convincingly in a famous experiment (Aguayo *et al.*, 1991). In a damaged CNS area when a peripheral nerve stump containing Schwann cells is introduced, lesioned CNS axons grow into this stump and keep on growing over considerable time. Schwann cells and their basal membranes apparently provide a stimulus to grow, which is not offered by CNS glial cells.

Remyelination following demyelination occurs not only in the PNS but also in the CNS. When the demyelinating agent is not present or active anymore, the first attempts at remyelination can be seen after about a week, and if necessary oligo-dendrocytes with the capacity to remyelinate can migrate within the white matter or along blood vessels towards the demyelinated area. The new myelin sheaths are functionally and biochemically equal to the original sheaths, but they do not attain the same thickness as the original, however (Ludwin, 1995).

White matter lesions due to small vessel disease

The term *small vessel disease*, when used in the context of ICTDs, refers to an angiopathy of vessels smaller than arteriae. This sense of the term is used by Jenette and Falk (1994) for a category of vasculitides. Small vessel vasculitis occurs also in the CNS, and it creates great diagnostic difficulties because it cannot be visualized by angiography in contrast to vasculitis of middle and large vessels (arteries).

For many neurologists, the designation small vessel disease refers, in particular, to a disorder of perforating arterioles in the basal ganglia and internal capsule or in the subcortex. These latter vessels provide blood to the hemispheric white substance. Small vessel disease of this type is related to hypertension and arteriosclerosis, and is responsible for lacunar infarcts (< 1.5 cm), intracerebral haematoma in the basal ganglia and surroundings, and for similar small infarcts in the hemispheric white matter and so-called *leuko-araiosis* or confluent white matter lesions.

Small vessel disease is assumed to be one of the causes of confluent white matter lesions or leuko-araiosis because of its association with vascular risk factors and because of the results of histopathological studies (Fig. 2.9) (Hijdra *et al.*, 1990; van Swieten *et al.*, 1991). Confluent white matter disease may be clinically silent, or associated with mental slowness and other features of subcortical dementia (see *Cognitive Disorders and Dementia*); *e.g.*, urinary incontinence; gait and balance disturbances with falls; and resurgence of primitive reflexes (Ghika and Bogousslavsky, 1996). It has been described in SLE (Chapter 7) and Sjögren's syndrome (Chapter 11).

Diagnosis and management. Hypertension- and arteriosclerosis-related white matter disease is diagnosed on the basis of clinical manifestations and CT or MRI. A specific therapy is not available.

White matter lesions due to an immune-mediated inflammatory process

Multiple sclerosis (MS) and acute demyelinating encephalomyelopathy (ADEM) are the two prototype acquired auto-immune demyelinating disorders of the CNS. MRI, which is the method of choice for evaluation of white matter lesions (Gilman, 1998b), does not distinguish between MS and ADEM. MS lesions are localized predominantly periventricular in the cerebral hemispheres but occur also at many other places in the white matter, including the optic nerves and the spinal cord. The lesions appear as hyperintense spots or areas on T2-weighted images and have to be differentiated from similar lesions occurring normally in individuals of 50 years

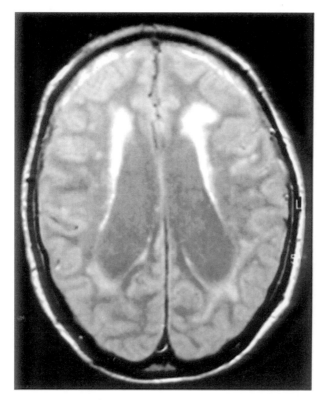

Figure 2.9 Periventricular, confluent white matter areas of hyperintensity (leuko–araiosis) in a 75-year old woman. MRI, T2-Wi (PD) image. Leuko–araiosis may be observed in SLE. (Courtesy of Dr. Lino Ramos.)

and older (Fig. 2.10). Acute lesions show contrast enhancement indicating breakdown of the blood-brain barrier. The pathology of acute MS lesions is characterized by demyelination, loss of oligodendrocytes and large numbers of CD4+ T-cells and B-cells. The actual stripping of the myelin from the nerve fibres is done by microglia cells (Pender, 1995). Symptoms of auto-immune white matter lesions depend on the extent of the lesions and the localization. Subcortical dementia has been described in MS. White matter lesions in SLE and Sjögren's syndrome may closely resemble those in MS/ADEM (see Chapters 7 and 11).

White matter lesions of viral origin: multifocal leuko–encephalopathy (MFL)
Multifocal leuko–encephalopathy (MFL) is a rare demyelinating disorder caused by an opportunistic infection by the JC strain of the papovavirus, in immune-compromised individuals. Imaging of the CNS in infected individuals shows multiple, in part confluent, areas of demyelination, mostly in the hemispheric white matter but also in the brainstem and spinal cord. The onset of clinical symptoms is either subacute or chronic. The clinical signs are variable and depend on the localization of the lesions. The disease is diagnosed by polymerase chain reaction of DNA of the JC virus in the CSF or by brain biopsy (Aksamit Jr, 1997). Results of treatment with

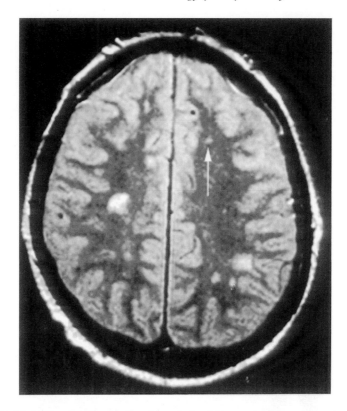

Figure 2.10 Multiple, mostly small, subcortical white matter hyperintensity areas in a case of multiple sclerosis (MS). MRI, T2-Wi (PD) image. The small punctate lesions as shown here (arrow) of increased signal intensity at T2-Wi images are often observed in aged subjects and in MS, SLE, Hughes' syndrome, primary Sjögren's syndrome, and mixed connective tissue disease. The larger hyperintensity areas are compatible with somewhat larger demyelinated plaques. (Courtesy of Dr. Lino Ramos.)

cytarabine have been disappointing and those with alpha interferon remain to be evaluated. The course of the disease is commonly progressive and outcome unfavourable within a year or shorter. MFL has been suggested as possible cause for white matter lesions in some patients with SLE (see Chapter 7).

OPTIC NEURITIS AND NEUROPATHY

Optic neuritis is characterized by loss or partial loss (scotoma, parascotoma, dimness of vision, colour desaturation) of vision usually in one eye with or without concomitant papilloedema. It develops in a few days or approximately a week. When associated with papilloedema one refers to the condition with the term *papillitis*, and when ocular changes are not present the condition is labelled as *retrobulbar neuritis*. Absence of the pupillary light reflex in the affected eye confirms that the lesion is located in the optic nerve. Patients often complain at onset about pain behind the eye, which increases during eye movement. The protein content and the immunoglobulin-G (IgG) index of the CSF may be raised and there may be oligo-clonal bands in the CSF at immuno–electrophoresis. When using appropriate tech-niques, MRI may reveal swelling of the optic nerve and contrast enhancement (Guy *et al.*, 1992) (Fig. 2.11).

Optic neuritis is presumably an immune–mediated inflammatory condition and occurs in isolation or with MS. The isolated form generally recovers spontaneously, at least in part, but there is a risk of relapse and some of these patients develop MS in due time (Beck *et al.*, 1993). The risk of MS is highest in patients who, during an episode of visual loss, have periventricular white matter lesions on MRI. Studies of human leukocyte antigen (HLA) indicate that there is a genetic predisposition for reacting to external stimuli with optic neuritis and MS. The external stimulus may be an infection, presumably a viral infection, but definite associations have not been established (see Jacobson, 1997).

Optic neuritis of this type has to be differentiated from *ischaemic optic neuropathy* and other ophthalmologic conditions. Ischaemic optic neuropathy differs from optic neuritis by a more sudden onset and lack of spontaneous recovery (Table 2.5).

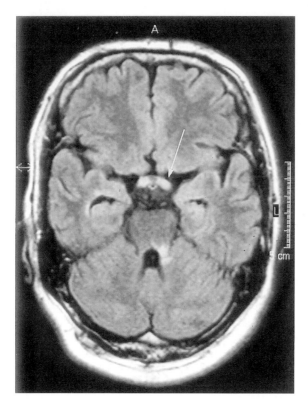

Figure 2.11 High signal of optic nerves near chiasma (arrow) in a case of bilateral optic neuritis. There is also a high signal lesion in the right cerebellar peduncle. Axial fast fluid attenuated inversion recovery (FLAIR). (Courtesy of Dr. Lino Ramos.)

Table 2.5 Clinical features of optic neuropathy or neuritis

	Optic nerve infarcts	*Optic neuritis/Retrobulbar neuritis*
Onset	Acute	Within days or a week
Associated symptoms		Pain
Field defects	Altitudinal, centrocecal	Central/paracentral scotoma
Pupillary light reflex	Afferent defect	Afferent defect
Papil	Oedema	Oedema; not in retrobulbar neuritis
Course	Irreversible	Spontaneous recovery

Isolated optic neuritis occurs mostly in adults of 20–40 years or in children, while ischaemic optic neuropathy affects individuals of middle or old age.

Optic neuritis is a manifestation of SLE and has been described in few patients with Sjögren's syndrome (see Chapters 7 and 11). In some of the SLE patients, antiphospholipid antibodies were found, thereby raising the question whether these patients were not more likely to have ischaemic optic neuropathy instead of optic neuritis. Another possibility might be that ischaemia of the optic nerve is due to SLE vasculitis. It is of interest that optic neuritis or neuropathy is associated in several patients with transverse myelitis, as in Devic's syndrome (see Harada *et al.*, 1995). Optic neuritis and compression neuropathy have been reported in patients with orbital cellulitis and Graves' ophthalmopathy (see Chapter 6). Ischaemic optic neuropathy or neuritis has been reported in patients with vasculitis (see Chapter 5).

Diagnosis and management. The results of the Optic Neuritis Treatment Trial show that antinuclear antibodies are positive in approximately 20% of isolated patients with optic neuritis, but this does not predict that they will develop an ICTD (Optic Neuritis Study Group, 1991). Patients treated with intravenous infusions of methyl-prednisolone recover more rapidly than others, but after one year there is no differ-ence between treated and placebo groups (Beck *et al.*, 1992). Treatment with intravenous methylprednisolone infusions delays onset of MS (Beck *et al.*, 1993).

TRANSVERSE MYELITIS OR MYELOPATHY

Transverse myelitis or *myelopathy* (TM) should be in the differential diagnosis when a spinal cord syndrome develops, within hours or days, with progression perhaps during weeks. TM is presumed to be inflammatory in origin but the dis-tinction with a vascular cause may create difficulties (Ropper and Poskanzer, 1978; Jeffrey *et al.*, 1993;). TM is a feature of SLE, Sjögren's syndrome and Hughes' syndrome.

The first symptom is often back pain or neck pain and is followed by weakness, sensory disturbances and bladder dysfunction. Weakness may involve only the lower limbs, or lower and upper limbs, dependent on the level of the cord that is affected. The lower limbs are initially flaccid and become gradually spastic; the upper limbs may show signs of both lower and upper motor neuron involvement. The sensory disturbances have an upper level, as usual in spinal cord syndromes. In most cases, motor and sensory symptoms are symmetrical, in contrast to the clinical signs of myelopathy in MS, which are usually asymmetrical (Scott *et al.*, 1998). In some but not all cases, MRI reveals swelling of part of the spinal cord or even the whole cord with a hyper-intense signal at T2-weighted images and with contrast enhancement (Fig. 2.12). MRI lesions of the spinal cord in MS are often smaller and multifocal (Fig. 2.13) (Scott *et al.*, 1998). Abnormalities in the CSF are described in case reports and concern pleocytosis with lymphocyte predominance and a raised protein content (Stone, 1997). Oligoclonal bands were not present in any of 12 patients tested (Scott *et al.*, 1998). Antecedent infections have been observed in many cases, but whether there is indeed a relation with the inflammatory process of TM is not clear (Krupp, 1997; Stone, 1998). The course of the disease is mostly monophasic, although relapses occur in some patients (Tippett *et al.*, 1991). The percentage of patients with TM that develop MS is probably less than 10%, although initially much higher percentages were reported (Berman *et al.*, 1981; Jeffrey *et al.*, 1993; Scott *et al.*, 1998).

The differential diagnosis is quite comprehensive, even if one takes the development time of TM into consideration (see Table 2.6). Anterior spinal artery infarcts resemble TM with their similar rapid onset, but differ from TM because they spare the posterior tracts and preserve gnostic sensibility.

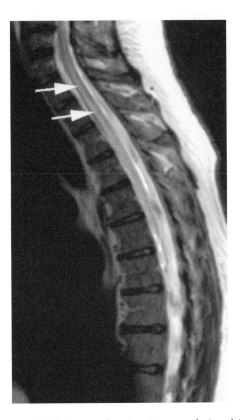

Figure 2.12 Sagittal T2-Wi (PD) image showing increased signal in the lower cervical and thoracic cord (arrows) in a case of myelitis. (Courtesy of Dr. Lino Ramos.)

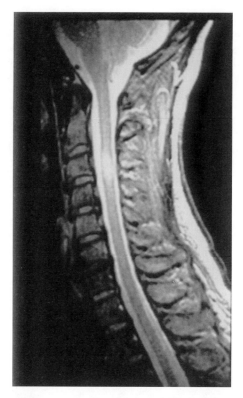

Figure 2.13 Sagittal T2-Wi (PD) image showing focal, poorly marginated, increased signal intensity area at level C3 in patient with multiple sclerosis. (Courtesy of Dr. Lino Ramos.)

Diagnosis and management. Diagnosis is based on (1) the clinical picture, (2) the presence of pleocytosis in the CSF, (3) imaging by MRI, (4) exclusion of other causes and (5) establishing whether ICTDs or any other associated diseases are involved. If no other cause and no associated disease can be detected, TM is considered as idiopathic. Management depends in the first instance on the cause, or the involvement of associated disorders. Immunosuppression is often applied in view of the presumed auto-immune origin of the condition, but whether it is really effective is

Table 2.6 The differential diagnosis of transverse myelitis

Compression of the spinal cord by whatever cause
Intramedullary haemorrhage due to arteriovenous malformation or another cause
Anterior spinal cord infarct
Vasculitis
Multiple sclerosis
Devic syndrome

questionable. In a related disorder, optic neuritis, patients treated with methylprednisolone infusions recovered somewhat faster but were not different from placebo treated patients after one year (see *Optic Neuritis*). At present, for treatment of transverse myelitis one chooses mostly intravenous infusions of methylprednisolone or cyclophosphamide (see Chapter 4). The prognosis is approximately 75% fair or good and 20–25% poor (Berman *et al.*, 1981; Stone, 1997).

CHOREA

Chorea is 'a state of excessive spontaneous movements, irregularly timed, non-repetitive, randomly distributed, and abrupt in character' (Lakke, 1981). It is encountered in a number of entirely different diseases, including SLE, Hughes' syndrome and acute rheumatic fever (Weindl *et al.*, 1993; Fahn, 1995). Chorea has been related to disorders in the basal ganglia, notably the corpus subthalamicum, caudate nucleus, and putamen, and to a lesser degree the ventral nucleus of the thalamus and brain stem. The underlying disorder may be diffuse, with loss of a specific neuronal population, or focal or multifocal with one or several infarcts. In Huntington's disease, imaging first reveals a phase of hypo-metabolism of the striatum, as demonstrable by positron emission tomography (PET), followed by atrophy of putamen and caudate nucleus (Gilman, 1998b). Post-mortem investigations demonstrate a diffuse neuronal disorder in the striatum and elsewhere. In *Sydenham chorea*, PET shows increase of striatal glucose metabolism; MRI shows, in some cases, enlargement of the caudate nucleus, putamen and globus pallidum (Goldman *et al.*, 1993; Weindl *et al.*, 1993; Gied *et al.*, 1995). Post-mortem investigations of Sydenham's chorea have not often been performed as patients in general survive. They show widespread neuronal changes, perivascular cellular infiltrates, and in some cases vasculitis (see Nausieda, 1986). In a case of progressive chorea, marked neuronal loss perhaps related to chronic use of phenitoin was found in the corpus subthalamicum (Sinard and Hedreen, 1995). Hemichorea or hemiballism, resulting from a vascular lesion of the contralateral corpus subthalamicum may occur in middle and old age (Fahn, 1995). This summary shows that both diffuse neuronal loss in nuclei in the striatum and haemorrhages or infarcts in the same region may underlie chorea in young and old individuals.

Diagnosis and management. Diagnosis of chorea is by visual inspection. Patients should refrain as much as possible from motor activity as this furthers choreic movements. They may benefit from sedatives, and if these are not sufficiently effective, from valproate. Medical treatment, however, does not succeed in general to suppress the choreic movements completely. The best option, as far as the effect on the abnormal movements is concerned, is haloperidol. As nearly all other neuroleptics, haloperidol is associated with the risk of tardive dyskinesia. These movements are located in the tongue, jaw, face and limbs and are choreiform or rhythmic in character. *Tardive dyskinesia* is a serious complication because it does not disappear spontaneously and because effective treatment is not available. The cumulative incidence after one year of treatment with neuroleptics (including haloperidol) is 5%, and after two years 10% (see Kane, 1995). Surveys on the prevalence of tardive dyskinesia indicate that the risk increases with age. For more detailed description of Sydenham's chorea and its treatment, see the section on rheumatic fever in Chapter 9.

TRIGEMINAL NEUROPATHY

Neuropathy of the n. trigeminus is entirely or almost entirely sensory. It is often associated with scleroderma, mixed connective tissue disease (MCTD), or undifferentiated connective tissue disease (UCTD). Less often, it is seen in patients with SLE, Sjögren's syndrome and RA. It has been reported at least twice in patients with dermatomyositis (Hagen *et al.*, 1990; see Hughes, 1993), and at least once in Churg–Strauss syndrome. In approximately 10% of patients no cause or associated disease can be detected. However, trigeminal neuropathy may precede development of symptoms of MCTD (Hagen *et al.*, 1990).

Onset of trigeminal neuropathy is gradual in the large majority of cases, though subacute or even acute onset (less than a week) has been described. Symptoms are usually unilateral, though they may be bilateral. Patients complain of numbness comparable to the anaesthesia induced by the dentist and, in varying degrees, of paraesthesia, painful itching, electric-shock-like experiences when touched at the cheek, an aching or stabbing pain, a lancinating pain several times daily, or a burning sensation. Examination shows that all sensory modalities are involved. Hypaesthesia is present usually in the territories of 2 or 3 branches of the nerve, rarely in only one. The tongue and the inner side of the cheek can also be affected and taste can be impaired. When sensibility is markedly reduced in the territory of the first branch, the cornea reflex is diminished and the blink reflex can not be elicited. Two of 81 retrospectively reviewed cases had, according to Hagen *et al.* (1990), weakness at mastication, and Hughes (1993) states that 'motor function is rarely affected'. Definite involvement of other nerves has not been reported, though Hagen *et al.* (1990) mention 'suggestive involvement of other cranial nerves' in 7 cases (numbness of posterior pharynx, unilateral weak palate, EMG evidence of abnormalities in facial nerve innervated muscles, and mild drooping of a corner of the mouth). Teasdall *et al.* (1980) mention facial weakness in some cases, and hypaesthesia in territory innervated by the n. glossopharyngeus. In view of these communications, it is likely that trigeminal neuropathy is not always purely sensory, and that neighbouring cranial nerves are not always entirely spared. The CSF is mostly normal, but protein is mildly raised in some cases and the number of lymphocytes may be slightly increased (Lecky *et al.*, 1987). Some patients apparently improve somewhat after a variable time period (Hagen *et al.*, 1990).

Electrophysiological investigations and MRI point to a disorder of the ganglion Gasseri (Förster *et al.*, 1996; Rorick *et al.*, 1996). Hughes (1993) describes sections of the trigeminal ganglion showing cell loss, lymphocytic infiltration, fibrosis and hyaline degeneration. Exploration in three patients with 'chronic trigeminal neuropathy', 1–12 years after onset, revealed reduction of the sensory root to 'a few wisps of nerve fibre' (Hughes, 1993).

This short review shows that trigeminal neuropathy is most likely an inflammatory disorder of the ganglion Gasseri. The association with ICTDs points to an autoimmune mediated mechanism.

Diagnosis and management. Diagnosis is based on sensory symptoms developing within days or weeks in the area innervated by one or two trigeminal nerves and is supported by the presence of an ICTD. No effective therapy is known. Corticosteroids have been attempted, but according to Hughes (1993) 'rather halfheartedly'. Patients with impairment of sensation of the cornea should protect their eyes by wearing glasses, preferably with protective side pieces, and should inspect their eyes daily for signs of inflammation.

ASEPTIC MENINGITIS AND INFLAMMATORY MENINGEAL SYNDROMES

Aseptic meningitis refers to a syndrome of meningitis for which no fungal or bacterial cause can be detected. The term was introduced in the 1920s and was used mainly or exclusively for viral meningitis until recently. Now that virus infections can be detected reliably in the laboratory, the term aseptic meningitis is not really necessary anymore, but it is still used in a loose fashion, for instance, for the meningeal syndrome induced in some patients treated with gammaglobulins. Inflammatory processes of the meninges are not rare in the ICTDs, for instance in Sjögren's syndrome. Although such processes might perhaps best be denoted as inflammatory meningeal syndromes or pachymeningitis, they are sometimes referred to as aseptic meningitis or meningoencephalitis (Alexander and Alexander, 1983). Meningismus is not always among the clinical symptoms in this kind of aseptic meningitis. The main meningeal syndromes in the ICTDs are summarized in Box 2.2. (See also Chapter 12, relapsing polychondritis and mixed connective tissue disease).

Box 2.2 Meningeal syndromes in the inflammatory connective tissue diseases

---

- *Sjögren's syndrome*: perivascular infiltrates in the meninges consisting of lymphocytes, plasma cells, macrophages and polymorphonuclear granulocytes. Symptoms: none at all, or one or more of the following: diffuse pain in the limbs and elsewhere, headache, meningismus, episodes of fever, confusion, delirium, dementia, epilepsy, cranial nerve palsies, transverse myelitis (Chapter 11).
- *Rheumatoid arthritis*: plaque-like diffuse inflammation or rheumatic nodules with lymphocytes and plasma cells. Symptoms: organic brain syndrome, severe headache, seizures, cranial nerve palsies, paresis, agnosia or aphasia; other symptoms of focal lesions due to compression of the meningeal process on the brain tissue and meningovasculitis; myelopathy due to pressure on the cord, or radiculopathy (Chapter 9).
- *Wegener's granulomatosis*: diffuse, focal, plaque-like thickening of the meninges with granulomata, multinucleated giant cells and lymphocytic infiltrations. Symptoms: headache, cranial nerve palsies, seizures, encephalopathy, diabetes insipidus, spastic paraparesis (Chapter 5).
- *Behçet's disease*: meningismus, meningomyelitic syndrome, lymphocytic pleocytosis with a significant number of polymorphonuclear leukocytes (Chapter 5).
- *Medication associated*: intravenously administered gammaglobulins, isoniazid, trimethoprim-sulfamethoxazole, azathioprine, OKT3, non-steroidal anti-inflammatory agents. Symptoms: self limiting, often with resolution of symptoms despite continuation of therapy. Headache, nausea, vomiting, fever, neck stiffness, increased protein content and increased number of white blood cells (mainly neutrophils) in the CSF (Garagusi *et al.*, 1976; Haas, 1984; Martin *et al.*, 1988; see also Chapter 4).

THE PERIPHERAL NERVOUS SYSTEM (PNS)

INTRODUCTION

The PNS extends from the brainstem and spinal cord to the most out of the way corners of the body and is only comparable to the vascular system in its extensiveness. The structure of the somatic PNS is relatively simple. It consists largely of nerve fibres, arranged in tubes or fascicles that connect peripheral target cells with neuronal cell bodies located near or in the CNS. The walls of the fascicles, *the perineurial sheaths*, together with the endothelium of the small blood vessels in the fascicles constitute the blood-nerve barrier, which is considered to preserve a more or less constant 'milieu interne' in the fascicles (Thomas *et al.*, 1993). At a few places this blood-nerve barrier is lacking: there is no perineurial sheath at the end of the motor nerve fibres or at and near the neuromuscular junctions, and there is also no blood-nerve barrier around the dorsal root ganglia, which puts these ganglia in a vulnerable position. Antigenetically, peripheral nerves differ from nerve fibres in the CNS. This is not surprising as some of the major peripheral nerve myelin proteins are entirely lacking in the CNS and as some of the CNS myelin proteins do not occur in the myelin sheath of the peripheral nerve fibres. Lesions in the PNS disconnect target cells from the CNS and this results in a loss of function of the target cells. Similar symptoms occur when the target cells themselves are affected. The peripheral autonomous system has, in contrast to the somatic PNS, many of its neuronal cell bodies in the periphery.

DIFFERENT TYPES OF PERIPHERAL NEUROPATHY IN INFLAMMATORY CONNECTIVE TISSUE DISEASES

In the acquired diseases of the PNS, not all nerves will be affected simultaneously, at least not at onset. The clinical symptoms differ according to the structure that is affected; in some cases, the nature and distribution of the symptoms allow us to infer the kind of process that is responsible. Table 2.7 offers a summary of the structures in the PNS that may be affected in the ICTDs and the types of neuropathies that result from this. The table shows that disorders of the lower motor neuron cell bodies are not included and that peripheral sensory neuron cell bodies (dorsal root ganglia cells) are only affected in Sjögren's syndrome. This is in contrast to the peripheral sensory cell bodies of the trigeminal nerve, which may become affected in a series of ICTDs (see *Trigeminal Neuropathy*). Symptoms of *sensory neuronopathy* or *ganglionitis* (dorsal root ganglia cells) differ in several respects from sensory polyneuropathy as is explained in more detail in the section on sensory neuronopathy.

Symptoms of *mononeuritis multiplex* are mostly localized in distal parts of the limbs, for instance the fingers of one hand and the distal part of a lower limb. During the course of the disease, the neurological changes may gradually progress and become first asymmetrical and finally symmetrical as in the polyneuropathies. Vasculitis is the most frequent cause of mononeuritis (or mononeuropathy) multiplex, but there are several other causes as well, *e.g.* diabetes mellitus, leprosy, Lyme neuroborreliosis, and hereditary neuropathy due to liability of pressure palsies.

Polyneuropathies are mostly symmetrical and involve the distal parts of the limbs preferentially. There are, however, many variations on this theme, the most

Table 2.7 Peripheral neuropathies in the inflammatory connective tissue diseases

Structure	Type of neuropathy	Type of nerve fibre degeneration	ICTD
Peripheral sensory cell bodies	Sensory neuronopathy or ganglionitis	Axonal	Sjögren's syndrome
One single nerve	Mononeuropathy	Axonal and demyelinative	Compression or entrapment in RA, vasculitis
Several nerves	Mononeuritis multiplex	Axonal	Vasculitis, also in SLE, Sjögren's syndrome, systemic sclerosis, RA, MCTD
System diseases of the PNS	Polyneuropathy	Axonal, demyelinative or both	Vasculitis, SLE, RA, systemic sclerosis, MCTD, Sjögren's syndrome
System diseases of the PNS, predominantly sensory nerve fibres	Sensory polyneuropathy	Mostly axonal	Vasculitis, SLE, RA, systemic sclerosis, MCTD, Sjögren's syndrome
Autonomic Nervous System	Autonomic neuropathy, usually combined with sensory polneuropathy	Axonal	Systemic sclerosis, Sjögren's syndrome, SLE

Abbreviations: RA, Rheumatoid Arthritis; SLE, Systemic Lupus Erythematosus; MCTD, Mixed Connective Tissue Disease.

striking one being the Fisher syndrome, a variant of the Guillain-Barré syndrome, in which weakness does not develop in upper or lower limbs first, but in ocular and bulbar muscles.

HISTOPATHOLOGY AND ELECTRONEUROGRAPHY OF PERIPHERAL NEUROPATHIES

When the continuity of a nerve fibre is interrupted, a series of changes occurs in a stereotypical fashion in the distal nerve stump (Griffin and Hoffman, 1993; Griffin *et al.*, 1995). By lesioning the axolemma, an influx of Ca^{++} ions takes place into the interior of the axon. The rise in the axonal Ca concentration activates Ca-sensitive proteases and depolymerization of axonal tubuli and neurofilaments, and granular degeneration is brought about. Fragmentation of the axolemma follows. Axonal debris is rapidly cleared, but it takes several weeks before macrophages succeed in removing the myelin breakdown products (but not a year, as in the CNS). The nerve conduction velocity changes little as long as the axon in the distal stump is pre-served, which in humans is no longer than a few days. The loss of conducting nerve fibres gives rise to a decrease of the nerve action potential, denervation of muscle fibres and a decrease of the compound (the total) muscle action potential (Table 2.8). This *Wallerian degeneration* is the main type of degeneration in nerve ischaemia and forms part of the spectrum of changes in nerve compression.

Other forms of axonal degeneration exist as well. In some conditions, axons become progressively atrophic and nodes of Ranvier widen, while other parts of the myelin segments are preserved (Dyck *et al.*, 1993a and b). Conduction along atrophic axons with wide nodes of Ranvier is slowed but not to the same degree as in demyelinating neuropathies (see Table 2.8). In yet another form of axonal degen-eration, antibodies bind to epitopes in the axonal membrane at or nearby nodes of Ranvier (Yeung *et al.*, 1991). Some of these antibodies may activate complement and thus cause axolemma damage and interruption of axons, as has been described in axonal forms of acute inflammatory neuropathy (Griffin *et al.*, 1996) (see this Chapter, *Inflammatory Neuropathies*).

Demyelination in ICTDs is either due to entrapment or to inflammatory processes. In entrapment, the myelin sheaths are pushed away to nearby areas where the pressure is somewhat less. How demyelination is induced and how it evolves in inflammatory demyelinating neuropathy is not entirely clear. One con-

Table 2.8 Electrophysiology of axonal degeneration and demyelination

	CV	NAP	CMAP	TD	CB
Wallerian degeneration	Approximately normal	Decreased	Decreased	Approximately normal	No
Axonal atrophy	Moderately decreased	Decreased	Decreased	Increased	No
Demyelination	Markedly decreased	Decreased	Decreased	Increased markedly	In some cases

Abbreviations: CV, conduction velocity; NAP, nerve action potential; CMAP, compound muscle action potential; TD, temporal dispersion (uneven innervation and contraction of motor-units); CB, conduction blocking

cept is that a complement activating antibody binds to the abaxonal Schwann cell surface and causes a vesicular type of myelin degeneration (Hafer-Macko *et al.*, 1996). Demyelination in inflammatory neuropathies is mostly widespread, but it is multifocal in some cases. Demyelination causes marked slowing of nerve conduction; uneven arrival of nerve fibre action potentials at the target muscle; uneven innervation and contraction of motor units (temporal dispersion); blocking of conduction along some nerve fibres (conduction block) (Fig. 2.14); loss of innervation of motor units; and decrease of the total number of contracting motor units, which is revealed by decrease in amplitude and in area of the compound (total) muscle action potential (see Table 2.8).

REPAIR OF PERIPHERAL NERVE FIBRES AND THE EFFECTS FOR CONDUCTION AND INNERVATION

Regeneration of the original nerve fibres after Wallerian degeneration is a slow and tedious process that often only partly succeeds (Bisby, 1995; Kreutzberg, 1995). When some of the regenerating nerve fibres succeed in reaching the muscle, they will re-innervate as many muscle fibres as possible, which means that the motor units are large. Whether the compound muscle action potential becomes as large as the original depends on the number of nerve fibres that reach the muscle and re-innervate motor units.

Abnormal functioning of axons due to ligand binding to epitopes at nodes of Ranvier is likely to be rapidly reversible as long as the continuity of the axons has not been compromised. Re-myelination, after demyelination and recovery of conduction and of innervation of the target cells, occurs when this is not prohibited by the underlying cause of the demyelinating process anymore.

THE INFLAMMATORY NEUROPATHIES

Acute inflammatory neuropathy (AIP or Guillain-Barré syndrome)

The acute form of inflammatory neuropathy has a monophasic course and reaches its nadir before the 30th day after onset. Weakness is at onset, most often approximately symmetrical in the limbs, not rarely proximal more than distal, and associated with areflexia or hyporeflexia. The nerves of the trunk and the cranial nerves also become involved and respiratory insufficiency is not seldom. Pain, paraesthesia, hypaesthesia and autonomic symptoms are present to a variable degree. In some exceptional cases, AIP presents not with limb weakness but with ophthalmoplegia, ataxia and areflexia (Miller-Fisher syndrome) (Ropper, 1994). Following a plateau phase a variable degree of improvement follows. Repeat attacks occur, in some cases after many years, but are rare. Table 2.9 lists the clinical features of AIP.

In approximately 33% of all cases, AIP is preceded by an infection with *Campylobacter jejuni et coli* (CJC) or other agents. There is evidence that antibodies directed against CJC cross-react with epitopes of peripheral nerve proteins, indicating that molecular mimicry may play a role in the pathogenesis of this form of inflammatory neuropathy (Jacobs *et al.*, 1995; Oomes *et al.*, 1995).

Recent findings suggest strongly that subgroups of Guillain-Barré syndrome exist. Mixed motor-sensory Guillain-Barré encompasses not only a demyelinating but also an axonal form (Feasby *et al.*, 1986; Feasby, 1994; Griffin *et al.*, 1996). A pure motor form of Guillain-Barré differs from the mixed motor-sensory form by onset of

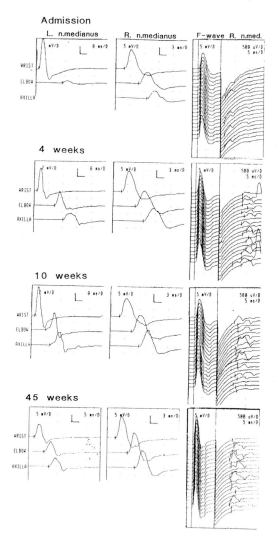

Figure 2.14 Nerve conduction block in a case of Lyme borreliosis neuropathy. At admission, stimulation of the left median nerve at the wrist results in a compound muscle action potential (CMAP) in the abductor pollicis muscle (1 mv/D). Stimulation at the right side results in a CMAP of higher amplitude (5 mv/D). Stimulation at the elbow at the left side shows only a very shallow CMAP. At the right side, the CMAP after stimulation at the elbow is slightly lower than after stimulation at the wrist. Stimulation at the axilla produces no response in the abuctor pollicis muscle at the left side, and a slightly lower CMAP than after stimulation at the elbow and wrist at the right side. Similar investigations at 4, 10 and 45 weeks show a gradual recovery at both sides. An F-wave response is at admission not obtainable. Recovery is expressed by return of F-wave responses after 4 weeks and decrease in F-wave latencies at subsequent investigations. (An F-wave is a late response to a supramaximal electric shock delivered to a nerve; the impulse travels first to the spinal cord and returns due to back-firing of motor neurons). (Courtesy of Dr. PL Oey.)

weakness usually distal at the limbs, and less serious weakness of the respiratory muscles, and muscles innervated by cranial nerves (Visser *et al.*, 1995). The classic Guillain-Barré syndrome has been described in SLE and MCTD, and Miller-Fisher syndrome in patients with SLE (see Chapters 7 and 12).

Diagnosis and management. Differential diagnosis usually is not a great problem as there are only few other polyneuropathies with acute or subacute onset (see Table 2.9). The diagnostic criteria for Guillain-Barré syndrome need updating in view of recent developments concerning subgroups (Arnason and Soliven, 1993).

Severely weak patients or patients with rapidly progressive weakness should be monitored in an intensive care unit. Special attention should be given to possible respiratory insufficiency, cardiovascular disorders and other dysregulations due to autonomic neuropathy. Treatment of the more severe cases (those with more than just limb muscle weakness) is with intravenous infusion of gammaglobulin, according to the guidelines in chapter 4. This has a favourable effect on the course of the disease and improvement starts earlier (van der Meché *et al.*, 1992; van der Meché, 1998). Overall, about 65% of patients recover fully (de Jager and Minderhoud, 1991), though this percentage may now be higher because of the introduction of intravenous gammaglobulins in treatment programmes.

Table 2.9 Clinical features of Guillain-Barré syndrome (GBS or AIP)

Events preceding onset	3 to 40 days before onset: infection (*Campylobacter jejuni et coli*, 30%; cytomegalovirus, 15%; Epstein-Barr virus, few cases; mycoplasma pneumoniae, few cases), vaccination, trauma.
Symptoms at onset	Tingling, weakness
Main clinical signs	Absent or decreased tendon reflexes, symmetrical weakness of limbs and trunk, involvement of cranial nerves, variable degree of sensory changes, variable degree of autonomic disturbances including tachycardia or bradycardia, orthostatic hypotension, hypertension, disturbance of micturition.
Other signs	Papilloedema when CSF protein is high. Seldom Babinski reflexes
Course	Onset acute or subacute; nadir before 30th day; plateau phase mostly less than 90 days; gradual improvement during next two years; death in 5%; persistent functional deficit, predominantly distal, at lower limbs in approximately 15%.
Cerebrospinal fluid	Raised CSF protein from 1 week after onset; no or slight increase in white blood cells.
EMG	Compatible with demyelination in the majority, in some cases pointing to axonal degeneration.
Associated diseases	HIV, lymphoma, sarcoidosis, SLE
Differential diagnosis	Porphyric and toxic neuropathies, poliomyelitis, acute myositis, hyperkaliaemia

See Arnason and Soliven, 1993; van der Meché, 1994;

Chronic inflammatory demyelinating polyneuropathy (CIDP)

CIDP does not reach its nadir before the eighth week after onset and has a chronic or relapsing course (Barohn *et al.*, 1989). It is an approximately symmetrical mixed motor and sensory neuropathy, though a predominantly sensory variant exists as well (Oh *et al.*, 1992; van Dijk *et al.*, 1996). CIDP is occasionally associated with MS-like lesions in the CNS (Feasby *et al.*, 1990). Table 2.10 lists the clinical features of CIDP.

Diagnosis and management of chronic inflammatory neuropathies. Diagnosis is based on the clinical features and on clinical laboratory investigations (raised protein content in the CSF without pleocytosis and evidence of demyelination at EMG in most cases). At present, there is uncertainly about the preferred treatment. Both corticosteroids and intravenous gammaglobulins are effective. Repeat infusions of intravenous gammaglobulins are often needed to keep patients in a reasonable condition (Dyck *et al.*, 1994). The long-term prognosis of patients with CIDP is insufficiently known (see Vermeulen, 1998).

SENSORY NEURONOPATHY OR GANGLIONITIS VERSUS SENSORY POLYNEUROPATHIES

The *sensory polyneuropathies* are in general symmetrical, and present at onset with symptoms distal at the limbs. Small and large sensory nerve fibre qualities may be equally involved or, alternatively, one of these may dominate in the clinical picture.

Table 2.10 Clinical features of chronic inflammatory demyelinating polyneuropathy

Events preceding onset	None definitely established
Course of the disease	Does not reach its nadir before the 8th week after onset; the course is progressive, stepwise progressive, or relapsing
Symptoms at onset	Tingling, weakness, mostly distal at the limbs, often initially at the upper limbs
Clinical signs	Symmetrical variable degree of weakness; variable degree of sensory disturbance, mainly of thick sensory nerve fibre qualities; absent or decreased tendon reflexes; cranial nerves may be involved
Other signs	Papilloedema when protein content of the CSF is high; postural tremor
Cerebrospinal fluid	Protein content raised above 0.50 g/l in 90% of cases, often more than 1 g/l; CSF white cells <30.10⁶/l
EMG	Compatible with demyelination
Other lab findings	White matter lesions upon MRI investigations in minority of patients; inflammatory cell infiltrates in 50% of sural nerve biopsies
Associated diseases	SLE, MS, myasthenia gravis, colitis ulcerosa, diabetes mellitus, psoriasis, Hodgkin's disease, hyperthyroidy, HIV

See Dyck *et al.*, 1993a; Franssen *et al.*, 1997 for review and diagnostic criteria.

Symptoms progress from distal to proximal, but the trunk and face are mostly spared. There is no weakness, or almost no weakness, except perhaps in advanced stages. Signs of autonomic neuropathy are frequent however, especially in the small sensory nerve fibre polyneuropathies. The causes of the sensory polyneuropathies are manifold. Some disturb processes in the cell bodies in the dorsal root ganglia, others are considered to affect the sensory nerve fibres. *Cisplatin neuropathy* is an example of the first category and *sensory diabetic neuropathy* of the second.

Ganglionitis or *sensory neuronopathy* is an inflammatory disorder, probably immune-mediated, of the dorsal root ganglia and often the autonomic ganglia. Ganglionitis occurs in association with small lung cell carcinoma and several other malignancies (lung, breasts, ovary), immunoglobulin-M (IgM) paraproteinaemia and Sjögren's syndrome. In some cases no associated disorder has been discovered. Onset is acute, subacute or gradual. It is mainly or exclusively sensory and auto-nomic, similar to sensory polyneuropathy. However, it has a few distinctive characteristics (Windebank *et al.*, 1990; Chalk *et al.*, 1992; Sobue *et al.*, 1993; Hainfeller *et al.*, 1996; Lee *et al.*, 1996; Wanschitz *et al.*, 1997). These are:

1. Sensory neuronopathy is often at onset and for some time during the course of the disease, asymmetrical or even unilateral (Kaplan and Schaumburg, 1991).
2. Sensory neuronopathy often presents with numbness, painful dysaesthesia, or painful paraesthesia distal in the limbs and often in the fingers. It may also start with symptoms in the face or with band-like feelings around the trunk or neck, and it may progress from the face towards the trunk.
3. Symptoms at the trunk may already be present from an early stage of the disease.
4. Though all sensory modalities may be disturbed, a severe degree of sensory ataxia is one of the most striking features of the syndrome.
5. Though an effective therapy is not available, the course of the disorder is not steady or progressive. When patients survive, some degree of improvement follows after some time (Griffin *et al.*, 1990; Wada *et al.*, 1997).

Diagnosis and management. Electrophysiology is of little use in differentiating gan-glionitis from sensory polyneuropathy. Usually, it shows that sensory nerve action potentials are not measurable, while motor nerve conduction is not markedly impaired. MRI may reveal gadolinium enhancement of the posterior spinal roots thus confirming the proximal localization of the process (Wada *et al.*, 1997). The pro-tein content of the CSF may be raised and there may be some degree of pleocytosis, but this is not so in all cases. The histopathology of spinal root ganglia is character-ized by loss of sensory nerve cell bodies and inflammatory infiltration by either pre-dominantly CD8+ T-cells (Hainfeller *et al.*, 1996) or T-cells, B-cells and plasma cells (Wanschitz *et al.*, 1997). The pathogenesis of sensory ganglionitis is not clear and may be heterogeneous. At present, there is evidence for both humoral and cellular immune processes (Dalakas and Quarles, 1996; Hainfeller *et al.*, 1996; Willison *et al.*, 1994; van Dijk *et al.*, 1997).

Reputedly, prednisone is not of much help, and though improvement following some form of therapy has been reported (Wada *et al.*, 1997), no effective form of therapy can be recommended as yet.

DISORDERS OF NEUROMUSCULAR TRANSMISSION

INTRODUCTION

Nerve fibres innervating muscle fibres divide just before arriving at the endplates in a number of delicate branches (Fig. 2.15). Each of these branches ends in a slight swelling (the axon terminals) and each fits nicely into a transversely ribbed groove on the surface of the muscle fibre. Nerve terminals, grooves, and areas of the muscle fibre immediately below the grooves constitute the neuromuscular synapse, also known as the junction or endplate. At higher magnification, it becomes clear that the transverse ribs in the grooves are the secondary clefts and foldings. The primary cleft is the shallow space in between the nerve terminals and tops of the folds. The folding of the postsynaptic membrane is unlike anything seen at other synapses and is a characteristic feature of neuromuscular junctions. The synaptic basal lamina in the primary and secondary clefts contain several proteins that do not occur elsewhere in the extracellular matrix of the muscle fibre. Acetylcholinesterase is one of these proteins. The neurotransmitter acetylcholine is stored in synaptic vesicles in the axon terminals. the dense lining at the top of the folds indicates where the

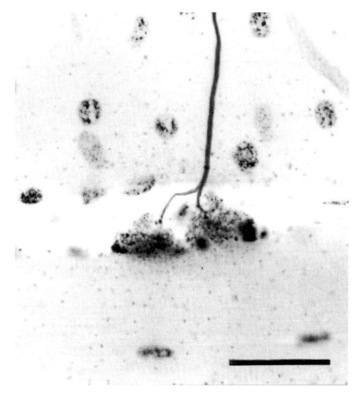

Figure 2.15 Preterminal motor axon and endplates, stained according to the silver cholinesterase method of Pestronk and Drachman (1978). Two endplates ('duplex endplate') on one muscle fibre. [From Hesselmans *et al.* (1992) *Acta Neuropathol* **83**, 202–206.]

acetylcholine receptors are located in the postsynaptic membrane. Neuromuscular transmission in auto-immune myasthenias is endangered by antibody-induced dysfunction or loss of three different types of ion channels (Fig. 2.16).

MYASTHENIA GRAVIS

Myasthenia gravis (MG) is a disease of all ages (Engel, 1994a; McCombe, 1995). Females are affected more frequently than males, at least in adolescence and adulthood. MG is frequently associated with other auto-immune diseases, including SLE, RA, systemic sclerosis, and Sjögren's syndrome. In affected muscles, weakness increases by activity (Table 2.11). The extraocular muscles, including the *m. levator palpebrae*, are more frequently affected than any other muscles. The bulbar musculature is second in frequency of involvement, and upper limb and respiratory muscles third. In a small minority of the patients, weakness starts in the lower limb muscles.

Ninety percent of patients with the clinical features of MG have antibodies against acetylcholine receptors (AChRs) and are classified as seropositive. Immuno-electronmicroscopy of endplates from these patients reveals IgG and complement at the postsynaptic membrane (Engel, 1994a). The membrane is often severely damaged and the number of AChRs is reduced. Why these antibodies that are directed against AChRs are produced is not clear at present, though the thymus is probably involved (DeBaets and Kuks, 1993). The thymus contains muscle-like myoid cells

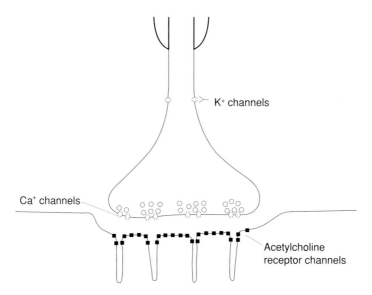

Figure 2.16 Diagram of neuromuscular junction showing the localization of three different types of ion channels: acetylcholine receptors at the postsynaptic membrane, Ca^{++} channels at the presynaptic membrane and potassium channels in the axonal membrane just before the terminal axon bulb. These channels are targets of auto-antibodies in three different auto-immune disorders, occasionally associated with inflammatory connective tissue diseases.

Table 2.11 Clinical features of myasthenia gravis (MG), Lambert-Eaton myasthenic syndrome (LEMS), and acquired neuromyotonia (ANM)

	Myasthenia gravis	Lambert-Eaton	Acquired neuromyotonia
Symptoms	Variable weakness, abnormal fatiguability	Weakness, some abnormal fatiguability, dry mouth	Muscle twitching, aching, excessive cramps, pseudo-myotonia
Distribution weakness	Variable, in order of frequency of involvement: extraocular muscles, bulbar, upper limbs, respiratory, lower limbs	Mostly proximal limb muscles, mild degree of ocular and bulbar muscle weakness, respiratory muscles	Generalized
Tendon reflexes	Preserved	Decreased or absent	Preserved
Autonomic disturbance	None	Decreased salivation, lacrimation, and sweating; impotence, orthostatic hypotension	Excessive sweating
Electromyography	Decrement of CMAP at slow nerve stimulation	Low CMAP at supramaximal nerve stimulation; increasing by voluntary contraction or tetanic stimulation	Abnormal spontaneous discharges of single motor units, as doublets, triplets or prolonged bursts
Antibodies	Against acetylcholine receptors in 90% of patients	Against voltage gated P/Q channels in 85% of patients	Against voltage gated K channels
Associated diseases	Many auto-immune diseases, including SLE, RA, systemic sclerosis, Sjögren's syndrome	Small-cell lung cancer (70%), SLE, other auto-immune diseases	Myasthenia gravis with thymoma, lung-cancer, SLE, juvenile chronic arthritis

Abbreviation: CMAP, compound muscle-action potential.

that express AChRs at its surface. In approximately 70% of the seropositive patients thymic abnormalities are present. The thymus of MG patients contains an increased number of differentiated T-cells and AChR-specific T-cells. Investigation of *bcl-2* expression has provided evidence for inhibition of apoptotic cell death in the medulla of the thymus, presumably of auto-reactive thymocytes (Onodera *et al.*, 1996). In 20% of patients with MG, a thymoma is detected and has to be removed because it occupies space and tends to metastasize in the thoracic cavity.

Ocular myasthenia which is confined to extraocular muscle, is in approximately 50% of patients AChR negative (seronegative). Damage to postsynaptic membranes and reduction of AChRs in seronegative myasthenia has been reported but has not been sufficiently investigated yet (McCombe, 1995).

Diagnosis and management. Clinical diagnosis is confirmed by:

1. Improvement of weakness when breakdown of acetylcholine is inhibited by intramuscular injection of neostigmine or intravenous injection of edrophonium. The effect of edrophonium is rapid, short (≤5 min), and dramatic but carries the risk of cholinergic side effects. The effect of intramuscular injection of neostigmine is slower, less dramatic, and is maintained longer (hours). The risk of cholinergic side effects is less (Oosterhuis, 1997). In our view the use of intravenous edrophonium is not advisable.
2. Decrease of the muscle-action potential at slow repetitive stimulation of the innervating nerve, thus demonstrating insufficiency of neuromuscular transmission. This test is slightly painful but reproducible, reliable, and not risky.
3. The auto-immune origin of the disorder is confirmed by the demonstration of a raised titre of anti-AChR antibodies.

In the AChR negative cases, diagnosis depends on the clinical and electomyographic findings. CT of the mediastinum should be made to establish or exclude the presence of thymoma.

The four steps that can be distinguished in the treatment of MG are:

1. In a newly diagnosed patient, pyridostigmine should be prescribed (up to 5–6 times/day 20–90 mg) for symptomatic treatment, and sulfas atropini should be supplied if required (1/8–1/4th mg, up to three-times daily).
2. In patients between 10 and 45 years, thymectomy should be performed, unless spontaneous remission occurs within six months after onset. A thymoma should be removed because it occupies space and may metastasize in the thorax (Oosterhuis, 1997). Thymomectomy has no special advantage for the course of MG. In approximately 14% of patients, myasthenic symptoms increase within the first six months after operation. In few patients, SLE develops with a variable time interval after thymectomy or thymomectomy (see Chapter 7).
3. When symptoms do not disappear with these measures, immunosuppression is indicated. It is common practice to start with prednisone and to give either a high dose (approximately 1 mg/kg/day) or a starting dose of 15–20 mg and thereafter a gradual increase until a dose of 1 mg/kg/day is reached. This high dose is maintained for approximately 4 weeks and slowly tapered off thereafter. Corticosteroid treatment of MG is very effective in general, but has the drawback of a transient increase of symptoms during the first 2–3 weeks of

medication. Starting with a low dose regimen and then a gradual increase may make the increase less troublesome. This has, however, not been demonstrated in a prospective study. Many patients need a low-maintenance dose of corticosteroids for a prolonged period. Azathioprine is prescribed by some from the beginning, or not long after the beginning, to spare on the corticosteroids as much as possible. For more data on dosages and side-effects, see Chapter 4.

4. Plasma exchange is an extremely valuable addition to the foregoing treatment in an emergency situation. Its effect is temporary but its advantage is that it may induce a rapid improvement of patients in a crisis. (See Chapter 4.)

THE LAMBERT-EATON MYASTHENIC SYNDROME (LEMS)

LEMS was initially discovered in patients with small-cell lung cancer (SCLC), but subsequently appeared to be associated occasionally with other malignancies and to occur in approximately 30% of patients without any malignancy (O'Neil *et al.*, 1988; Engel, 1994b; McCombe, 1995). In general, LEMS is a disease of elderly people although young people and even children may become affected. Occasionally, LEMS is associated with other autoimmune diseases (*e.g.*, SLE).

LEMS presents with muscle weakness or autonomic dysfunction (see Table 2.11). Weakness is mostly located in the proximal muscles of the lower limbs and causes difficulties in walking and climbing stairs. Weakness of ocular and bulbar muscles occurs but does not dominate the clinical picture. The main symptoms of autonomic dysfunction are dry mouth, constipation and impotence. At examination, tendon reflexes are often low or not elicitable. However, they may reappear after 15 s of forceful continuous muscle contraction. Electromyography reveals low muscle-action potentials, increasing after sustained muscle contraction of 15 s (not painful) or after indirect tetanic stimulation (20–50 Hz) (painful). The mean increment of the compound muscle-action potential after tetanic stimulation in a group of 50 patients was 890%.

Auto-antibodies against voltage-gated Ca P/Q channels in the presynaptic membrane are detectable in 85% of patients, but not in controls or in patients with other neurological disorders (Motomura *et al.*, 1995; Newsome-Davis, 1998). There is evidence that these antibodies are induced in patients with SCLC by voltage-gated Ca cells in the membrane of the tumour cells. The antibodies bind to the P/Q channels in the presynaptic membrane and promote their clustering and possibly breakdown, thus impeding the Ca-stimulated neurotransmitter release. Complement activation has not been observed and the presynaptic membrane is otherwise not damaged. *In vitro* and *in vivo* electrophysiology have confirmed that the release of transmitter is insufficient. The presynaptic release of acetylcholine in the autonomic system is impaired also.

Diagnosis and treatment. Proximal muscle weakness and morning stiffness in patients with a 'dry mouth' and other evidence of autonomic disturbance is typical for LEMS and allows the diagnosis with a high degree of probability. The increase of CMAP after sustained muscle contraction confirms the clinical diagnosis.

Comparable to MG, four steps have to be distinguished in the management of LEMS.

1. The presence of SCLC or other malignancies should be established or ruled out. Successful treatment of SCLC is beneficial for LEMS (Chalk *et al.*, 1990).

2. Symptomatic relief is provided by 3,4 di-aminopyridine (3,4 DAP), a potassium channel antagonist that increases the release of acetylcholine (McEvoy *et al.*, 1989). 3,4 DAP is to be preferred to 4 aminopyridine because this enters the CNS less readily. Treatment is started with an oral daily dose of 3 times 5 mg 3,4 DAP; this dose is titrated upward if required until a maximum of 80 mg/day is reached. Side effects are paraesthesia in the perioral region and at the digits, some epigastric discomfort, and seizures at high doses (> 80 mg).
3. Corticosteroids or corticosteroids in combination with azathioprine (see this Chapter – *Diagnosis and management of MG* and Chapter 4) are necessary in some cases.
4. Plasma exchange can be applied in emergencies (Newsome-Davis, 1998; Newsome-Davis and Murray, 1984).

ACQUIRED NEUROMYOTONIA

Acquired neuromyotonia is characterized clinically by muscle twitching, aching or cramps, and myotonia-like features. These forms of abnormal muscle activity are absent at rest; they appear at activity and may be painful. Electromyography in such patients reveals evidence of spontaneous repetitive firing of motor units. Patients with this syndrome have antibodies against voltage-gated potassium channels in the membrane of the terminal part of the axon. A decrease in these functional channels increases the number of acetylcholine quanta released by nerve impulses, which may explain the abnormal firing pattern. Acquired myotonia has been reported in patients with MG and thymoma, and also in association with lung cancer, SLE and juvenile chronic arthritis (see Chapters 7 and 9) (Newsome-Davis, 1998).

Diagnosis and management. The typical spontaneous firing pattern observed at electromyography confirms the clinical diagnosis. Patients are treated with carbamazepine or phenytoin. When neuromyotonia is severe and anticonvulsants are insufficiently effective, treatment with immunosuppression should be considered (see Newsome-Davis, 1998).

REFERENCES

Aarli JA (1993) Immunological aspects of epilepsy. *Brain Development* **15**, 41–50.
Adams HP, Brott TG, Furlan AJ *et al.* (1996) Guidelines for thrombolytic therapy for acute stroke: A supplement to the guidelines for the management of patients with acute ischaemic stroke. *Stroke* **27**, 1711–1718.
Aguayo AJ, Rasminsky M, Bray GM *et al.* (1991) Degenerative and regenerative responses of injured neurons in the central nervous system of adult mammals. *Phil Trans R Soc Lond B* **331**, 337–343.
Aksamit Jr AJ (1997) Cerebrospinal fluid in the diagnosis of central nervous system infections. In: Roos KL (ed) *Central Nervous System Infectious Diseases and Therapy*, pp 731–745. New York: Marcel Dekker Inc.
Alexander EL and Alexander GE (1983) Aseptic meningoencephalitis in primary Sjögren's syndrome. *Neurology* **33**, 593–598.
Arnason BGW and Soliven B (1993) Acute inflammatory demyelinating polyradiculoneuropathy. In: Dyck PJ, Thomas PK, Griffin JW *et al.* (eds). *Peripheral Neuropathy*, Vol. 2, 3ed, pp 1437–1497. Philadelphia: WB Saunders.
Bär PR (1996) Apoptosis – the cell's silent exit. *Life Sci* **59**, 369–378.
Bähr M and Bonhoeffer F (1994) Perspectives on axonal regeneration in the mammalian CNS. *Trends Neurosci* **11**, 473–479.

Barohn RJ, Kissel JT, Warmolts JR *et al.* (1989) Chronic inflammatory demyelinating polyneuropathy: Clinical characteristics, course, and recommendations for diagnostic criteria. *Arch Neurol* **46**, 878–884.

Beatty WW, Paul RH, Wilbanks SL *et al.* (1995) Identifying multiple sclerosis patients with mild or global cognitive impairment using the Screening Examination For Cognitive Impairment (SEFCI). *Neurology* **45**, 718–723.

Beck RW, Cleary PA, Anderson MM *et al.* (1992) A randomized controlled trial of corticosteroids in the treatment of acute optic neuritis. *N Engl J Med* **326**, 581–588.

Beck RW, Cleary PA, Trobe JD *et al.* (1993) The effect of corticosteroids for acute optic neuritis on the subsequent development of multiple sclerosis. *N Engl J Med* **329**, 1764–1769.

Berman M, Feldman S, Alter M *et al.* (1981) Acute transverse myelitis: incidence and etiologic considerations. *Neurology* **31**, 966–971.

Bisby MA (1995) Regeneration of peripheral nervous system axons. In: Waxman SG, Kocsis JD and Stys PK (eds) *The Axon: Structure, Function and Pathophysiology*, pp 553–578. New York: Oxford University Press.

Bredesen DE (1995) Neural apoptosis. *Ann Neurol* **38**, 839–851.

Bousser MG, Ross Russell R (1997) *Cerebral Venous Thrombosis.* London: WB Saunders Ltd.

Caplan LR (1992) Intracerebral haemorrhage. *Lancet* **339**, 656–658.

Caplan LR, Mohr JP, Kistler JP *et al.* (1997) Thrombolysis – not a panacea for ischemic stroke. *N Engl J Med* **337**, 1309–1310.

Castillo J, Dayalos A and Noya M (1997) Progression of ischaemic stroke and excitotoxic aminoacids. *Lancet* **349**, 422–425.

Chalk CH, Murray NM, Newsom-Davis J *et al.* (1990) Response of the Lambert-Eaton myasthenic syndrome to treatment of associated small-cell lung carcinoma. *Neurology* **40**, 1552–1556.

Chalk CH, Windebank AJ, Kimmel DW *et al.* (1992) The distinctive clinical features of paraneoplastic sensory neuronopathy. *Canadian J Neurol Sci* **19**, 346–351.

Chen J, Zhu R, Basta K *et al.* (1996) Inhibition of *bcl-2* protein expression by antisense S-oligodeoxynucleotides treatment exacerbates neuronal death after cerebral ischaemia in rats. *Neurology* **46**, A270.

Cserr HF and Knopf PM (1992) Cervical lymphatics, the blood-brain barrier and the immunoreactivity of the brain; a new view. *Immunology Today* **13**, 507–512.

Dai J, Swaab DF and Buys RM (1998) Recovery of axonal transport in 'dead neurons'. *Lancet* **351**, 499–500.

Dalakas MC and Quarles RH (1996) Autoimmune ataxic neuropathies (sensory ganglionopathies): Are glycolipids the responsible autoantigens? *Ann Neurol* **39**, 419–422.

De Baets MH and Kuks JJM (1993) Immunopathology of myasthenia gravis. In: DeBaets MH and Oosterhuis HJGH (eds) *Myasthenia Gravis*, pp 147–202. Boca Raton: CRC Press.

De Jager AFJ and Minderhoud JM (1991) Residual signs in severe Guillain-Barré syndrome. *J Neurol Sci* **104**, 151–156.

de Keyser J (1998) Antipyretics in ischaemic stroke. *Lancet* **352**, 6–7.

Dichter MA (1994) Emerging insights into mechanisms of epilepsy: Implications for new antiepileptic drug development. *Epilepsia* **35** (suppl), S51–S57.

Doble A (1995) Excitatory amino acid receptors and neurodegeneration. *Thérapie* **50**, 319–337.

Dreifuss FE and Henriksen O (1992) Classification of epileptic seizures and the epilepsies. *Acta Neurologica Scandinavica* **86** (suppl 140), 8–17.

Dyck PJ, Giannini C and Lais A (1993) Pathologic alterations of nerves. In: Dyck PJ, Thomas PK, Griffin JW *et al.* (eds) *Peripheral Neuropathy*, Vol. 1. 3ed, pp 514–595. Philadelphia, WB Saunders.

Dyck PJ, Prineas J and Pollard J (1993a) Chronic inflammatory demyelinating polyradiculoneuropathy. In: Dyck PJ, Thomas PK, Griffin JW *et al.* (eds) *Peripheral Neuropathy*, Vol. 2, 3ed, pp 1498–1517. Philadelphia: WB Saunders.

Dyck PJ, Litchy WJ and Kratz KM (1994) A plasma exchange versus immune globulin infusion trial in chronic inflammatory polyneuropathy. *Ann Neurol* **36**, 838–845.

Engel AG (1994a) Acquired autoimmune myasthenia gravis. In: Engel AG and Franzini-Armstrong C (eds). *Myology*, Vol. 2, 2ed, pp 1769–1797. New York. McGraw-Hill Inc.

Engel AG (1994b). Myasthenic syndromes. In: Engel AG and Franzini-Armstrong C (eds) *Myology*, Vol. 2, 2ed, pp 1798–1835. New York: McGraw-Hill Inc.

Fahn S (1995) Sydenham and other forms of chorea. In: Rowland LP (ed) *Merritt's Textbook of Neurology* 9ed, pp 699–705. Baltimore: Williams-Wilkins.

Feasby TE (1994) Axonal Guillain-Barré syndrome. *Muscle Nerve* **17**, 678–679.

Feasby TE, Gilbert JJ, Brown WF *et al.* (1986) An acute axonal form of Guillain-Barré polyneuro-pathy. *Brain* **109**, 1115–1126.

Feasby TE, Hahn AF, Koopman WJ *et al.* (1990) Central lesions in the chronic inflammatory demyelinating polyneuropathy: An MRI study. *Neurology* **40**, 476–478.

Feigin VL, Rinkel GJE, Algra A, Vermeulen M, van Gijn J (1998) Calcium antagonists in patients with aneurysmal haemorrhage. A systematic review. *Neurology* **50**, 876–883.

Feldmann E (1991) Intracerebral hemorrhage. *Stroke* **22**, 684–691.

Förster C, Brandt T, Meinck HM *et al.* (1996) Trigeminal neuropathy in connective tissue disease: evidence for the site of the lesion. *Neurology* **46**, 270–271.

Franssen H, Vermeulen M and Jennekens FGI (1997) Chronic inflammatory neuropathy. In: Emery A (ed) *Diagnostic Criteria of Neuromuscular Diseases*, 2ed, pp 53–56. London: Royal Society of Medicine Press.

Garagusi VF, Neefe LI and Mann O (1976) Acute meningoencephalitis associated with isoniazid administration. *JAMA* **235**, 141–142.

Gied JN, Rapoport JL, Kruesi MJP *et al.* (1995) Sydenham's chorea: Magnetic resonance imaging of the basal ganglia. *Neurology* **45**, 2199–2202.

Gilman S (1998a) Imaging the brain: First of two parts. *N Engl J Med* **338**, 812–820.

Gilman S (1998b) Imaging the brain. Second of two parts. *N Engl J Med* **338**, 889–896.

Ginsberg MD and Busto R (1998) Combating hyperthermia in acute stroke: A significant clinical concern. *Stroke* **29**, 529–534.

Ghika J and Bogousslavsky J (1996) White matter disease and vascular dementia. In: Prohovnik I, Wade J, Knezevic S *et al.* (eds) *Vascular Dementia*, pp 113–141. Chichester: John Wiley and Sons.

Goldman SE, Amron D, Szilowoski HB *et al.* (1993) Reversible striatal hypermetabolism in a case of Sydenham's chorea. *Movement disorders* **8**, 355–358.

Gorelick DA and Balster RL (1995) Phencyclidine (PCP). In: Bloom FE and Kupfer DJ (Eds) *Psychopharmacology: The Fourth Generation of Progress*, pp 1767–1776. New York: Raven Press, Ltd.

Griffin JW and Hoffman PN (1993) Degeneration and regeneration in the peripheral nervous system. In: Dyck PJ, Thomas PK, Griffin JW *et al.* (eds). *Peripheral Neuropathy*, Vol. 1, 3ed, pp 361–376. Philadelphia: WB Saunders.

Griffin JW, Cornblath DR, Alexander E *et al.* (1990) Ataxic sensory neuropathy and dorsal root ganglionitis associated with Sjögren's syndrome. *Ann Neurol* **27**, 304–315.

Griffin JW, George EB, Hsieh S-T *et al.* (1995) Axonal degeneration and disorders of the axonal cytoskeleton. In: Waxman SG, Kocsis JD and Stys PK (eds) *The Axon. Structure, Function and Pathophysiology*, pp 375–390. New York: Oxford University Press.

Griffin JW, Li CY, Ho TW *et al.* (1996) Pathology of the motor-sensory axonal Guillain-Barré syndrome. *Ann Neurol* **39**, 17–28.

Guy J, Mao J, Bidgood WD *et al.* (1992) Enhancement and demyelination of the intraorbital optic nerve. Fat suppression magnetic resonance imaging. *Ophthalmology* **99**, 713–719.

Haas EJ (1984) Trimethoprim-sulfamethoxazole: another cause of recurrent meningitis. *JAMA* **252**, 345–346.

Hafer-Macko CE, Sheikh KA, Li CY *et al.* (1996) Immune attack on the Schwann cell surface in acute inflammatory demyelinating polyneuropathy. *Ann Neurol* **39**, 625–635.

Hagen NA, Stevens JC and Michet CJ Jr (1990) Trigeminal sensory neuropathy associated with connective tissue diseases. *Neurology* **40**, 891–896.

Hainfeller JA, Kristoferitsch W, Lassmann H *et al.* (1996) T-cell mediated ganglionitis associated with acute sensory neuronopathy. *Ann Neurol* **39**, 543–547.

Harada T, Ohashi T, Miyagishi R *et al.* (1995) Optic neuropathy and acute transverse myelopathy in primary Sjögren's syndrome. *Jpn J Ophthalmol* **39**, 162–165.

Hesselmans LFGM, Jennekers FGI, Kartman J *et al.* (1992) Secondary changes of the motor endplate in Lambert-Eaton myasthenic syndrome: a quantitative studies. *Acta Neuropathol* **83**, 203–206.

Hosford DA (1995) Models of primary generalized epilepsy. *Curr Opin Neurol* **8**, 121–125.

Hughes RAC (1993) Diseases of the fifth cranial nerve. In: Dyck PJ, Thomas PK, Griffin JW *et al.* (eds) *Peripheral Neuropathy*, Vol. 2, 3ed, pp 801–817. Philadelphia: WB Saunders.

Hijdra A, Verbeeten B Jr and Verhulst JA (1990) Relation of leukoaraiosis to lesion type in stroke patients. *Stroke* **21**, 890–894.

Jacobs BC, Endtz HPH, van der Meché FGA *et al.* (1995) Serum anti-GQ$_{1b}$IgG antibodies recognize surface epitopes on *Campylobacter jejuni* from patients with Miller-Fisher syndrome. *Ann Neurol* **37**, 260–261.

Jacobson DM (1997) Optic neuritis. In: Rolak LA and Harati Y (eds) *Neuro-Immunology for The Clinician*, pp 133–154. Boston: Butterworth-Heinemann.

James J (1994) Celveroudering en celdood. Amsterdam: Amsterdam University Press.

Javitt DC and Zukin SR (1991) Recent advances in the phencyclidine model of schizophrenia. *Am J Psychiatry* **148**, 1301–1308.

Jeffrey DR, Mandler RN and Davis LE (1993) Transverse myelitis (retrospective analysis of 33 cases, with differentiation of cases associated with multiple sclerosis and parainfectious events). *Arch Neurol* **50**, 532–536.

Jennekens-Schinkel A, Laboyerie PM, Lanser JBK and van der Velde EA (1990). Cognition in patients with multiple sclerosis: After four years. *J Neurol Sci* **99**, 229–247.

Jennett B and Teasdale G (1977) Aspects of coma after severe head injury. *Lancet* **1**, 878–881.

Jenette JC and Falk RJ (1994) Small-vessel vasculitis. *N Engl J Med* **337**, 1512–1523.

Kane JM (1995) Tardive dyskinesia: Epidemiological and clinical presentation. In: Bloom FE and Kupfer DJ (eds) *Psychopharmacology: The Fourth Generation of Progress*, pp 1485–1495. New York: Raven Press Limited.

Kaplan JE and Schaunburg HH (1991) Predominantly unilateral sensory neuronopathy in Sjögren's syndrome. *Neurology* **41**, 948–949.

Kreutzberg GW (1995) Reaction of the neuronal cell body to axonal damage. In: Waxman SG, Kocsis JD and Stys PK (eds) *The Axon: Structure, Function and Pathophysiology*, pp 355–374. New York: Oxford University Press.

Krupp LB (1997) Postinfectious neurological syndromes. In: Roos KL (ed) *Central Nervous System Infectious Diseases and Therapy*, pp 455–480. New York: Marcel Dekker.

Kuehnen J, Schwartz A, Neff W *et al.* (1998) Cranial nerve syndrome in thrombosis of the transverse/sigmoid sinuses. *Brain* **121**, 381–388.

Kwa VIH, Limburg M, Voogel AJ *et al.* (1996) Feasibility of cognitive screening of patients with ischaemic stroke using the CAMCOG: A hospital-based study. *J Neurol* **243**, 405–409.

Lakke PWF (1981) Classification of extrapyramidal disorders. *J Neurol Sci* **51**, 311–327.

Lampl Y, Gilad R, Eshel Y *et al.* (1995) Neurological and functional outcome in patients with supratentorial hemorrhage. A prospective study. *Stroke* **26**, 2249–2250.

Lai EC (1997) Paraneoplastic syndromes. In: Rolak LA and Harati Y (eds) *Neuroimmunology for the Clinician*, pp 377–391. Boston: Butterworth-Heinemann.

Lecky BRF, Hughes RAC and Murray NMF (1987) Trigeminal neuropathy. *Brain* **110**, 1463–1485.

Lee HC, Coulter CL, Adickes DO *et al.* (1996) Autonomic ganglionitis with severe hypertension, migraine and episodic but fatal hypotension. *Neurology* **47**, 817–821.

Lezak MD (1995) Neuropsychological Assessment, 3ed. New York: Oxford University Press.

Linnik MD, Zobrist RH and Hatfield MD (1993) Evidence supporting a role for programmed cell death in focal cerebral ischemia in rats. *Stroke* **24**, 2002–2009.

Lipton SA and Rosenberg PA (1994) Excitatory amino acids as a final common pathway for neurologic disorders. *N Engl J Med* **330**, 613–622.

Lowenstein DH and Alldredge BK (1998) Status epilepticus. *N Engl J Med* **338**, 970–976.

Ludowyk PA, Willenborg DO and Parish CR (1992) Selective localization of neurospecific T lymphocytes in the central nervous system. *J Neuroimmunol* **37**, 237–250.

Ludwin SK (1995) Pathology of the myelin sheath. In: Waxman SG, Kocsis JD and Stys PK. *The Axon. Structure, Function and Pathophysiology*, pp 412–437. New York: Oxford University Press.

Mano Y, Nakamuro T, Tamura R *et al.* (1995) Central motor reorganization after anastomosis of the musculocutaneous and intercostal nerves following cervical root avulsion. *Ann Neurol* **38**, 15–20.

Martin MA, Massanari M, Nghiem DD *et al.* (1988) Nosocomical aseptic meningitis associated with administration of OKT3. *JAMA* **259**, 2002–2005.

Martinou JC, Dubois-Dauphin M, Staple JK *et al.* (1994) Overexpression of BCL-2 in transgenic mice protects neurons from naturally occurring cell death and experimental ischaemia. *Neuron* **13**, 1017–1030.

Mayberg MR, Batjer HH, Dacey R *et al.* (1994) AHA medical/scientific statement special report. Guidelines for the management of aneurysmal subarachnoid hemorrhage. A statement for healthcare professionals from a special writing group of the Stroke Council, American Heart Association. *Stroke* **25**, 2315–2328.

McCombe PA (1995) Autoimmune disease of the neuromuscular junction and other disorders of the motor unit. In: Pender MP and McCombe PA (eds). *Autoimmune Neurological Disease*, pp 257–303. Cambridge: Cambridge University Press.

McEvoy KM, Windebank AJ, Daube JR *et al.* (1989) 3,4-Diaminopyridine in the treatment of Lambert-Eaton myasthenic syndrome. *N Engl J Med* **321**, 1567–1571.

McKerracher L, Julien J-P and Aguayo AJ (1995) Role of cellular interactions in axonal growth and regeneration. In: Waxman SG, Kocsis JD and Stys PK (eds). *The Axon. Structure, Function and Pathophysiology*, pp 579–589. New York: Oxford University Press.

McNamara JO (1994) Cellular and molecular basis of epilepsy. *J Neurosci* **14**, 3413–3425.

Motomura M, Johnston I, Lang B *et al.* (1995) An improved diagnostic assay for Lambert-Eaton myasthenic syndrome. *J Neurol Neurosurg Psychiat* **58**, 85–87.

Nausieda PA (1986) Sydenham's chorea, chorea gravidarum and contraceptive induced chorea. *Handbook of Clinical Neurology* **49**, 359–367.

NINDS (The National Institute of Neurological disorders) rt-PA Stroke Study Group (1995) Tissue plasminogen activator for acute ischaemic stroke. *N Engl J Med* **335**, 1581–1587.

Newsome-Davis J (1998) Neuromyotonia and the Lambert-Eaton syndrome. In: Latov N, Wokke JHJ and Kelly JJ Jr (eds) *Immunological and Infectious Diseases of the Peripheral Nerves*, pp 238–250. Cambridge: Cambridge University Press.

Newsom-Davis J and Murray NMF (1984) Plasma exchange and immunosuppressive drug treatment in the Lambert-Eaton syndrome. *Neurology* **34**, 480–485.

Oh SJ, Joy JI and Kuruoglu R (1992) Chronic sensory demyelinating neuropathy: Chronic inflammatory demyelinating polyneuropathy presenting as a pure sensory neuropathy. *J Neurol Neurosurg Psychiat* **55**, 667–680.

Olney JW (1978) Neurotoxicity of excitatory amino acids. In: McGeer EG, Olney JW and McGeer PL (eds) *Kainic Acid As A Tool in Neurobiology*, pp 95–112. New York: Raven Press.

Olney JW and Farber NB (1995) Glutamate receptor dysfunction and schizophrenia. *Arch Gen Psychiatry* **52**, 998–1007.

O'Neil JH, Murray NMF, Spiro SG *et al.* (1988) The Lambert-Eaton myasthenic syndrome. A review of 50 cases. *Brain* **111**, 577–596.

Onodera J, Nakamura S, Nagano I *et al.* (1996) Upregulation of *bcl-2* protein in the myasthenic thymus. *Ann Neurol* **39**, 521–528.

Oomes PG, Jacobs BC, Hazenberg MPH *et al.* (1995) Anti-GM$_1$ IgG antibodies and campylobacter bacteria in Guillain-Barré syndrome: evidence of molecular mimicry. *Ann Neurol* **38**, 170–175.

Oosterhuis HJGH (1997) *Myasthenia Gravis*. Groningen: Groningen Neurological Press.

Optic Neuritis Study Group (1991) The clinical profile of optic neuritis. Experience of the optic neuritis treatment trial. *Arch Opthalmol* **109**, 1673–1678.

Pender MP (1995) Multiple sclerosis. In: Pender MP and McCombe PA (eds) *Autoimmune Neurological Disease*, pp 89–154. Cambridge: Cambridge University Press.

Plum F and Posner JB (1982) The diagnosis of stupor and coma, 3ed. Philadelphia: FA Davis Company.

Powers WJ (1993) Acute hypertension after stroke: The scientific basis for treatment decisions. *Neurology* **43**, 461–467.

Pulsinelli W (1992) Pathophysiology of acute ischaemic stroke. *Lancet* **339**, 533–536.

Reese TS and Karnowsky MJ (1967) Fine structural localization of a blood brain barrier to exogenous peroxidase. *J Cell Biol* **34**, 207–217.

Ropper AH (1994) Miller-Fisher syndrome and other acute variants of Guillain-Barré syndrome. In: McLeod JG (ed). *Inflammatory Neuropathies*, pp 95–106. London: Baillière Tindall.

Ropper AH and Poskanzer DC (1978) The prognosis of acute and subacute transverse myelopathy based on early signs and symptoms. *Ann Neurol* **41**, 51–59.

Rorick MB, Chandar K and Colombi BJ (1996) Inflammatory trigeminal sensory neuropathy mimicking trigeminal neurinoma. *Neurology* **46**, 1455–1457.

Rosen DR, Siddique T, Patterson D *et al.* (1993) Mutations in Cu/Zn superoxide dismutase gene are associated with familial amyotrophic lateral sclerosis. *Nature* **362**, 59–62.

Ross CA and Pearlson GD (1996) Schizophrenia, the heteromodal association neocortex and development: Potential for a neurogenetic approach. *Trends Neurosci* **19**, 171–176.

Sedvall G and Farde L (1995) Chemical brain anatomy in schizophrenia. *Lancet* **346**, 743–749.

Scott TF, Bhagavatula K, Snyder PJ *et al.* (1998) Transverse myelitis. Comparison with spinal cord presentations of multiple sclerosis. *Neurology* **50**, 429–433.

Smith JL, Finley JC, Lennon VA *et al.* (1988) Autoantibodies in paraneoplastic cerebellar degeneration bind to cytoplasmic antigens of Purkinje cells in humans, rats, and mice and are of multiple immunoglobulin classes. *J Neuroimmunol* **18**, 37–48.

Sobue G, Yasuda T, Kachi T *et al.* (1993) Chronic progressive sensory ataxic neuropathy: Clinicopathologic features of idiopathic and Sjögren's syndrome-associated cases. *J Neurol* **240**, 1–7.

Stam J (1997) Cerebrale veneuze thrombose. Voordracht nascholingscursus Neurologie, Cerebrovasculaire ziekten.

Sinard JH and Hedreen JC (1995) Neuronal loss from the subthalamic nuclei in a patient with progressive chorea. *Movement Disorders* **10**, 305–311.

Stone LA (1997) Transverse myelitis. In: Rolak LA and Harati Y (eds) *Neuroimmunology for The Clinician*, pp 155–165. Boston: Butterworth-Heinemann.

Stroke Prevention In Reversible Ischaemia Trial (SPIRIT) Study Group (1997) A randomized trial of anticoagulants versus aspirin after cerebral ischaemia of presumed arterial origin. *Ann Neurol* **42**, 857–865.

Stys PK, Ransom BR, Black JA *et al.* (1995) Anoxic/ischemic injury in axons. In: Waxman SG, Kocsis JD and Stys PK (eds) *The Axon. Structure, Function and Pathophysiology*, pp 462–479. New York: Oxford University Press.

Teasdall RD, Frayha RA and Shulman LE (1980) Cranial nerve involvement in systemic sclerosis (scleroderma): a report of 10 cases. *Medicine* **59**, 149–159.

The Dutch TIA Study Group (1994) A comparison of two doses of aspirin (30 mg vs 283 mg a day) in patients after a transient ischaemic attack or minor stroke. *N Engl J Med* **325**, 1261–1266.

Thomas PK, Ochoa J, Berthold CH *et al.* (1993) Microscopic anatomy of the peripheral nervous system. In: Dyck PJ, Thomas PK, Griffin JW *et al.* (eds) *Peripheral Neuropathy*, vol 1, 3ed, pp 28–91. Philadelphia: WB Saunders.

Tippett DS, Fishman PS and Panitch HS (1991) Relapsing transverse myelitis. *Neurology* **41**, 703–706.

Van der Meché FGA (1994) The Guillain-Barré syndrome. In: McLeod JG (ed.). *Inflammatory neuropathies*, pp 73–94. London: Baillière Tindall.

Van der Meché FGA (1998) Guillain-Barré syndrome and variants. In: Latov N, Wokke JHJ and Kelly Jr (eds) *Immunological and Infectious Diseases of The Peripheral Nerves*, pp 99–110. Cambridge: Cambridge Unversity Press.

Van der Meché FGA, Schmitz PIM and The Dutch Guillain-Barré Study Group (1992) A randomized trial comparing intravenous immune globulin and plasma exchange in Guillain-Barré syndrome. *N Engl J Med* **326**, 1123–1129.

Van Dijk GW, Wokke JHJ, Notermans NC *et al.* (1997) Indications for an immune-mediated etiology of idiopathic sensory neuronopathy. *J Neuroimmunol* **74**, 165–172.

Van Dijk GW, Notermans NC, Franssen H *et al.* (1996) Response to intravenous immunoglobulin treatment in chronic inflammatory demyelinating polyneuropathy with only sensory symptoms. *J Neurol* **243**, 318–322.

Van Swieten JC, Van den Hout JHW, Van Ketel BA *et al.* (1991) Periventricular lesions in the white matter on magnetic resonance imaging in the elderly. *Brain* **114**, 761–774.

Vermeulen M (1998) Chronic inflammatory demyelinating polyneuropathy. In: Latov N, Wokke JHJ and Kelly JJ Jr (eds) *Immunological and Infectious Diseases of The Peripheral Nerves*, pp 111–125. Cambridge: Cambridge University Press.

Visser LH, van der Meché FGA, van Doorn PA *et al.* (1995) Guillain-Barré syndrome without sensory loss (acute motor neuropathy). A subgroup with specific clinical, electrodiagnostic and laboratory features. *Brain* **118**, 841–847.

Wada M, Kato T, Yuki N *et al.* (1997) Gadolinium-enhancement of the spinal posterior roots in acute sensory ataxic neuropathy. *Neurology* **49**, 1470–1471.

Wardlaw JM, Warlow CP and Counsell C (1997) Systematic review of evidence on thrombolytic therapy for acute ischaemic stroke. *Lancet* **350**, 607–614.

Wanschitz J, Hainfeller JA, Kristoferitsch W *et al.* (1997) Ganglionitis in paraneoplastic subacute sensory neuronopathy: A morphologic study. *Neurology* **49**, 1156–1159.

Weindl A, Kuwert T, Leenders KL *et al.* (1993) Increased striatal glucose consumption in Sydenham's chorea. *Movement Disorders* **8**, 437–444.

Weir CJ, Murray GD, Dyker AG *et al.* (1997) Is hyperglycaemia an independent predictor of poor outcome after acute stroke? Results of a longterm follow-up study. *BMJ* **314**, 1303–1306.

Willison HJ, Almemar A, Veitch J and Thrush D (1994) Acute ataxic neuropathy with cross-reactive antibodies to GD_{1b} and GD_3 gangliosides. *Neurology* **44**, 2395–2397.

Windebank AJ, Blexrud MD, Dyck PJ *et al.* (1990) The syndrome of acute sensory neuropathy: clinical features and electrophysiologic and pathologic changes. *Neurology* **40**, 584–591.

Wyllie AH and Duvall E (1992) Cell death. In: McGee JO, Isaacson P and Wright NA (eds) *Oxford Textbook of Pathology*, vol 1, pp 141–157. Oxford: Oxford University Press.

Yeung KB, Thomas PK, King RHM *et al.* (1991). The clinical spectrum of peripheral neuropathies associated with benign monoclonal IgM, IgG and IgA paraproteinaemia. Comparative clinical immunological and nerve biopsy findings. *J Neurol* **238**, 383–391.

Zivin JA (1998) Factors determining the therapeutic window for stroke. *Neurology* **50**, 599–603.

3

Auto-antibodies in Inflammatory Connective Tissue Diseases: Clinical Value and Limitations of Laboratory Tests

INTRODUCTION

The main function of the immune system is to discriminate between self and non-self antigens. It enables identification and reaction with foreign antigens from bacteria, viruses or other agents without causing self damage. Initially it was suggested that tolerance to self was associated with the absence of auto-antibodies. However, during the last decades it has become clear that the immune system of almost all vertebrates is able to produce antibodies to auto-antigens that are preserved highly during evolution, such as histones and ribonuclear acids. The production of self-structure recognizing antibodies (auto-antibodies) is not necessarily related to overt disease. For example, auto-antibodies are often present in healthy relatives of patients with auto-immune disease (Buskila and Shoenfeld, 1995). Non-pathogenic auto-antibodies are found after tissue injury resulting from causes like trauma, ischaemia and inflammation. In these latter circumstances, it is suggested that antigenic epitopes that are usually not seen by the immune system are exposed. The production of such auto-antibodies is usually self-limited. Apparently, qualitatively different factors are needed in order to develop clinically manifest auto-immune diseases. T-lymphocytes from normal individuals may also react to auto-antigens, at least *in vitro*.

Some of the factors that contribute to the development of auto-immune disease have been identified (*e.g.*, immunoregulatory defects, deficiency of complement components, genetic background, environmental factors and sex hormones). The genetic background factors concern, in particular, human leukocyte antigen (HLA) class II genes, as for instance HLA-DR2, DR3 and DR4, which bear an increased risk on certain auto-immune diseases. Most auto-immune diseases are significantly more frequent in females in their reproductive period than in other females and males, apparently because of the high oestrogen levels during the reproductive period. A suitable trigger, such as an environmental factor, may give rise to auto-immune disease if the individual concerned has the proper immunological, immunogenetic and hormonal make-up.

AUTO-IMMUNE DISEASE AND ANTIBODIES

The term *auto-immune disease* is used for a wide spectrum of disorders in which the immune system damages normal components of the individual by virtue of auto-immune reactivity. Lambert-Eaton myasthenic syndrome (LEMS) serves as an example. Approximately 3% of patients with small-cell bronchus carcinoma produce antibodies against an epitope in the cell membrane of the tumour cells. This antibody cross-reacts with a Ca-channel protein in the presynaptic membrane of the neuromuscular junctions, and this hampers neurotransmitter release and causes muscle weakness (see Chapter 2). In most auto-immune diseases, especially the non-organ specific disorders, there is no clear cut evidence for a direct role of auto-antibodies, even if these are of high affinity and present in high titres in the circulation. In this respect, we must confess that the contribution of auto-antibodies to disease processes often is not understood well, and that their presence serves only as a diagnostic phenomenon. This holds for the auto-antibodies in most of the inflammatory connective tissue diseases (ICTDs) described here.

AUTO-ANTIBODIES AND DIAGNOSTIC LABORATORY TESTS

Laboratory investigations have demonstrated the presence of a variety of auto-antibodies in practically all patients with systemic lupus erythematosus (SLE) and Sjögren's syndrome. As well, tests have demonstrated their presence in high percentages of patients with polymyositis, dermatomyositis, diffuse and limited systemic sclerosis and Wegener's granulomatosis. Some of the auto-antibodies are designated as 'disease specific'. High-affinity anti-dsDNA and anti-Sm (named after patient Smith, in whom this antibody was discovered) are strongly associated with SLE (Tan, 1989); anti-Mi-2 occurs in dermatomyositis and only occasionally in other diseases (polymyositis, panniculitis) (Seelig *et al.*, 1995); anti-Jo-1 occurs in patients with myositis (either dermatomyositis or polymyositis) and not in other ICTDs unless there is overlap with myositis (Vazquez-Abad and Rothfield, 1996; see Chapter 12). Other examples are: anti-centromere antibodies in limited systemic sclerosis (previously known as CREST); anti-Scl70 in diffuse and limited systemic sclerosis (Rothfield, 1992; Seibold, 1997); and antineutrophil cytoplasmic antibodies (ANCA) directed against proteinase-3 in Wegener's granulomatosis (Kallenberg *et al.*, 1992). Some antibodies occur in several ICTDs; examples are anti Ro/SS-A and La/SS-B in Sjögren's syndrome, SLE and polymyositis (Tan, 1989; Targoff, 1993); anti-U1RNP in SLE, dermatomyositis and systemic sclerosis (Tan, 1989); and are anti-PM/Scl in polymyositis and systemic sclerosis (Targoff, 1993). Although these antibodies are not disease specific, some of them have been shown to detect specific subsets of diseases (*e.g.*, anti-Ro/SS-A and La/SS-B in subacute cutaneous lupus erythematosus featured by photosensitivity, in neonatal lupus, and in infants with isolated congenital heartblock). As such, these antibodies have proven their value in early diagnosis and recognition of subsets.

In this chapter we review the diagnostic value of the examination of auto-antibodies in the ICTDs.

AUTO-ANTIBODY TESTS FOR INFLAMMATORY CONNECTIVE TISSUE DISEASES AND HOW TO USE THEM

For most of the diseases discussed in this book, classification criteria have been developed and this has made it possible to calculate the specificity and the sensitivity of various laboratory tests. One should always realize that a single positive laboratory test does not allow a diagnosis and that a negative laboratory test does not necessarily exclude one, because sensivity and specificity is rarely absolute.

ANTINUCLEAR ANTIBODIES (ANAs)

Antibodies against antigens of cell nuclei probably occur regularly in the blood of most human beings. Only when ANAs occur in significantly elevated levels is the test considered positive. A test for ANAs is the most frequently used assay for the detection of ICTDs. Using human tissue culture lines (Hep-2 cells, fibroblasts, etc.) as substrate and an indirect immunofluorescent technique, significant levels of ANA will be detected in more than 95% of patients with SLE, in approximately 90% of patients with Sjögren's syndrome and scleroderma, and in 50% of patients with polymyositis and dermatomyositis (Tan, 1989; Rothfield, 1992; Targoff, 1993). However, if heterologous tissue (mouse liver) is used instead of human tissue culture lines, ANAs can be negative in 5–10% of patients with SLE. In these ANA-negative SLE patients, one or more auto-antibodies against nuclear antigens may often be detected using other sensitive techniques. An example is anti-Ro/SS-A nuclear antibody directed specifically against human epitopes, which is missed when mouse livers are used as substrate (Reichlin and Reichlin, 1989). ANAs can also be found in various titres in other ICTDs and in 4–25% of elderly controls. The percentage of positive controls increases with the mean age of the control group.

The distribution of the antigen in the nucleus demonstrated by immunofluorescent staining is also of diagnostic value (Fig. 3.1). A speckled type of staining points to the presence of antinuclear antibodies directed against Sm, nRNP (U1RNP) or La/SS-B but is not sufficiently sensitive for the detection of these special forms of ANAs. A homogenous pattern signifies that antibodies against nucleoprotein (the LE cell factor) or antihistone antibodies are present. This pattern is typical for drug-induced LE. A peripheral (ring) staining pattern fits with antibodies against dsDNA. Antinucleolar antibodies are seen in patients with scleroderma. These antibodies are directed against a variety of nuclear antigens including RNA-polymerase and PM/Scl antigen (Reichlin *et al.*, 1984; Reimer *et al.*, 1987).

Clinical significance. The ANA test is very valuable when screening for ICTDs. It is sensitive, but lacks specificity. If the test is positive, specification tests are necessary as these may provide information to the nature of the underlying disease (Table 3.1).

ANTI-DOUBLE STRANDED DNA (dsDNA) ANTIBODIES

Anti-dsDNA antibodies are highly specific for SLE and are detected in approximately 40% of patients by enzyme-linked immunosorbent assay (ELISA) and

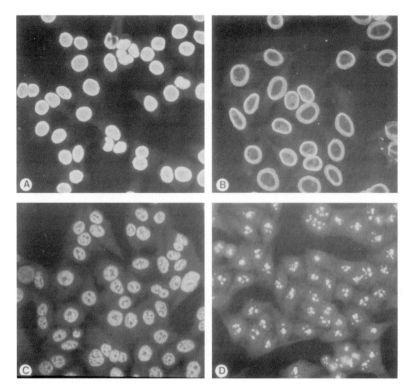

Figure 3.1 Four different patterns of immunohistochemical antinuclear antibody stainings. *A.* Homogeneous pattern compatible with presence of antibodies against nucleoproteins (LE cell factor) or against histones. *B.* Peripheral ring staining, fitting in with antibodies against dsDNA. *C.* Speckled staining pointing to the presence of antibodies against small ribonuclear proteins. *D.* Antinuclear antibodies directed against a variety of other nuclear antigens, occurring in scleroderma.

radioimmunoassay. They can also be demonstrated by an indirect immunofluorescent assay using *Crithidia luciliae* as substrate, which carries dsDNA in its kinetoplast. The antibody against dsDNA in the patient's serum will react with the kinetoplast (Aarden *et al.*, 1975) (Fig. 3.2). For quantification of anti-dsDNA, a radioimmunoassay (usually Farr assay) is used. This assay detects only anti-dsDNA antibodies of relatively high affinity that are very specific for SLE. An increase in levels of anti-dsDNA within a few weeks and a lowering of complement levels are indicative of impeding disease activity. We have shown that early treatment with 30 mg prednisone prevents these exacerbations (Bootsma *et al.*, 1995).

Clinical significance. Antibodies to high affinity dsDNA are highly specific for SLE. The titres fluctuate with disease activity, and these changes in levels can be used to monitor treatment.

Table 3.1 Antinuclear antibodies in the diagnosis of systemic lupus erythematosus

Antibody	Frequency %	Clinical relevance
Antinuclear antibody (ANA)	>98 (SLE)	Excellent screening test for SLE; highly sensitive, low specificity
Anti-dsDNA	40 (SLE)	Highly specific for SLE
Anti-ssDNA	70 (SLE)	Not specific, also in cutaneous LE, especially those at risk to develop SLE
Anti-histones	70 (SLE)	Induced LE; not specific; occur in 100% of procainamide induced LE
Anti-Sm	20 (SLE)	Highly specific for SLE; occur mostly together with anti-U1 RNP
Anti-U1RNP	35 (SLE)	SLE patients with increased frequency of Raynaud's syndrome, sclerodactyly, oesophageal dysmobility and pulmonary disease; not specific; also present in up to 95% of patients with MCTD and in 5–10% of patients with myositis and scleroderma
Anti-Ro/SS-A	40–45 (Sjögren's syndrome) 25–30 (SLE)	Tend to be especially positive in Sjögren's with extraglandular manifestations; not specific, also associated with photosensitive cutaneous LE, late onset SLE, neonatal SLE (including congenital heart block) (98% of mothers are positive), 10% of patients with polymyositis
Anti-La/SS-B	15 (Sjögren's syndrome) 10 (SLE)	Nearly always found together with anti-Ro/SS-A; in at least 60% of children and mothers of neonatal lupus patients
Anti-ribosomal P	12–16 (SLE)	SLE associated with lupus psychosis?

Abbreviations: see sections on specific antibodies in this chapter.
From Provost and Kater (1995), with permission.

ANTI-SINGLE STRANDED DNA (ssDNA) ANTIBODIES

Anti-ssDNA antibodies occur in about 70% of patients with SLE, but also in patients with many other ICTDs, such as rheumatoid arthritis (RA) and cutaneous lupus, and especially in those at risk to develop systemic features like fatigue, arthralgia and myalgia (Rothfield, 1992).

Clinical significance. Since they lack specificity, detection of anti-ssDNA has no direct significance as a diagnostic tool.

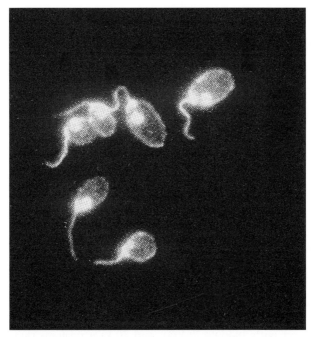

Figure 3.2 High magnification of positive *Crithidia luciliae* assay. Screening for antibodies against dsDNA is often done with an immunofluorescent technique using the trypanosome *Crithidia luciliae*. These prokaryotic cells contain DNA in a kinetoplast located near the flagellum. Positive results of screening require confirmation by an ELISA or radioimmunoassay.

ANTIBODIES TO HISTONES AND NUCLEOSOMES

Many SLE patients produce antibodies against DNA-binding proteins, particularly against various histones (Tan, 1989). The homogenous antinuclear antibody immunofluorescence pattern that often occurs when testing SLE sera is caused both by antibodies against nucleoproteins (LE cell factor) and by antihistone antibodies reacting with nucleosomes.

Antibodies to histones occur in approximately 70% of patients with SLE. A close association exists between antihistone antibodies and drug-induced lupus. Drug-induced lupus and the idiopathic form of SLE can be distinguished serologically. Drug-induced lupus (*e.g.*, procainamide or hydralazine lupus) is characterized by antihistone antibodies and by the absence of anti-dsDNA, anti-Sm and other SLE related antibodies.

The *nucleosome* is a basic structure of chromatine and has an important function in the compaction of DNA in the nucleus of the cell. Recent evidence indicates that the nucleosome is the principle auto-antigen in SLE (Tax *et al.*, 1995). The classical assumption was that anti-DNA antibodies form complexes with DNA either in the circulation or *in situ* in vessel walls. Now, there is evidence that whole nucleosomes are involved in immune complex formation (Kramer *et al.*, 1993). Nucleosomes are composite particles of histones and DNA; they are released upon apoptosis (Bell and Morrison, 1991). In SLE, nucleosomes are either complexed with anti-DNA antibodies in the circulation or directly deposited in basal membranes and subsequently complexed with the antibody (van Bruggen *et al.*, 1997).

Clinical significance. Drug-induced ANAs are almost exclusively of the antihistone type, which is helpful to differentiate between drug-induced lupus and SLE.

ANTI-Sm (SMITH) ANTIBODIES

Anti-Sm antibodies belong to the category of antibodies against small ribonuclear proteins (RNP) (Lerner and Steitz, 1979) and are directed against polypeptides (29-, 28-, 16- and 13-kDa) of spliceosomes. They are specific for SLE and occur in about 20% of patients. They are mostly found in association with anti-nRNP (U2RNP).

Clinical significance. The value of anti-Sm and anti-dsDNA antibodies is that they are not seen in other ICTDs and therefore are recognized as highly diagnostic for SLE (Tan *et al.*, 1982).

ANTI-nRNP ANTIBODIES

Just like anti-Sm antibodies, anti-nRNP antibodies belong to the category of small anti-ribonuclear protein antibodies and are directed against proteins of the spliceosomes. They react with 33-kDa, 22-kDa, and 70-kDa proteins (Lerner and Steitz, 1979). They are found in high titres in about 35% of patients with SLE and in up to 95% of patients with mixed connective tissue diseases (MCTD) (Sharp *et al.*, 1972; see Chapter 12). These patients have a heterogeneous clinical picture. Anti-nRNP (U1RNP) antibodies have been detected in 12% of patients with cryptogenic fibrosing alveolitis (Chapman *et al.*, 1984) and in some cases of neonatal lupus syndrome (Reichlin *et al.*, 1984), but not in patients with congenital heartblock.

Clinical significance. Anti-nRNP (U1RNP) antibodies occur in high titre in about 95% of patients with MCTD. Although not specific, they are helpful for the diagnosis of MCTD.

ANTI-Ro/SS-A ANTIBODIES

Anti-Ro/SS-A (Sjögren's syndrome A) antibodies (Robair is the patient in whom the antibody was discovered) belong with anti-Sm and anti-nRNP antibodies in the category of small anti-ribonuclear proteins, and occur in about 25–30% of SLE patients and 40–45% of patients with Sjögren's syndrome. Most anti-Ro/SS-A antibodies containing sera appear to react with either 60-kDa or 52-kDa proteins (Itoh and Reichlin, 1992). Auto-antibodies against 52-kDa occur more frequently in patients with Sjögren's syndrome; those directed against the 60-kDa protein are generated more often in SLE (Ben-Chetrit *et al.*, 1990).

Anti-Ro/SS-A are generally found in lupus patients with photosensitive cutaneous disease and in subacute cutaneous lupus erythematosus characterized by distinctive annular polycyclic or psoriatiform photosensitive skin lesions. Late onset SLE, beginning after the age of 55, in patients with Sjögren's syndrome is strongly associated with anti-Ro/SS-A. In one small cohort, about 90% of these anti-Ro/SS-A positive late onset SLE patients had neuropsychiatric manifestations, pulmonary disease, and photosensitive cutaneous disease, but no nephritis (Catoggio *et al.*, 1984). In almost all mothers giving birth to children with neonatal lupus syndrome and/or congenital heart block, anti-Ro/SS-A have been found, especially anti-52-kDa Ro/SS-A and anti-48-kDa La/SS-B (Petri *et al.*, 1989; Watson *et al.*, 1984). The mothers may be asymptomatic at the time of the birth of the affected child, or have features of Sjögren's syndrome, lupus, or both. Anti-Ro/SS-A positivity is much more frequent in Chinese, Korean and Japanese patients suspected of having lupus than in Caucasian patients (Kim *et al.*, 1987; Boey *et al.*, 1988). Anti-Ro/SS-A positive neonatal lupus mothers, female Sjögren's syndrome patients, female late onset lupus patients, and female subacute cutaneous lupus patients share an increased frequency of HLA-B8, DR3, DQ2 and Drw52 phenotypes (Provost *et al.*, 1988a; Provost *et al.*, 1988b; Alexander *et al.*, 1989; Provost and Watson, 1993; Reveille *et al.*, 1991; Simmons-O'Brien *et al.*, 1995).

Clinical significance. See anti-La/SS-B antibodies.

ANTI-La/SS-B ANTIBODIES

Anti-La/SS-B antibodies are also small anti-ribonuclear protein antibodies. They are named for patient Lapière and Sjögren's syndrome B, and occur in about 10% of patients with SLE and 15% of patients with Sjögren's syndrome. They occur almost always together with anti-Ro/SS-A and have the same clinical associations. La/SS-B antigen is a ribonucleoprotein particle of 50-kDa, which is transiently associated with all RNA polymerase III transcripts (Gottlieb and Steitz, 1989a; 1989b). The La/SS-B macromolecule also binds to the Ro/SS-A associated hy1-5RNAs, thus providing evidence that at least one of the Ro/SS-A molecules is physically associated with the La/SS-B macromolecule.

Clinical significance. Elevated levels of anti-Ro/SS-A and anti-La/SS-B are present in a minority of patients with Sjögren's syndrome and SLE, the association with Sjögren's syndrome is higher than with SLE. One of the criteria in the proposed European criteria for Sjögren's syndrome (see Chapter 11) concerns the presence of auto-antibodies, and among these are anti-Ro/SS-A and anti-La/SS-B.

ANTI-RIBOSOMAL P ANTIBODIES (ANTI-P)

Anti-P antibodies are directed against three phosphoproteins, P0, P1, and P2, and have been detected in 12–16% of patients with SLE (Harris and Hughes, 1985). These three phosphoproteins are located in the 60S subunit of eukaryotic ribosomes and have molecular weights of 38-kDa, 18-kDa and 17-kDa respectively. Ribosomal P proteins share a common linear determinant that is present in the carboxyl terminal 22 amino-acid sequence (Elkon *et al.*, 1986). An association of anti-P antibodies with neuropsychiatric manifestations of SLE has been reported. However, results of further investigation into this association show considerable discrepancies (see Chapter 7). It appears that anti-P is significantly elevated in serum of patients with organic brain syndrome or psychosis but not in their CSF, which is in contrast to expectations had there been a relation (Isshi *et al.*, 1996; Watanabe *et al.*, 1996).

Clinical significance. Additional studies are required to establish whether anti-P antibodies are markers for a distinct class of disorder in SLE.

ANTIPHOSPHOLIPID ANTIBODIES

Since the description of anticardiolipin antibodies (ACAs) by Harris *et al.* in the eighties (Harris *et al.*, 1983), research on the antiphospholipid (APL) antibodies and the thrombotic manifestations associated with them has grown enormously. Lupus anticoagulants (LACs) and ACAs are both APL antibodies. The antigenic targets of ACAs and LACs are phospholipid binding plasma proteins, notably β_2-glycoprotein I (β_2GPI) and prothrombin, or complexes of these proteins with phospholipids (see Roubey, 1996). LACs and ACAs overlap only partially. In the laboratory, LACs are measured as a pathobiologic haemostatic effect, giving prolonged coagulation *in vitro*. ACAs are measured by an enzyme-linked immunoabsorption assay (ELISA) procedure. LACs are peculiar because *in vivo* they are not associated with bleeding but with thrombosis, despite their *in vitro* anticoagulant activity.

Although recent evidence points to a role of APL antibodies in the pathogenesis of placental infarcts (see Chapter 8), a causal relationship has not been demonstrated yet between the presence of APL antibodies and thrombosis in other organs. APL antibodies can be used however as markers for thrombotic disorders with a high chance of recurrence (see Chapter 8).

APL antibodies in SLE are associated with arterial and venous thrombosis, thrombocytopenia and fetal wastage. APL antibodies occur also in patients with complete absence of an SLE disease process.

Clinical significance. APL antibodies are associated strongly with a set of clinical manifestations designated as Hughes' syndrome or antiphospholipid syndrome (see Chapter 8).

ANTIBODIES IN PATIENTS WITH MYOSITIS

There are two kinds of auto-antibodies in polymyositis (PM) and dermatomyositis (DM). One kind is designated as *myositis specific* (MSA) and the other as *myositis associated* (MAA). The MAAs occur in low percentages of patients with myositis (approximately 20–30%) and are related to myositis subgroups or other ICTDs. To this category belong, for example, anti-U1RNP, anti-Ro/SS-A and anti-PM/Scl (polymyositis/scleroderma) (Table 3.2).

MSAs occur predominantly or almost exclusively in PM or DM and only occasionally (or not at all) in the other main ICTDs. Whether they occur in other muscular diseases has not been sufficiently investigated. MSAs are found in approximately 30–40% of patients with PM or DM (Targoff, 1993; Mimori, 1996; Provost and Kater, 1995). The two MSAs of clinical relevance are anti-Jo-1 and anti-Mi-2. Four other antibodies with similar characteristics also belong to the category of the MSAs, but their incidence is so low that we shall not discuss them. Still another MSA is directed against the signal recognition particle (anti-RSP) and occurs in approximately 5% of patients with PM or DM, and is associated with severe and progressive myositis in some patients (Table 3.3). Different MSAs rarely occur simultaneously.

Table 3.2 Myositis associated antibodies

Antibody	Frequency (%)	Disease
Anti-PM/Scl	8–10	Polymyositis/scleroderma overlap syndrome, polymyositis or scleroderma, or undifferentiated inflammatory connective tissue disease
Anti-Ku	20–30	Polymyositis/scleroderma in Japanese patients, also in white patients with SLE
Anti-DNA-PK	<5	Polymyositis/scleroderma overlap, polymyositis
Anti-U1RNP	12	MCTD, polymyositis overlap with scleroderma and SLE
Anti-U2RNP	<5	Same as anti-U1RNP antibodies
Anti-Ro/SS-A	10	Polymyositis or dermatomyositis in overlap with Sjögren's syndrome and SLE

Data from Mimori (1996) and Provost and Kater (1995) with permission.

Table 3.3 Myositis specific antibodies

Antibody	Frequency (%)	Disease
Anti-Jo-1 (anti-histidyl transfer RNA synthetase)	20	Antisynthetase syndrome: myositis, interstitial pulmonary fibrosis, arthritis, fever, mechanic's hands, Raynaud's phenomenon
Anti-PL-7 (another anti-synthetase)	<5	Same as anti-Jo-1
Anti-PL-12 (another anti-synthetase)	<5	Same as anti-Jo-1
Anti-OJ (another anti-synthetase)	<5	Same as anti-Jo-1
Anti-EJ (another anti-synthetase)	<5	Same as anti-Jo-1
Anti-SRP	<5	Severe therapy resistant polymyositis
Anti-Mi-2	15–20	In adult dermatomyositis
Anti-KJ	<1	Polymyositis with lung fibrosis
Anti-Fer	<1	Nodular myositis
Anti-Mas	<1	Alcoholic rhabdomyolysis

Data from Targoff *et al.* (1997) with permission.

Anti-Jo-1

This antibody is directed against histidyl transfer RNA synthetase. Interstitial pulmonary fibrosis occurs in about 70% of patients with anti-synthetase syndrome; about 90% have arthritis and about 60% have Raynaud's phenomenon. Not all elements of the anti-synthetase syndrome are always present. Some patients have interstitial lung disease and no myositis or vice versa. Anti-Jo-1 antibodies have been detected in approximately 20% of patients with PM or DM, but not in RA and SLE without polymyositis. In one investigation, none of 213 patients with systemic sclerosis had anti-Jo-1 antibodies (Vazquez and Rothfield, 1996).

Clinical significance. The diagnostic criteria used by Bohan and Peter (1975) for PM and DM are in need of revision. Several groups have now suggested that anti-Jo-1 antibodies should be included in the new criteria (Tanimoto *et al.*, 1995; Targoff *et al.*, 1997). This would require that the laboratory method guarantees high specificity and reproducibility. Targoff *et al.* (1997) propose therefore that two methods – immunodiffusion and ELISA – should be used and that the results should confirm each other.

Anti-Mi-2

Anti-Mi-2 is directed against a nuclear helicase. It occurs in approximately 15–20% of adult DM cases and in 0–3% of patients with PM. It seldom occurs in childhood DM. Anti-Mi-2 is very rarely encountered in patients with other ICTDS. Whether it occurs in other inflammatory disorders or in other muscle diseases has been examined insufficiently.

Clinical significance. Inclusion of anti-Mi-2 in new classification criteria for DM has been suggested (Tanimoto *et al.* 1995; Targoff *et al.* 1997).

ANTIBODIES ASSOCIATED WITH SYSTEMIC SCLEROSIS

ANAs of different types are present in more than 90% of patients with systemic sclerosis and in many with localized scleroderma (see Chap. 10) (Table 3.4). Two of these ANAs are characteristic for systemic sclerosis. An antibody directed against DNA-topoisomerase I (anti-Scl70) occurs in 20–40% of patients with systemic sclerosis, and is hardly found in patients with SLE, Sjögren's syndrome and MCTD (Seibold, 1997). At indirect immunofluorescence assay, another group of antibodies stains the centromere region of the chromosomes and is present in 50–96% of patients with limited systemic sclerosis (previously CREST and in 10% of patients with diffuse systemic sclerosis (Fig. 3.3). Anticentromere (ACeA) antibodies are rare in SLE, RA or Sjögren's syndrome (Seibold, 1997). The role of these antibodies in the pathogenesis of systemic sclerosis is not known, and a relation of the antibody titres to the stage or progression of the disease has not been established.

Clinical significance. The detection of anti-Scl70 in serum supports the diagnosis of systemic sclerosis, and that of anticentromere antibodies supports the diagnosis of

Table 3.4 Scleroderma associated antibodies

Antibody	Frequency (%)	Disease
Anti-Scl70	20–40	Systemic sclerosis
Anti-PM/Scl	8–10	Polymyositis/scleroderma overlap, Polymyositis, or scleroderma
Anti-U1RNP	12	Polymyositis/scleroderma and SLE overlap, MCTD, scleroderma
Anticentromere (ACeA)	50–96	Limited systemic sclerosis (CREST), 10% of diffuse sclerosis

Data from Seibold, 1997 with permission.

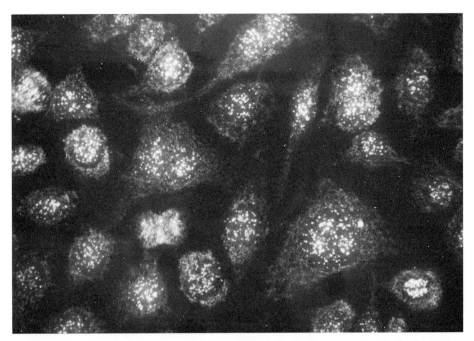

Figure 3.3 Staining by immunofluorescence of centromere region of chromosomes revealing the presence of anticentromere antibodies. Note the typical speckled staining pattern. Anticentromere antibodies occur in 50–96% of patients with limited systemic sclerosis (previously CREST) and in 10% of patients with diffuse systemic sclerosis. [From Provost and Kater (1995), with permission.]

limited sclerosis. Patients with Raynaud's phenomenon and anticentromere antibodies in serum, but without other clinical manifestations, are likely to be in the first stage of limited systemic sclerosis and should remain under observation.

ANTINEUTROPHIL CYTOPLASMIC ANTIBODIES (ANCA)

It is customary to distinguish primary idiopathic vasculitides from vasculitides secondary to other disorders (see Chapter 5). ANCAs are associated with some of the primary vasculitides (Table 3.5). Using the common indirect immunofluorescence technique, two ANCA staining patterns may be observed. cANCA is characterized by a specific cytoplasmic staining and its target antigen is proteinase 3 (PR3), a proteinase of human myeloid cells. pANCA is characterized by a specific perinuclear staining, and most commonly represents reactivity against myeloperoxidase (MPO) (Fig. 3.4). The ANCA staining patterns are manifest only after ethanol fixation of the neutrophils and must be considered as artifacts. PR3-ANCA and MPO-ANCA are now differentiated in most laboratories by ELISA.

cANCA is present in more than 90% of patients with Wegener's granulomatosis, particularly at active stages of the disease. It occurs also in microscopic polyangiitis and other primary vasculitides but at much lower incidences (Duna and Calabrese, 1995; Savage *et al.*, 1997). Increase in titres of cANCA may be predictive for an

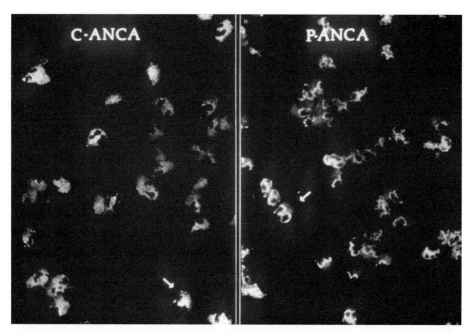

Figure 3.4 Antineutrophil cytoplasmic antibodies (ANCA). cANCA is characterized by cytoplasmic staining and is present in more than 90% of patients at active stages of Wegener's granulomatosis and in a few other conditions. pANCA stains the perinuclear region and lacks specificity. c- and p-ANCAs are usually not distinguished anymore by immunofluorescence but rather by an ELISA.

ensuing relapse of the disease, although this is not universally accepted (see Chapter 5, *Wegener's Granulomatosis*)

Clinical significance. cANCA is a sensitive and relatively specific marker of Wegener's granulomatosis in its active stages. Levels of cANCA fluctuate with

Table 3.5 ANCAs in primary vasculitides

	PAN	MPA	CSS	WG LTD	WG SYS
cANCA	–	Majority ANCA +; minority of these cANCA +	Occ +	Occ +	> 90% +
pANCA	Appr. 10% or less +	Majority ANCA +; majority of these pANCA +	Appr 70% +	Occ +	–

Abbreviations: cANCA, cytoplasmic antineutrophil cytoplasmic antibodies; pANCA, perinuclear antineutrophil cytoplasmic antibodies; PAN, polyarteritis nodosa; MPA, microscopic polyangiitis; CSS, Churg-Strauss syndrome; WG, Wegener's granulomatosis; Occ, Occasional; Appr, approximal; LTD, limited; Sys, systemic. Data for PAN, MPA and CSS from Guillevin *et al.* (1997); for WG from Kerr *et al.* (1993), Kallenberg *et al.* 1994), Jayne *et al.* (1995) Rao *et al.* (1995), Franssen *et al.* (1996).

disease activity and may be helpful in monitoring therapy effects. pANCA lacks specificity and has only limited value as a screening test for vasculitis.

RHEUMATOID FACTORS

Rheumatoid factors (RFs) are auto-antibodies directed against antigenic-determinants located on the Fc fragments of immunoglobulins, mainly IgG. Most tests for the detection of RF have a bias for IgM antibodies (IgM-RF) because an agglutination test is employed. RFs occur also in other immunoglobulin classes, particularly IgG and IgA.

IgM-RFs occur in serum of about 80% of patients with RA. However, in contrast to what the name suggests, they are also found in other ICTDs and in a variety of other diseases, such as Sjögren's syndrome (100%), SLE (40%), scleroderma (25–35%), sarcoidosis, mixed cryoglobulinaemia, monoclonal gammopathy, and infectious diseases. They occur also in healthy individuals of older age, ranging from 5% in middle age to 20% in old age.

Clinical significance. High titres of RFs are usually indicative for disease but lack specificity. Low titres RFs occur in a significant number of healthy individuals.

CONCLUSION

Considering the diagnostic usefulness of auto-antibodies in the ICTDs reviewed in this chapter, one should be aware that determination of these auto-antibodies is significant only in the context of the patient's symptomatology.

When should one apply for an investigation of auto-antibodies and for what should one ask? In patients with features of ICTD, a positive ANA test supports the diagnosis. A negative ANA test makes the diagnosis of ICTD much less likely. If positive, more specific assays are warranted for differential diagnostic purposes, *e.g.* anti-dsDNA for the diagnosis of SLE, anti-Scl70 for systemic sclerosis, etc. A similar reasoning is applicable for the examination of cANCA to confirm the diagnosis of Wegener's granulomatosis, for lupus anticoagulant (LAC) or anticardiolipin antibodies (ACAs) in patients suffering possibly from Hughes' syndrome (antiphospholipid syndrome), or for anti-Jo-1 in patients suspected of polymyositis.

Besides their diagnostic significance, auto-antibodies are of interest for two other clinical purposes. Levels of some auto-antibodies correlate with disease activity and are helpful in monitoring therapy. Examples are anti-dsDNA levels in SLE and cANCA levels in Wegener's granulomatosis. Some auto-antibodies serve as predictors of serious complications, *e.g.* anti-Jo-1 signalizes that there is a fair chance of interstitial lung fibrosis, which is associated with an unfavourable prognosis.

REFERENCES

Aarden LA, deGroot ER and Feltkamp TEW (1975) Immunologic factors and clinical activity in systemic lupus erythematosus. *Ann NY Acad Sci* **254**, 505–515.
Alexander EL, McNicholl J, Watson RM *et al* (1989) The immunogenetic relationship between anti-

Ro/SS-A/La/SS-B antibody positive Sjögren's syndrome/lupus erythematosus overlap syndrome and the neonatal lupus syndrome. *J Invest Dermatol* **93**, 751–756.

Bell DA and Morrison B (1991) The spontaneous apoptotic cell death of normal human lymphocytes in vitro: The release of, and immunoproliferative response to, nucleosomes in vitro. *Clin. Immunol. Immunopathol* **60**, 13–26.

Ben-Chetrit E, Fox RI and Tan EM (1990) Dissociation of immune response to the SS-A (Ro) 52-kD polypeptides in systemic lupus erythematosus and Sjögren's syndrome. *Arthritis Rheum* **33**, 349–355.

Boey ML, Peebles CL, Tsay G *et al* (1988) Clinical and autoantibody correlations in orientals with systemic lupus erythematosus. *Ann Rheum Dis* **47**, 918–923.

Bootsma H, Spronk P, Derksen RHWM *et al* (1995) Prevention of relapses in systemic lupus erythematosus. *Lancet* **345**, 1595–1599.

Bruggen MCJ van, Kramers C, Walgreen B *et al* (1997) Nucleosomes and histones are present in glomeral deposits in human lupus nephritis. *Nephrol Dial Transplant* **12**: 57–66

Bohan A and Peter JB (1975) Polymyositis and dermatomyositis. *N Engl J Med* **292**, 343–347.

Buskila D and Shoenfeld Y (1995) Disorders of the immune system leading to auto-immunity. In: Kater L and Baart de la Faille H (eds) *Multisystemic Auto-Immune Diseases: An Integrated Approach*, pp 1–15. Amsterdam: Elsevier.

Catoggio LF, Skinner RP, Smith G *et al* (1984) Systemic lupus erythematosus in the elderly: clinical and serologic characteristics. *J Rheumatol* **11**, 175–181.

Chapman JR, Charles PJ, Venables PJW *et al* (1984) Definition and clinical relevance of antibodies to nuclear/ribonuclear protein and other nuclear antigens in patients with cryptogenic fibrosing alveolitis. *Am Rev Resp Dis* **130**, 439–443.

Duna GF and Calabrese LH (1995) Limitations of invasive modalities in the diagnosis of primary angiitis of the central nervous system. *J Rheumatol* **22**, 662–667.

Elkon KB, Skelly S, Parnassa A *et al* (1986) Identification and chemical synthesis of a ribosomal protein antigenic determinant in systemic lupus erythematosus. *Proc Natl Acad Sci USA* **83**, 7419–7423.

Franssen CFM, Cohen Tervaert JW, Stegeman CA *et al* (1996) c-ANCA as marker of Wegener's disease. *Lancet* **347**, 115–116.

Gottlieb E and Steitz JA (1989a) The RNA binding protein La influences both the accuracy and efficiency of RNA polymerase III transcription in vitro. *Eur Mol Biol Organ J* **8**, 841–850.

Gottlieb E and Steitz JA (1989b) Function of the mammalian La protein: Evidence for its action in transcription termination by RNA polymerase III. *Eur Mol Biol Organ J* **8** 851–862.

Guillevin L, Lhote F and Gherardi R (1997) Polyarteritis nodosa and Churg-Strauss syndrome: Clinical aspects, neurologic manifestations and treatment. *Neurol Clin* **15**, 865–886.

Harris EN and Hughes CRV (1985) Cerebral disease in systemic lupus erythematosus. *Springer Seminar Immunopathol* **8**, 8251–8266.

Harris EN and Gharavi AE, Boey ML *et al* (1983) Anticardiolipin antibody detection by radioimmunoassay and association with thrombosis in systemic lupus erythematosus. *Lancet* **2**, 1211–1214.

Harris EN and Hughes CRV (1985) Cerebral disease in systemic lupus erythematosus. *Springer Seminar Immunopathol* **8**, 251–266.

Isshi K and Hirohata S (1996) Associations of antiribosomal P protein antibodies with neuropsychiatric systemic lupus erythematosus. *Arthritis Rheum* **39**, 1483–1490.

Itoh Y and Reichlin M (1992) Autoantibodies to the Ro/SSA antigen are conformation dependent. I Anti-60 KD antibodies are mainly directed to the native protein; anti-52 KD antibodies are mainly directed to the denaturated protein. *Autoimmunity* **14**, 57–65.

Jayne DR, Gaskin G, Pusey CD *et al* (1995) ANCA and predicting relapse in systemic vasculitis. *Q J Med* **88**, 127–133.

Kallenberg GCM, Mulder AHL and Cohen Tervaert JW (1992) Antineutrophil cytoplasmic antibodies: A still growing class of autoantibodies in inflammatory disorders. *Am J Med* **93**, 675–682.

Kallenberg GCM, Brouwer E, Weening JJ *et al* (1994) Antineutrophil cytoplasmic antibodies: Current diagnosis and pathophysiological potential. *Kidney Int* **46**, 1–15.

Kerr GS, Fleisher TA and Hallahan CW (1993) Limited prognostic value of changes in antineutrophil cytoplasmic antibody titer in patients with Wegener's granulomatosis. *Arthritis Rheum* **36**, 365–371.

Kim HY, Park DJ, Lee KS *et al* (1987) The frequencies and clinical significances of autoantibodies to extractable nuclear antigens in systemic lupus erythematosus. *Korean J Int Med* **32**, 172–180.

Kramer K, Hylkema M, Termaat RM *et al* (1993) Histones in lupus nephritis. *Exp Nephrol* **1**, 224–228.

Lerner NR and Steitz JA (1979) Antibodies to small nuclear RNAs complexed with proteins are produced by patients with systemic lupus erythematosus. *Proc Natl Acad Sci USA* **76**, 5495–5497.

Mimori T (1996) Structures targeted by the immune system in myositis. *Curr Opin Rheumatol* **8**, 521–527.

Petri M, Watson R and Hochberg M (1989) Anti-Ro antibodies and neonatal lupus. *Rheum Dis Clin N Amer* **15**, 335–360.

Provost TL, Talal N, Harley JB *et al* (1988a) The relationship between anti-Ro/SS-A antibody positive Sjögren's syndrome and anti-Ro/SS-A antibody positive lupus erythematosus. *Arch Dermatol* **124**, 63–71.

Provost TT, Talal N, Bias W *et al* (1988b) Ro/SS-A positive Sjögren's syndrome lupus erythematosus overlap patients are associated with the HLA-DR3 and/or DRw6 phenotypes. *J Invest Dermatol* **91**, 359–371.

Provost TT and Watson RM (1993) Anti-Ro/SS-A HLA-DR3 positive women: The interrelationship between some ANA negative, SS, SCLE and NLE mothers and SS/LE overlap female patients. *J Invest Dermatol* **100**, 14s–20s.

Provost TT and Kater L (1995) Guidelines for the clinical application of immunologic laboratory investigations. In: Kater L and Baart de la Faille H (eds) *Multisystemic Autoimmune Disease: An Integrated Approach*, pp 61–84. Amsterdam: Elsevier.

Rao JK, Allen NB, Feussner JR *et al* (1995) A prospective study of antineutrophil cytoplasmic antibody (cANCA) and clinical criteria in diagnosing Wegener's granulomatosis. *Lancet* **346**, 926–931.

Reichlin M and Reichlin MW (1989) Auto-antibodies to the Ro/SS-A particle react preferentially with the human antigen. In: Talal N (ed) *Second International Symposium on Sjögren's Syndrome*, pp 51–57. London: Academic Press.

Reichlin M, Maddison PJ, Targoff IN *et al* (1984) Antibodies to a nuclear/nucleolar antigen in patients with polymyositis-overlap syndrome. *J Clin Immunol* **4**, 40–44.

Reimer G, Rose KM, Scherr U *et al* (1987) Autoantibody to RNA polymerase I in scleroderma sera. *J Clin Invest* **79**, 65–72.

Reveille JD, MacLeod MJ, Whitingham K *et al* (1991) Specific amino acid residues in the second hypervariable region of HLA-DQA1 and DQB1 chain genes promote the Ro/SS-A/La/SS-B autoantibody responses. *J Immunol* **146**, 3871–3876.

Rothfield NF (1992) Autoantibodies in scleroderma. *Rheum Dis Clin N Amer* **18**, 483–498.

Roubey RAS (1996) Immunology of the antiphospholipid antibody syndrome. *Arthritis Rheum* **39**, 1444–1454.

Savage COS, Harper L and Adu D (1997) Primary systemic vasculitis. *Lancet* **349**, 553–558.

Seelig HP, Moosbrugger IU, Ehrfeld H *et al* (1995) The major dermatomyositis-specific Mi-2 autoantigen is a presumed helicase involved in transcriptional activation. *Arthritis Rheum* **38**, 1389–1399.

Seibold JR (1997) Scleroderma. In: Kelley WN, Ruddy S, Harris ED Jr *et al* (eds) *Textbook of Rheumatology*, 5 ed, pp 1133–1162. Philadelphia: WB Saunders.

Sharp GC, Irvin WS, Tan EM *et al* (1972) Mixed connective tissue disease: an apparent distinct rheumatic disease syndrome associated with a specific antibody to an extractable nuclear antigen (ENA). *Am J Med* **52**, 148–159.

Simmons-O'Brien E, Chen S and Watson R (1995) One hundred anti-Ro (SS-A) antibody-positive patients: A 10 year follow-up. *Medicine* **74**, 109–130.

Tan EM (1989) Antinuclear antibodies: diagnostic markers for auto-immune diseases and probes for cell biology. *Adv Immunol* **44**, 93–151.

Tan EM, Cohen AS, Fries JF *et al* (1982) The 1982 revised criteria for the classification of systemic lupus erythematosus. *Arthritis Rheum* **25**, 1271–1277.

Tanimoto K, Nakano K, Kano S *et al* (1995) Classification criteria for polymyositis and dermatomyositis. *J Rheumatol* **22**, 668–674.

Targoff IN (1993) Humoral immunity in polymyositis/dermatomyositis. *J Invest Dermatol* **100**, 116S–123S.

Targoff IN, Miller FW, Medsger TA *et al* (1997) Classification criteria for the idiopathic myopathies. *Curr Opin Rheumatol* **9**, 527–535.

Tax WJM, Kramers C, van Bruggen MCJ *et al* (1995) Apoptosis, nucleosomes and SLE nephritis. *Kidney Int* **48**, 666–673.

Vazquez-Abad D and Rothfield NF (1996) Sensitivity and specificity of anti-Jo-I antibodies in autoimmune diseases with myositis. *Arthritis Rheum* **39**, 292–296.

Watanabe T, Sato T, Uchiumi T *et al* (1996) Neuropsychiatric manifestations in patients with systemic lupus erythematosus. *Lupus* **57**, 178–183.

Watson RM, Lane AT, Barnett NK *et al* (1984) Neonatal lupus erythematosus: a clinical, serological and immunogenetic study with review of the literature. *Medicine* **63**, 362–378.

4

Guidelines for Immunotherapy

INTRODUCTION

In general, therapy for patients with inflammatory connective tissue diseases (ICTDs) can be directed at one or several of the following:

1. Suppression of disease activity as expressed in clinical symptoms and in laboratory parameters (*e.g.*, erythrocyte sedimentation rate (ESR), C-reactive protein (CRP), levels of serum complement, decrease of anti-dsDNA, etc.). *Disease activity* is defined as a reversible process due to an inflammatory event secondary to immunological abnormalities.
2. Eradication of causative pathogenic substances, *e.g.*, infectious agents in systemic lupus erythematosus (SLE).
3. Prevention of irreversible organ damage by the disease or by side-effects of therapy *e.g.*, treatment of hypertension due to renal SLE, of microscopic angiitis to prevent cerebral infarcts or haemorrhages, of osteoporosis for patients receiving corticosteroids, etc..
4. Palliative therapy, *e.g.* symptomatic treatment of pain for patients with cervical radicular nerve compression.
5. Rehabilitation, *e.g.* following cerebral infarct in SLE.

Though every one of these forms of treatment is essential for patients, we cannot deal with all of them given the scope of the present book. Therefore, we shall confine ourselves to immunotherapy and its side-effects, which is the most crucial part of treatment of the ICTDs. The kind of treatment applied in any given situation should always emanate from an accurate diagnosis, as is illustrated in the example described by Kallenberg (1998):

> A 25-year-old lady was under control for recurrent episodes of exacerbations of SLE. She visited her physician because of fever, jumping polyarthritis and muscle pains. She had been previously, and was still, anti-dsDNA positive; ANA was strongly positive and CRP was strongly elevated. She was treated with antiphlogistic therapy and 30 mg prednisone per day. As she did not improve, she was sent to a hospital. It appeared that her temperature was

raised to 38.5°C and that she had a holosystolic murmur (II/VI). ESR was 120 mm after one hour; CRP 125 µg/l; rheumatoid factors (RFs) were positive and the urine contained erythrocytes and casts, leukocytes, and 2.0 g/l protein. She was considered to have an exacerbation of her disease activity but because of the pansystolic murmur and the strikingly elevated CRP, blood was sent to the laboratory for culturing, resulting in a positive culture of non-haemolytic *Streptococcus viridans*. Echocardiography revealed mitral regurgitation and valve vegetations. Infective endocarditis was diagnosed and the patient was treated with proper antibiotics.

THE CHOICE OF AN AGENT FOR IMMUNOTHERAPY

There are two difficulties in choosing an immunosuppressive or an immunomodulating agent for a patient with ICTD. Their effects usually can not be predicted using the results of adequate clinical studies, as only a few clinical trials have been performed in this field, and they cannot be predicted easily from theoretical considerations, as knowledge about the pathogenesis of the ICTDs and their complications is insufficient. Therefore, the choice is often determined by the experience of clinical experts, by the conclusions of retrospective analyses, or by what is considered customary. This applies not only to strategies for treatment of the diseases, but also to measures taken to prevent, alleviate or treat side effects of medication.

CHAPTER AIM

This chapter aims to give general guidelines for immunological treatment of neurological complications. The agents used for the treatment of ICTDs are summarized in Table 4.1, and the putative immunological actions of the main agents are summarized in Table 4.2. The use of immunosuppressive cytostatic agents for patients with serious manifestations of ICTDs has become quite common, and to a lesser extent, so has the use of immunoglobulins. We shall refrain from extensive discussions about the pharmacology of the different agents, as these are dealt with at many other places in the literature, and shall concentrate on dosages, side effects, prevention of side effects, and other new potentially interesting developments. Tailored therapies for individual diseases are given in relevant chapters in this book. For general aspects of treatment of the ICTDs, the reader is referred to handbooks (Kelly *et al.*, 1997; Klippel and Dieppe, 1997; Wallace and Hahn, 1997).

Table 4.1 Immunomodulating agents and interventions reviewed in this chapter

Antimalarials and non-steroidal anti-inflammatory drugs (NSAIDs) (only side effects)	Haemapheresis
	Total lymphoid irradiation
	New immunosuppressive drugs
Corticosteroids	Other new immunosuppressants
Azathioprine	Monoclonal antibodies
Cyclophosphamide	Bone marrow transplantation
Chlorambucil	Dehydroepiandrosteron (DHEA)
Methotrexate	Oral tolerance
Cyclosporine	Dietary fish oils
Intravenous immunoglobulins	

Table 4.2 Putative immunological effects of corticosteroids, azathioprine, cyclophosphamide, methotrexate, cyclosporine and intravenous immunoglobulin

Agent	Action
Corticosteroids	Decreased number of lymphocytes in blood (redistribution)
	Reduced proliferation and differentiation of lymphocytes
	Decreased synthesis of pro-inflammatory cytokines (IL-1, IL-2, TNF)
	Inhibition of antigen presenting cell functions
	Modulation of T-helper phenotype
Azathioprine	Influence of cell-mediated immunity more than humoral immunity
	Decrease of non-specific immune function (K-cell and NK-cell activity)
Cyclophosphamide	Inhibition of humoral and cellular immune response (primary > cellular response)
	Disruption of DNA replication
Methotrexate	Poorly understood; low doses show only marginal effects on humoral and cellular immune responses; a mainly anti-inflammatory effect is suggested
Cyclosporine	Inhibition of T-helper (CD4+) cell activation and IL-2 production
	Inhibition of *in vivo* transcription of genes coding for IL-2 and IFN-γ
	Reversible inhibition of calcium dependent T-cell activation
	Blocks action of calcineurin
Intravenous immuno-globulin (IVIG)	Rapid short term blockade of phagocytosis by cells of the mononuclear phagocytic system
	Binding to activated complement component C4b and C3b receptors
	Down regulation of antibody production
	Stimulation of suppression mechanisms
	Decrease in NK cell activity
	Interference with antigen presentation by down regulation of Fc-receptors
	Suppression of auto-antibody production against disease associated antibodies by anti-idiotypic mechanisms
	Modulation in function and release of cytokines
	Functional modulation of lymphocytes

Abbreviations: IL, interleukine; TNF, tumour necrosis factor; K-, killer; NK- natural killer; IFN, interferon. Data in part from Kater *et al.* (1995) with permission.

NON-STEROIDAL ANTI-INFLAMMATORY DRUGS (NSAIDs), ANTIMALARIALS, AND D-PENICILLAMINE

Since these substances only have limited value for therapy of the neurological or psychiatrical manifestations of the ICTDs, we shall review only the main un-warranted neurological side effects.

NSAIDs

All effects of NSAIDs can be attributed to the inhibition of the synthesis of prostaglandins. When used in moderate doses, and when idiosyncratic reactions are excluded, these substances are safe in general. Salicylates are used in low doses for their inhibitory effect on the aggregation of thrombocytes. The drawback of this effect is that salicylates occasionally cause haemorrhages, particularly in the gastro-intestinal tract but seldom elsewhere. Salicylism includes tinnitus, hearing loss, headache, hyperventilation, and dullness. Other NSAIDs may induce headache, fatigue, depression, occasionally confusion, convulsions, aseptic meningitis, and other central nervous system (CNS) manifestations.

ANTIMALARIALS

We shall restrict ourselves to the chinoline derivatives, chloroquine and hydroxy-chloroquine (Plaquenil). Therapeutic doses of chloroquine may cause a retinopathy after months or years. Patients therefore should be screened every six months for visual defects. The ocular toxicity of hydroxychloroquine is much less, probably because it does not break down the blood-retinal barrier. Authors now agree that patients who use a daily dose of hydroxychloroquine of 6.5 mg/kg lean body mass or less do not need regular ophthalmological control. A baseline ophthalmological evaluation after 6–12 months should be done, then no more controls until five years after onset are necessary (Levy *et al.*, 1997; Block, 1998).

Therapeutic doses of chloroquine (250–750 mg/day for several weeks and up to 4 years) in some patients cause a painless myopathy with proximal limb weakness due to autophagic degeneration and a mainly subclinical neuropathy (Kakulas and Mastaglia, 1992). Recovery slowly follows after cessation of chloroquine medication. A similar myopathy in patients using hydroxychloroquine is rare. Chinoline and its derivates have a slight deleterious effect on neuromuscular transmission, and therefore should preferably not be used by patients with myasthenia gravis (MG).

D-PENICILLAMINE

D-penicillamine (dimethylcystein) is a chelating agent. The mechanism underlying its effect in the rheumatic diseases is not clear. D-penicillamine acts as an anti-pyridoxin, which probably explains why patients occasionally develop a polyneuropathy or an optic neuropathy. One should therefore combine the use of d-penicillamine with pyridoxine (25 mg/day) (Hoogenraad, 1996). Two other rare side effects are MG and polymyositis (PM) (see Chou, 1992 and Chapter 6). Weakness due to these side effects disappears when drug administration is halted.

CORTICOSTEROIDS (GLUCOCORTICOIDS)

PHARMACOLOGY

Corticosteroids are synthesized in and secreted by the adrenal cortex. They are vital for the maintenance of life. They enable the resistance of noxious influences, which tend to break down the organism. The most important functions of the corticosteroids are summarized as follows: control of carbohydrate, lipid, and protein metabolism, balance of electrolytes and water, and modulation of inflammatory and immune reactivity. Corticosteroid receptors are distributed all over the body, including the musculoskeletal system and the CNS. The influence of various factors on pro-inflammatory phenomena and the potential of corticosteroids to influence these factors has been reviewed recently (Boumpas, 1996). The role of corticosteroids in the endogenous control of inflammation through the hypothalamic-pituitary-adrenal (HPA) axis is now well established (Chrousos, 1995; Morand, 1997).

The synthetic corticosteroids mostly used are prednisone and methylprednisolone. Prednisone itself is inactive and is converted by the liver to the active prednisolone.

USE AND ADMINISTRATION

Corticosteroids are traditionally the first choice for immunosuppressive therapy, and often, no other second line agent is required.

Oral prednisone

Oral prednisone is given usually in a single dose in the morning, thereby leaving the circadian rhythm of endogenous corticosteroids intact. An aggressive approach is advocated for the treatment of neurological and neuromuscular manifestations. According to Villalba and Adams (1996), most authors nowadays agree that a patient with newly diagnosed disease should be treated with a dose of more than 1 mg/kg/day. However, Machkhas *et al.*, (1997), Mastaglia *et al.*, (1997) and others prefer to start treatment with 1 mg/kg/day. We also prefer to start with 1 mg/kg/day. Children are often treated with 2 mg/kg/day, though not everyone agrees with this high-dose policy (Miller *et al.*, 1983).

Mastaglia *et al.* (1997) draw attention to a few exceptions to these general rules. They advise a higher initial dose for patients who receive drugs that induce hepatic enzymes, which increase the rate of metabolism of the corticosteroid. They prescribe lower doses to the elderly because in old age the chances of osteopenia and vertebral fractures are higher. Patients with hypoalbuminaemia have higher unbound serum levels of corticosteroids and therefore require a lower daily dose.

In general, we continue high dose treatment for approximately 5 weeks. If a therapeutic effect is reached after 3 weeks, we taper the daily dose with 5 mg/week, until a reduction of 50% of the original dose is reached. Subsequently, we continue to taper the dose at alternative days with up to 1.25 mg/week (total approximately 5 mg/month), dependent on the well-being of the patient. Once medication is given at alternative days only, tapering should continue more slowly. We prefer this scheme, in general, because a higher dose at onset and a more prolonged period of high-dose medication are not more beneficial but increase the chance of serious side effects. Mastaglia *et al.* (1997) advocate a comparable scheme of corticosteroid tapering. Machkhas *et al.* (1997) advise to continue the initial high dose for 3–4 months (!), and then to taper the second day dose by 10 mg/week until an alternate day regimen is reached.

In general, lack of a beneficial effect in the initial high-dose treatment period should be reason to consider the addition of a cytostatic agent, usually methotrexate, azathioprine or cyclophosphamide. For some diseases (*e.g.*, Wegener's granulomatosis), treatment from onset should be with the combination of a corticosteroid and a cytostatic agent (prednisone and cyclophosphamide if there is a life-threatening situation or prednisone and methotrexate in less seriously ill patients) (Langford and Sneller, 1997; Hoffman *et al.*, 1990).

Intravenous pulse therapy with methylprednisolone
Intravenous pulse therapy is advocated in serious and threatening situations, such as CNS manifestations in SLE, but also in more chronic conditions, such as dermatomyositis (DM) and PM. The effect of intravenous pulse therapy is said to be more powerful, and the time to clinical response is said to be shorter than in patients on oral medication (Villalba and Adams, 1996). Other advantages may be that a dose of oral prednisone given simultaneously can be lower and that there are fewer side effects (Chrousos *et al.*, 1993). The effectiveness of this form of administration has been demonstrated in the treatment of exacerbations in MS and, to a certain degree, in optic neuritis, but its effectiveness has not been shown in any of the ICTDs yet (Milligan *et al.*, 1987; see Chapter 2, *Optic Neuritis*). However, there are case reports and a small intervention study that suggest the effectiveness of intravenous pulse therapy on neurological and myological complications of ICTDs (Matsubara *et al.*, 1994). Interestingly, intravenous pulse therapy in MS has not been demonstrated to be superior to oral therapy (Alam *et al.*, 1993; Troiano *et al.*, 1984).

The dose of methylprednisolone given for intravenous administration ranges from 500–1000 mg/day on 3 consecutive days to once/1–3 weeks. The experience of the Optic Neuritis Study Group has shown that methylprednisolone infusions are generally safe (Chrousos *et al.*, 1993). Before onset, patients should be screened for infections and treated if any are present. Blood pressure during infusions, serum potassium levels, and glucose content of urine should be kept under control.

SIDE EFFECTS OF CORTICOSTEROID THERAPY

The side effects of corticosteroids are numerous and several of them have a considerable detrimental effect on the well-being of patients (Table 4.3). The clinician should be aware of the strategies available to prevent or alleviate them. First, we discuss the side effects that are the most relevant for the management of patients, and then the neurological complications. Hyperlipidaemia and hypertension are among the well recognized risk factors that we do not discuss. They may accelerate common vasculopathic processes and therefore long-term therapeutic planning should include the control of all factors contributing to vascular injury.

Osteoporosis
Long-duration treatment with daily doses of prednisone ≥ 7.5 mg is associated with loss of bone and an increased risk of fractures, particularly vertebral compression fractures (Lukert and Raisz, 1990). In this respect, alternate day treatment is not better than a daily-dose regimen [see American College of Rheumatology Task Force on Osteoporosis Guidelines (ACRTFOG), 1996].

The current view is that bone mineral density (BMD) of the lumbar spine and hip should be measured in patients starting corticosteroid treatment for longer than 6 months (ACRTFOG, 1996; Miller *et al.*, 1996). The method used mostly for this purpose is Dual Energy X-ray Absorptiometry (DXA). It is rapid, painless, and requires

Table 4.3. Side effects of corticosteroid therapy

Immunological	Ocular	Musculoskeletal	Cardiovascular
Impaired wound healing	Cataract	Osteoporosis	Hypertension
Increased susceptibility to infections	Glaucoma	Avascular necrosis Steroid myopathy	Sodium and fluid retention

Endocrinological and Metabolical	Neurological/ Psychiatrical	Gastrointestinal	Dermatological/ Allergic
Glucose intolerance/ diabetes	Euphoria	Peptic ulcer	Acne
Menstrual irregularities/ secondary amenorrhoea	Mania	Dyspepsia	Striae
	Depression	Pancreatitis	Ecchymoses
	Insomnia		Urticaria
Depression of HPA*	Psychosis		Anaphylaxis
Growth retardation in children	Pseudotumour cerebri		
Cushing appearance	Myelopathy (due to epidural lipomatosis)		
Obesity from increased appetite			
Hyperlipidaemia			
Hypokalaemic alkalosis			
Negative nitrogen balance			
Epidural lipomatosis			

*Hypothalamic-Pituitary Axis

a low radiation load. BMD measurement at the start of corticosteroid treatment provides a baseline with which results of subsequent measurements can be compared. The BMD value determines the patient's risk of osteoporotic fractures.

Patients starting with corticosteroids should be informed about the benefits as well as the potential side effects. They should know that daily weight-bearing exercise (*i.e.*, walking) for 30–60 minutes is advisable. A negative calcium balance should be prevented and hypovitaminosis-D should be prevented or corrected (Table 4.4).

For post-menopausal female patients with decreased BMD, hormone replacement therapy (HRT) is recommended with standard commercially available packages. HRT induces the return of menstrual bleeding and slightly increases the risk of endometrial carcinoma, breast carcinoma, deep venous thrombosis (DVT), and embolism. Favourable effects are prevention of bone loss and fractures, and reduction of the risk for ischaemic heart disease and dementia. For all other patients, intermittent therapy with biphosphanates and calcium is advisable (Diamond *et al.*, 1995; Eastell, 1998; Adachi, 1997; Eastell, 1995) (see Table 4.4). Biphosphanates increase death of osteoclasts and prevent bone loss. They are tolerated well (Adachi *et al.*, 1997; Dequeker, 1998).

Table 4.4 Proposal for prevention or treatment of osteoporosis at onset or during corticosteroid treatment

Category	Proposal
All patients	Adequate information about/for patients Weight bearing exercise for 30–60 minutes/day Dietary calcium intake of 1500 mg/day. If necessary supplementary calcium* 1000 mg/day Vitamin D supplementation if hypovitaminosis is likely (elderly patients, indoor patients): 400–800 IU vitamin D3.
At onset and during corticosteroid treatment; T-score > –1 and no fractures	At onset: perform DXA at onset of corticosteroid therapy and repeat after 6 months During chronic corticosteroid treatment: perform DXA and repeat after 1 year
T-score ≤ –1, or decrease in BMD since previous measurement, or fractures at X-ray investigation	Hormonal supplementation therapy in postmenopausal women: oestrogen in combination with progestagens as in standard packages Cyclical etidronate 400 mg/day during 2 weeks followed by calcium 500 mg during 11 weeks

* Calcium should be taken during the evening as bone resorption is fastest during the night.

The effect of these measures should be controlled by determination of calcium excretion in the urine, which should be < 300 mg/day, from one month after onset of corticosteroid treatment; by repeating BMD measurement of hip and spine; and by lateral X-ray investigation of the lumbar spine 6 months after onset. BMD measurement allows to determine the mean peak bone mass (T-score) and to compare T-scores at different time points. The T-score is a measure used to calculate the chance of fractures at the moment of measurement. If the T-score is ≤ –1 (more than 1 standard deviation below the mean peak bone mass of young adults), change of medication or supplementary medication is needed. Recently, the combination of etidronate with sodium fluoride 25 mg twice daily was reported to be superior to that of etidronate alone (Lems *et al.*, 1997).

Corticosteroid myopathy
Weakness and atrophy of proximal limb muscles, associated with weakness of the diaphragma and neck flexors, is a common complication of prolonged corticosteroid administration, and is probably more common with fluorinated steroids (dexamethasone, triamcinoline) than non-fluorinated steroids (prednisone, hydrocortisone) (Dropcho and Soong, 1991; Dekhuijzen and De Cramer, 1992). A relation between muscle weakness and cumulative doses of steroids is likely, which may explain why weakness develops not only in patients treated with high doses but also after prolonged treatment with low oral doses, as for instance in asthmatics

(Bowyer *et al.*, 1985; Weiner *et al.*, 1993; Batchelor *et al.*, 1997). The myopathic effect of the corticosteroids is attributed primarily to the inhibition of the synthesis of a number of specific muscle proteins, although changes in muscle energy metabolism occur also (Kakulas and Mastaglia, 1992).

Acute quadriplegic myopathy usually occurs in patients in intensive care departments who are treated concomitantly with corticosteroids and an agent that blocks neuromuscular transmission (Lacomis *et al.*, 1996; Rich *et al.*, 1996). Almost complete loss of myosin in biopsy material from patients with rapidly developing corticosteroid myopathy has been documented (Al-Lozi *et al.*, 1994).

Weakness of the respiratory muscles can develop in both acute and chronic forms of steroid myopathy, but this responds favourably to lowering of the steroid dose, as we observed in a patient who suffered from SLE and whose respiratory function improved markedly after a significant lowering of the steroid dose. Steroid-induced respiratory muscle weakness may or may not be accompanied by obvious symptoms of proximal limb weakness. Corticosteroid myopathy of the diaphragm and other respiratory muscles has to be differentiated from weakness due to MG or causes related to one of the ICTDs (Turner-Stokes and Turner-Warwick, 1982).

Glucose intolerance

Corticosteroid therapy can lead to glucose intolerance or even frank diabetes mellitus. In patients on long-term corticosteroid therapy, the urine should be tested regularly for excretion of glucose. Patients with pre-existing diabetes mellitus need careful control, preferably by a diabetes specialist.

Gastrointestinal side effects and peptic ulcers

There are no established guidelines for gastro-protective therapy in patients receiving corticosteroid therapy. It is disputed whether corticosteroid therapy really increases the risk of peptic ulcers. Healing of gastric and duodenal mucosal defects is probably delayed, and the chance of recurrence of mucosal defects may be increased. Though the effect of histamine H2 antagonists and famotidine on the prevention of gastric ulcers has not been proven, these agents are often prescribed for older patients, patients with a history of peptic ulcers or gastrointestinal haemorrhage, and patients using NSAIDs concomitantly. Misoprostol has been proven to prevent the development of NSAID-induced gastric and duodenal ulcers and to reduce the risk of ulcer-associated complications (Table 4.5). It may therefore be an appropriate choice for prophylaxis.

Increased susceptibility to infections

In particular, susceptibility increases to tuberculosis, parasitic infections and influenza. A careful medical history in the case of tuberculosis is needed. Vaccination against influenza is advisable for patients on long-term immuno-

Table 4.5 Proposal for prevention of gastric and duodenal ulcers and ulcer-associated complications

Misoprostol 400–800 µg/daily in divided doses (Silverstein *et al.*, 1995; Hawkey *et al.*, 1998)
Famotidine 40 mg/day, or
Histamine H2 receptor antagonist (omeprazole 20–40 mg/day)

suppressive therapy. Corticosteroid-treated patients with SLE or other ICTDs are at risk for opportunistic infections (see Chapter 7, *Neuro-Infections*).

Ocular side effects

Patients on long-term corticosteroid therapy run an increased risk of cataract, glaucoma, and occasionally exophthalmos. Changes in the water content of the lens may lead to visual blurring (see Delattre and Posner, 1989). Control by the opthalmologist is needed for patients with ocular complaints.

Neuropsychiatrical changes

Most individuals develop mood changes early in the course of therapy. They may become slightly manic or, less often, depressive. These changes are transient or improve when the dose is reduced. Occasionally, these mood changes are severe and require cessation of medication and treatment with antidepressants or antipsychotics. In a few patients, corticosteroids induce a schizophrenia-like psychotic condition, with delusions, hallucinations and paranoia, forcing cessation of corticosteroid therapy (Gelder *et al.*, 1996; see Chapters 2 and 7, sections on psychosis).

Rapid withdrawal of corticosteroids is not customary anymore, but previously has been responsible for *corticosteroid withdrawal syndrome*, which included lethargy, weakness, joint pain and delirium (see Walker and Brochstein, 1988; Delattre and Posner, 1989; Gelder *et al.*, 1996).

Pseudotumour cerebri

Increased intracranial pressure with papilloedema has been reported previously as a manifestation of the corticosteroid withdrawal syndrome (Walker and Adamkiewitcz, 1964).

Epidural fat accumulation

Increase of epidural fat is recorded in case histories and may cause spinal cord compression (George *et al.*, 1983).

MONITORING CORTICOSTEROID TREATMENT

Careful follow-up, once or twice monthly dependent on the dose, is important to assess the effect on the disease and to detect side effects. Regular examination is required for control of mood and behaviour, blood pressure, body weight, the skin (Cushings appearance, striae, acne), and the eyes (cataract, glaucoma). As well, laboratory check-ups should be done for control of glucose excretion in urine, glucose levels in blood, electrolytes, total blood counts and differentiation. At 6–12 month intervals, the degree of osteoporosis should be measured.

AZATHIOPRINE

PHARMACOLOGY

Azathioprine belongs to the class of antimetabolites. It is a purine analogue and is converted enzymatically in the body to 6-mercaptopurine, which is the active substance. The immunosuppressive effect is due to the incorporation of this substance in the DNA of dividing cells and the inhibition of the purine nucleotide synthesis. Its precise mode of action on the immune system is still not completely understood however. Azathioprine appears to influence cell-mediated immunity more than humoral immunity and also exerts anti-inflammatory effects (see Table 4.2). In general, it is tolerated well.

USE AND ADMINISTRATION

Azathioprine is mostly used as an adjunct to corticosteroids and as a steroid-sparing agent. As such, it is prescribed for MG, when the response to thymectomy is insufficient, and for PM and DM. It may take months before azathioprine effects become manifest (Buch *et al.*, 1980). Some authors have advocated its use in MG as the single immunosuppressive agent (Cosi *et al.*, 1993).

Commonly, azathioprine is used orally. It takes 2–3 months before the immuno-suppressive effects become noticeable. The usual dose is 2–3 mg/kg/day. One usually starts in the first 2 weeks with 50 mg/day to test the tolerance for the drug, and then gradually increases the dose under control of blood cell count (number of white blood cells, leukocyte differentiation and thrombocytes) and liver function. If white blood cells decrease to < 2500/µl, or neutrophils < 1000/µl, the medication should be stopped and reintroduced more slowly after normalization of the blood cell count, if required.

SIDE EFFECTS

Haematology
The main haematological side effect is bone marrow depression, which generally occurs early during medication and results in leukoeytopenia, thrombocytopenia and macrocytic anaemia.

Hepatotoxicity
Dose-dependent hepatotoxicity is frequent and usually improves with lowering of the dose. Allergic hepatotoxicity is associated with other signs of hypersensitivity (*e.g.*, skin rash) and necessitates stopping medication.

Susceptibility for infections
Azathioprine medication increases the risk of localized herpes zoster. There is no obvious increase in frequency of any other infection.

Malignancy
Azathioprine probably does not significantly increase the risk of malignancy in patients with systemic auto-immune diseases, though there seems to be an increased incidence of non-Hodgkin's lymphoma in patients receiving azathioprine after organ transplantation (Kinlen *et al.*, 1979; Clements and Davis, 1986).

Teratogenesis
Azathioprine can pass the placenta, but congenital defects and chromosome abnormalities only occur very occasionally (Williamson and Karp, 1981).

Drug interactions

Allopurinol blocks metabolization of 6-mercaptopurine (Kaplan and Calabresi, 1973). Therefore, the azathioprine dose should be reduced to 75% when patients are treated with allopurinol simultaneously.

Hypersensitivity

Malaise, fever and aseptic meningitis have been described. Skin rash is uncommon.

MONITORING AZATHIOPRINE TREATMENT

Following the first control after 2 weeks, a monthly control of bone marrow activity and liver function is advisable for the first three months. The frequency can be reduced thereafter to once/2–3 months.

CYCLOPHOSPHAMIDE

PHARMACOLOGY

Cyclophosphamide is a nitrogen mustard and belongs to the class of alkylating agents. Like azathioprine, it acts synergetically with corticosteroids; the effects on rapidly dividing cells, including B- and T-lymphocytes and other blood cells, are transient as well as dose and, probably, disease dependent (Vita *et al.*, 1991) (see Table 4.2).

USE AND ADMINISTRATION

Cyclophosphamide is one of the most powerful immunosuppressants and is used for many serious neurological complications of the ICTDs, notably those of SLE, Sjögren's syndrome, vasculitides, etc. There is only limited experience with cyclophosphamide in the inflammatory myopathies, though there are reports of effective treatment in patients with refractory PM and in PM with co-existing inter-stitial lung fibrosis (Al-Janadi *et al.*, 1989; Hirano *et al.*, 1993). In view of the dose-related serious side effects, particularly the increased risk of bladder cancer (Travis *et al.*, 1995), the use of cyclophosphamide should be restricted to life and organ threatening situations.

Oral administration: the dose range varies from 1–3 mg/kg/day.

Intravenous (bolus) administration: 0.5–1.0 g/m² in 150 ml physiological saline solution for 60 minutes. Following the infusion, 2–3 litres of fluid/24 h should be taken. The number of white blood cells should be maintained above 2500 cells/µl and lymphocytes should remain above 10% of white blood cells.

Bolus or pulse therapy with cyclophosphamide, mostly in combination with oral prednisone, is given to patients in whom irreversible organ damage due to an immunologically mediated process is imminent, *e.g.* encephalopathy in SLE, transverse myelitis in Sjögren's syndrome or SLE, serious lupus nephritis, etc. Pulse therapy doses exceed those of the regular regimes. Supposedly, the advantages are a more powerful immunosuppressive effect and a longer interval between administrations that allows the vital functions to recover. The pulse doses can be given orally or intravenously. Tolerance in both instances is comparable. Several dose regimen are employed, *e.g.* 0.5 g, 0.5 g/m^2–1 g/m^2, or 0.5 g/m^2–2.5 g/m^2 (de Vita *et al.*, 1991). Dependent on the nature or the severity of the disease and the view of the responsible physician, the pulses are given in the following frequencies: once/2–3 weeks, once monthly, or every 2–3 months as maintenance therapy. Pulse cyclophosphamide can be alternated with pulse methylprednisolone combined with a daily low dose of prednisone or prednisolone, or combined with plasma exchange. Maintenance pulse therapy, once/2–3 months is given in some cases when remission has been obtained.

SIDE EFFECTS

The side effects of cyclophosphamide are listed in Table 4.6.

Table 4.6 Side effects of cyclophosphamide

General	Malaise, weight loss
Genito-urinary	Haemorrhagic cystitis, bladder fibrosis, bladder carcinoma (Travis *et al.*, 1995; Talar-Williams *et al.*, 1996), gonadal failure, teratogenesis, infertility
Haematological	Myelotoxicity
Metabolical	Inappropriate antidiuretic hormone secretion
Gastrointestinal	Nausea, anorexia, diarrhoea, hepatotoxicity (Snijder *et al.*, 1993)
Respiratory	Interstitial pneumonitis (seldom)
Hypersensitivity	Seldom any (Knysak *et al.*, 1994)

Haemorrhagic cystitis
In 50% of unprotected patients, metabolites of cyclophosphamide cause a potentially severe haemorrhagic cystitis (Efros *et al.*, 1994). Cystitis may be prevented by vigorous oral or intravenous hydration and infusion of mercaptoethane sulphonic acid (MESNA) (Vose *et al.*, 1993).

Urinary bladder cancer
Cyclophosphamide is a mutagen and induces a dose-dependent increased risk of bladder cancer. The incidence of bladder cancer initially was suggested to be 3% (Stillwell *et al.*, 1988), but this percentage has now risen to 16% (Talar-Williams *et al.*, 1996). In a large number of patients, a cumulative dose of 20 g was associated with a non-significant 2.4 times the normal risk of bladder cancer. This increased to 14.5 times the normal risk after a cumulative dose of 50 g (Travis *et al.*, 1995).

Teratogenesis and infertility
Cyclophosphamide is a teratogen, and therefore contraception should be advised strongly to patients using it. Contraception should be used for 6 months after cessation of medication. Conception, months or years after cessation of therapy, may result in a normal pregnancy and infant. Sterility is slightly more frequent in males than females. Amenorrhoea has been noted in 40–70% of female users for up to five years after treatment. Amenorrhoea is more frequent in patients over 20 years and is related to the cumulative dose of cyclophosphamide (see Kater *et al.*, 1995).

Haematology
Myelotoxicity is a common complication of cyclophosphamide. It develops usually at a maximum of 7–14 days after therapy and is followed by a remarkable recovery at about the third week after pulse therapy. Prolonged oral use may lead to chronic myelosuppression.

Gastrointestinal tract
Acute nausea and vomiting are very common and can be controlled by the anti-emetics, ondansetron or granesetron. Delayed emesis, 24 h after administration is not influenced by these substances.

Side effects of intravenous pulse therapy
Data available so far suggest that intravenous administration is relatively safe and is associated with less short-term side effects than daily oral administration. The most common side effect is probably infection. Retrospective analysis of 451 monthly pulses given to 75 patients revealed 8 infectious episodes that required hospitalization. Interestingly, three of these 75 patients died unexpectedly and without explanation at home in the week following pulse therapy (Martin *et al.*, 1997).

MONITORING CYCLOPHOSPHAMIDE TREATMENT

Pre-treatment laboratory analysis should include routine blood counts, urine analysis, chemistry screening and chest roentgenography. In patients on oral therapy, monthly control of blood cell counts and urine analysis are required. The cumulative dose should be kept preferably under 20 g. This is the dose that is associated with a non-significant 2.4 the normal risk of bladder cancer (Travis *et al.*, 1995).

CHLORAMBUCIL

The mode of action of chlorambucil is similar to cyclophosphamide. There are few data on its use in neurological manifestations of the ICTDs. One report concerns its use in drug-resistant DM, and another on its therapeutic success in a case of inclusion body myositis (IBM) (Sinoway and Callen, 1993; Jongen *et al.*, 1995). Chlorambucil's advantage is that it does not cause haemorrhagic cystitis, however it does increase the incidence of leukaemia (Kaldor *et al.*, 1990), which has prevented its widescale use. The advised dose of chlorambucil is 0.1–0.2 mg/kg/day, to be increased gradually, while maintaining the white blood cell count at about 3000 cells/µl.

METHOTREXATE (MTX)

Excellent overviews have been published on the clinical pharmacology, mechanisms of action, and side effects of MTX (Cronstein, 1995; Furst, 1995; Sandoval *et al.*, 1995).

PHARMACOLOGY

MTX is a folic acid antagonist and belongs to the class of anti-metabolists. It binds to and effectively inhibits dihydrofolated reductase, thereby causing impaired synthesis of DNA and RNA by a partial depletion of tetrahydrofolate co-factors. These co-factors are crucial for the synthesis of purines and thymidylate (Calabresi and Chabner, 1990). As MTX is excreted in the urine, caution is necessary in patients with renal failure. The immunological effects are poorly understood, but are probably mainly anti-inflammatory.

USE AND ADMINISTRATION

As far as neurological disorders are concerned, MTX is best known for its use in inflammatory myopathies, mostly as a corticosteroid-sparing agent. Some authors consider the combination of prednisone and MTX as more effective than that of prednisone and azathioprine (Joffe *et al.*, 1993). It has been suggested that in some patients with inclusion body myositis (IBM), MTX in combination with azathioprine may be beneficial (Leff *et al.*, 1993), but most authors do not agree with this contention (Griggs *et al.*, 1995).

Orally MTX is given as tablets of 2.5 mg. Usually one starts with 7.5 mg/week, taken either in one single dose or in three fractional doses at 12 h intervals. This dosage is maintained for three weeks and then, if necessary, gradually increased by steps of 2.5 mg at intervals of 6–8 weeks, up to 25 mg/week (Newman and Scott, 1995).

For *intravenous or subcutaneous administration*, the dose at onset is 10 mg once a week. If required, the dose can be increased by 2.5 mg every 6–8 weeks until a maximum of 25 mg/week is reached. If remission has been obtained, the dose can be lowered by 2.5 mg every 3 weeks until the lowest effective dose has been reached. Subcutaneous administration is as good as intramuscular and avoids false elevation of serum creatine kinase activity (Jundt *et al.*, 1993).

SIDE EFFECTS

Side effects of MTX given in doses customary to the ICTDs are usually mild. For treatment of malignancies, much higher dosages and intrathecal administration are employed, which results in much more serious side effects.

Liver

Pre-treatment examination should include, according to the recommendations of the American College of Rheumatology, determination of liver-function tests (Kremer *et al.*, 1994). Liver abnormalities associated with low-dose MTX may vary from transient increase of serum transaminase activity to cirrhosis. Increase of transaminase activity occurs in the first three weeks of MTX administration, and this may normalize spontaneously after about 3 months (Lacki *et al.*, 1993). Liver cirrhosis occurs in 0.1%–1% of treated patients; the risk increases with the cumulative dose of MTX.

Gastrointestinal tract

Mucosal ulceration (stomatitis), nausea, diarrhoea and even intestinal perforation may occur.

Haematology

MTX toxicity may include bone marrow depression, *e.g.* leucopenia and thrombo-cytopenia. Pancytopenia is uncommon and occurs almost only in the following conditions: old age, renal failure, pre-existing bone marrow depression, and treatment with a combination of MTX and trimethoprim-sulfamethoxazole (Govert *et al.*, 1992). Cytopenias are usually mild and respond well to reduction of therapy. Severe MTX induced cytopenia can be managed by stopping MTX and with administration of leukovorin (10–20 mg intravenously ever 6 hours until cell counts are normalized). Megaloblastic anaemia also may occur; it reacts favourably to supplementation with folate. Continuous routine folate supplementation during MTX therapy reduces symptoms of the gastrointestinal tract and other side effects, but reduces MTX efficacy.

Lungs

MTX induces pneumonitis once every 276 patient years (Conaghan *et al.*, 1997). Pre-existing lung disease does not increase its occurrence. There are reports on MTX induced asthma and on hypersensitivity pneumonitis, which causes a sustained cough without evidence of underlying lung pathology (Hilliquin *et al.*, 1996; Schnabel *et al.*, 1996). Management consists of withdrawal of MTX.

Opportunistic infections

These occur mostly during a period of leukocytopenia or pancytopenia and only occasionally when blood counts are normal. Pneumocystis carinii is the most frequent of these infections, but mycobacterium avium cellulare, histoplasma capsulatum, and cytomegalovirus infections occur also, as seen in cellular immunodeficiencies including AIDS. MTX should be stopped when patients acquire an opportunistic infection and appropriate antibiotic treatment should be started.

Malignancy

There are case reports on lymphoma in MTX treated patients (Usman and Yunus, 1996; Viraben *et al.*, 1996).

Neurological complications

The main neurological side effects are aseptic meningitis, transverse myelitis and leukoencephalopathy. They occur mostly after intrathecal administration and in the setting of cranial radiation (see Walker and Brochstein, 1988).

A stroke-like syndrome, fluctuating from one side to the other, with mental alteration, hemiparesis, aphasia and other focal signs has been observed after high-dose intravenous administration. The condition develops in the second week after MTX therapy and resolves spontaneously in 48–72 h. MRI reveals changes indicative for white matter oedema (Gay *et al.*, 1994).

Leukoencephalopathy occurs not only after intrathecal administration but also after high-dose intravenous MTX treatment and occasionally even after low-dose MTX treatment (Worthley and McNeil, 1995). Patients develop personality changes and learning disabilities, or overt dementia, spasticity and death. CT scans show bilateral white matter low-density, and MRI of the brain reveals increased signal of the white matter on T2-weighted images. Microscopy reveals necrosis, axonal degeneration and loss of myelin, and sometimes fibrinoid necrosis of small vessels.

Mild evidence of CNS toxicity in low-dose oral treatment with MTX is not that infrequent and occurs in a variable degree in 20% of patients (Wernicke and Smith, 1989). The symptoms include alterations in mood and memory and unpleasant cranial sensations. Seizures are exceptional (Thomas *et al.*, 1993)

MONITORING MTX TREATMENT

Pre-treatment control of liver function tests and hepatitis B and C antibody tests are required before beginning treatment (Kremer *et al.*, 1994). Some doctors also require pre-treatment lung function tests. Constant surveillance and monitoring of the MTX dose are necessary in view of the large number of side effects. Liver function tests should take place every 4–8 weeks. A liver biopsy should be considered if MTX treatment leads to persistent abnormalities in liver function tests (Kremer *et al.*, 1994).

CYCLOSPORINE

PHARMACOLOGY AND EFFECTS ON THE IMMUNE SYSTEM

Cyclosporine is produced by a fungus, *Tolypocladium inflatum*. It is metabolized in the liver via cytochrome P-450 mediated oxydation and secreted through bile. Its half-life is approximately 20 h. Cyclosporine exerts its immunosuppressive effect mainly by blocking T-helper (CD4+) dependent production of cytokines, notably IL-2 (see Table 4.2) (Russel *et al.*, 1992; Thomson and Nield, 1992).

USE AND ADMINISTRATION

Experience with cyclosporine in the treatment of neurological manifestations of ICTDs is limited. It has a beneficial effect on MG, as demonstrated in a prospective double-blind placebo-controlled trial, but is considered a third-line drug (after corticosteroids and azathioprine) because of its side effects (Hohlfeld and Toyka, 1993; Tindall *et al.*, 1993). There are case reports on therapeutic successes of cyclosporine in PM and DM, but prospective studies and large retrospective investigations have not been performed (Alijotas *et al.*, 1990; Adams and Plotz, 1995)

The recommended dose in auto-immune disease is 5 mg/kg/day, preferably given in two doses of 2.5 mg/kg as this seems to reduce renal toxicity (Feutren and Mihatsch, 1992). More details about administration are given under 'monotoring cyclosporine treatment.'

SIDE EFFECTS

Kidneys
Renal dysfunction occurs in up to 30%, and is caused by vasoconstriction of afferent renal arterioles. It is usually reversible when medication is discontinued or reduced. Caution is needed when cyclosporine medication is combined with other nephrotoxic drugs, *e.g.* co-administration of cyclosporine with trimethoprim.

Hypertension
Hypertension is the most frequent side effect and occurs in 25–40% of patients. It is considered to be due to peripheral vascular resistance rather than to renal toxicity.

After discontinuation, blood pressure usually returns to normal (Feutren and Mihatsch, 1992).

Liver
Cyclosporine is hepatotoxic and may cause cholelithiasis.

Nervous system
There is a long list of neurological and myological complications, namely headache, seizures, altered sensorium, deafness, visual hallucinations, cortical blindness, dysphasia, akinetic mutism, hemiparesis, quadriparesis, intention tremor, ataxia, leukoencephalopathy, paraesthesias and burning dysaesthesias, muscle cramps, weakness and myopathy. The cyclosporine doses used for treatment of the inflammatory nervous system diseases rarely cause serious neurological manifestations.

Malignancy
The risk of malignancy is probably higher than in the general population, as shown in studies on transplanted patients treated with high doses and often with several drugs. The most reported malignancies are lymphoproliferative diseases and epithelial skin cancers (Frei *et al.*, 1993; Ritters *et al.*, 1994).

Other adverse drug reactions
These include nausea, anorexia, gingival hyperplasia, skin flushing and burning, hypertrichosis, decreased C1-esterase inhibitor levels, hyperkalaemia, and hypomagnesia.

Drug interactions
Concomitant use of erythromycine, doxycycline, fluconazole, ketonazole, diltiazem, sex hormones and high doses of methylprednisolone may cause rises in blood levels of cyclosporine. Concomitant use of phenotoine, rifampicine, carbamazepine, isoniazide, and intravenous sulfadimidine and trimethoprim may reduce cyclosporine levels. Special caution is needed when cyclosporine is used concomitantly with other nephrotoxic substances, like NSAIDs, aminoglycosides, and amfotericin B, and when combining cyclosporin with lovostatin or colchine because of muscle toxicity.

MONITORING CYCLOSPORINE TREATMENT

To identify patients at risk for nephrotoxicity, pre-treatment measures should include a careful medical history, special attention for concomitant medication, blood pressure registration, cell blood counts, renal and liver function tests, and urine analysis. The following guidelines may be helpful for monitoring cyclosporine medication:

  – Keep the initial dose below 5 mg/kg/day.
  – Maintain blood levels at or slightly below 200 ng/ml.
  – Reduce the dose if serum creatinine level rises more than 30% above baseline.

At follow up, kidney function (serum ureum and creatinine levels and urine analysis) should be tested at least monthly, and cell blood counts and routine clinical chemistry at least once every three months.

INTRAVENOUS IMMUNOGLOBULIN INFUSIONS (IVIG)

IMMUNOPHARMACOLOGY

Following its successful application in idiopathic thrombocytopenic purpura, IVIG has been demonstrated to be beneficial in a variety of other auto-immune disorders. In chronic disorders, the effect of IVIG is generally of limited duration, usually in the order of weeks (Dwyer, 1992). The mechanisms implicated in the action exerted by gammaglobulins are enumerated in Table 4.2 (Kater *et al.*, 1995).

USE AND ADMINISTRATION

Beneficial effects of IVIG have been demonstrated in Guillain-Barré syndrome, chronic inflammatory demyelinating neuropathy, multifocal motor neuropathy, and DM. In addition, IVIG is likely to be effective in remitting some cases of MS, stiff man syndrome, Lambert-Eaton myasthenic syndrome, MG, monoclonal gammopathies and several of the ICTDs (Van der Meché and Schmitz, 1992; Dalakas *et al.*, 1993; Van den Berg *et al.*, 1995; Hahn *et al.*, 1996; Mandell, 1996; Van der Meché and Van Doorn, 1997; Jongen *et al.*, 1998).

   In most clinical trials, IVIG is given intravenously in a dose of 0.4 mg/kg/day for 5 consecutive days. In many conditions, the beneficial effect is temporary. IVIG has to be regarded as an important adjunct therapy to the therapeutic repertoire, especially when regular treatment is insufficient or contraindicated. No consensus has been reached about doses for repeat treatments.

SIDE EFFECTS

IVIG is a relatively safe method but not entirely without risks, as discussed below.

Allergic reaction
Anaphylactic reactions are seldom. Serious anaphylaxias may occur in patients with IgA deficiency and are associated with the presence of anti-IgA antibodies (Koskinen *et al.*, 1995).

Heart
Fluid overload and increased serum viscosity are risk factors in patients with cardiac insufficiency and in elderly patients with coronary artery disease. Augmentation of serum viscosity may increase the risk of thromboembolic events (Dalakas, 1994).

Kidneys
IVIG has caused renal insufficiency in a few cases and for unknown reasons. The IVIG effect may vary from transient elevations of the creatinine level in serum without any symptoms to acute renal failure with severe and reversible tubular vacuolization (Cantu *et al.*, 1995).

Aseptic meningitis
Headache is common and judged as an innocent side effect of IVIG. In some patients, mostly those with a history of migraine, symptoms and signs of aseptic

meningitis with headache, nausea, vomiting, fever, and neck stiffness develop between 1 and 7 days after infusion (Sekul *et al.*, 1994). In the CSF, the protein content and number of neutrophils are raised and the glucose level is lowered, but there are no bacteria or viruses.

Cerebral infarction

Cerebral infarction has been reported in a few cases. The underlying mechanism has not been clarified but it may be that increased serum viscosity plays a role (Dalakas, 1994).

MONITORING IVIG THERAPY

Screening is recommended for renal and liver functions and for serum viscosity. The latter is recommended especially in elderly patients (Dalakas, 1994). As IVIG preparations are prepared commercially from human serum, one should be on the alert for the transmission of viruses, including hepatitis C, hepatitis B, and human immunodeficiency virus, dependent on the origin of the immunoglobulin products.

HAEMAPHERESIS

Plasmapheresis or plasma exchange is a technique by which blood cells are separated from plasma and plasma is removed or replaced by fresh plasma, albumin, or other replacement fluids. In case of leukalymphapheresis, leukocytes and lymphocytes are removed from the circulation. The rationale for plasmapheresis is the depletion of circulating antibodies, immune complexes or other high molecular weight substances from the body. The benefits are usually temporary. It can be used to remove antibodies from the circulation and thereby induce rapid improvement (*e.g.*, in hyperviscosity syndrome, MG, Lambert-Eaton myasthenic syndrome, or chronic polyneuropathy associated with monoclonal gammopathy). In the routine management of SLE, PM, DM, polyarteritis nodosa and other ICTDs, plasmapheresis in addition to corticosteroids and cytostatic agents proved of no benefit (Miller *et al.*, 1991; Guillevin *et al.*, 1992). However, plasmapheresis is useful in some specific conditions, such as SLE with thrombotic microangiopathic haemolytic anaemia or secondary thrombotic thrombocytopenic purpura. Synchronization of plasmapheresis and cyclophosphamide, based on the theory of 'stimulation depletion', which is the depletion of stimulated B-cells, is suggested to be effective in some cases of severe SLE (Euler *et al.*, 1994).

TOTAL LYMPHOID IRRADIATION

The immunosuppressive effect of total lymphoid irradiation is considered to be due to at least 4 mechanisms, which are: depletion of circulating and resting lymphocytes; alteration of the maturation steps of T-lymphocyte subsets; decrease of lymphocyte functions; and increase of T8/T4 ratios (Strober and Farinas *et al.*, 1989). The role of total lymphoid irradiation in various neurological disorders still has to be established. The method is not used often in view of the serious side effects

(Rubin *et al.*, 1992). However, it remains a last option for patients with intractable disease.

NEW IMMUNOSUPPRESSIVE DRUGS

INTRODUCTION

The search continues for a method that may induce long-term unresponsiveness to a specific antigen, while simultaneously leaving the response to other antigens intact. Several new immunosuppressive drugs are available, but their efficacy in the field of ICTDs is not demonstrated (Ten Berghe, 1997). Experience with these agents comes from transplant patients. The following is a short overview.

OVERVIEW OF NEW DRUGS

Tacrolimus (FK 506)

This drug is registered as Prograf®. Tacrolimus is an actinomycete macrolide that inhibits the Ca^{2+} dependent signal transduction from the T-cell receptor to the nucleus, thereby interfering with the transcription of cytokine genes (Kinto *et al.*, 1987). It inhibits lymphokine synthesis by a mechanism similar to that of cyclosporine, but it binds to a different set of intracellular proteins (immunophylin) and structurally is unrelated to cyclosporine (Kahan, 1996). Tacrolimus has been studied extensively in kidney and liver transplantation and has proven to be a potent immunosuppressive agent. It does not induce hypertension like cyclosporine, but is at least as nephrotoxic as cyclosporine and has serious diabeto-genic and neurotoxic side effects (Mayer *et al.*, 1997). There is still no experience with this drug in neurological disorders.

Mycophenolate mofetil

This drug is registered as Cellcept®. *In vivo* it is hydrolysed into its active metabolite, mycophenolic acid, which is an inhibitor of de novo purine synthesis and on which lymphocytes are fully dependent. It inhibits the proliferation of B-and T-lymphocytes and that of the monocyte lineage (van der Wouden, 1998). In studies performed in transplant patients, it has proven to be a more potent immunosuppressive agent than azathioprine and to have only mild side effects predominantly from the gastrointestinal tract. Data from controlled studies in auto-immune diseases are not available.

Sirolimus (rapamycin)

Sirolimus is a 31-member macrolipid that has a distinctly different mode of action than cyclosporin or tacrolimus, despite the fact that it is structurally homologous to tacrolimus and binds to the same immunophylin. Sirolimus does not inhibit calcineurin. It has a potent immunosuppressive effect at doses lower than those of cyclosporine. In several animal models of auto-immune diseases, sirolimus acts synergistically with cyclosporine to achieve powerful immunosuppression. There are indications that sirolimus has no nephrotoxic effects, though detailed studies are not available yet (Andoh *et al.*, 1997). Addition of sirolimus to sub-therapeutic concentrations of cyclosporine can potentiate the immunosuppressive activity

(Kahan, 1996). The toxicity spectrum of sirolimus overlaps with that of cyclosporine (Murgia *et al.*, 1996).

Cladribine

This purine analogue inhibits the proliferation of lymphocytes by inhibiting the enzyme adenosine deaminase, which is needed for the degradation of deoxyadeno-sine. Favourable results have been obtained with this drug in hairy-cell leukaemia, auto-immune haemolytic anaemia, lymphoma and progressive MS (Sipe *et al.*, 1994). Cladribine is well tolerated generally. Side effects include bone marrow depression, gastrointestinal disturbances, allergy (fever or skin rash), infections (herpes zoster), headache, mood changes (anxiety or depression), and confusion. In high doses, paraparesis, quadriparesis, amaurosis and severe neuropathy may be side effects (Cheson *et al.*, 1994).

Other new immunosuppressants

Mizoribine is an imidazole-nucleoside and is comparable in its mechanism to mycophenolate-nucleoside. Brequinar inhibits proliferation of lymphocytes by inhibition of de novo pyrimidine synthesis. Leflunomide is a synthetic analogue of isoxazole and has a strong immunosuppressive effect in experimental models of auto-immune diseases and transplantation.

SUMMARY

There is a whole series of new interesting immunosuppressants. Until now, none has demonstrated to be obviously preferable to those presently used.

IMMUNE INTERVENTION BY NEW BIOLOGICAL AGENTS

A series of new therapeutic modalities has been developed during the last several years. These drugs intervene with processes involved in the regulation of auto-immune processes, as illustrated in Fig. 4.1 (Amital *et al.*, 1996).

Cytokines play an important role in the development and control of immune responses and inflammatory reactions. The current view is that the specific cellular immune response is polarized into two subsets of T-cells with distinct cytokine secretion profiles and immunological functions (Fig. 4.2). T helper-1 (Th1) cells promote the proliferation of CD8+ and CD4+ T-cells by the secretion of IL-2 and IFN-γ. Th2 cells facilitate allergic reactions and contribute to the generation of immunoglobulins and secrete IL-4, IL-5, IL-6, IL-10 and IL-13. Interestingly, the cytokines of each subset have the potential to inhibit the functions and proliferation capacity of the other subset (Romagnani, 1995).

Different pathological conditions have been ascribed to either Th1 or Th2 dominant reactivity. Th1 cells would mediate MS and diabetes mellitus type 1, and Th2 cells mediate allergic disorders (Fruet *et al.*, 1995). Results of animal experiments indicate that Th1 cells might contribute to the pathogenesis of various organ specific auto-immune diseases, whereas Th2 cells would inhibit development of disease (Adorini *et al.*, 1996). The approach that seems most likely to be effective for therapy at present is the selective manipulation of Th1 and Th2 cells by cytokines (Kroemer *et al.*, 1996). The effect of such manipulations has been studied mainly in animal experiments (Table 4.7).

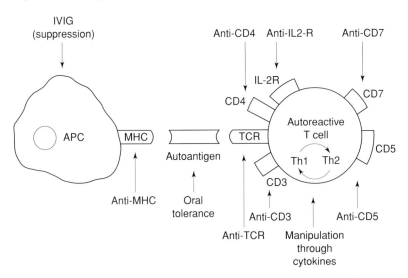

Figure 4.1 Intervention sites of immune therapy within the regulation of auto-immune processes. Abbreviations: APC, antigen presenting cell; IVIG, intravenous immunoglobulin; MHC, major histocompatibility complex class II; TCR, T-cell receptor; IL-2R, interleukine-2 receptor. The sites of intervention by new immunotherapeutic agents are given.

1. Monoclonal antibodies (MOABs) directed against cytokines and cytokine receptors interfere with the normal activation of T-cells, *e.g.* anti-CD3 interferes with normal activation of T-cells; anti-CD4 with function and behaviour of CD4+ T-cells; anti-CD5 and anti-CD7 are directed against the pan-T-cell antigens C5 and C7 and against CD5+ B cells; anti-IL-2R are directed against IL-2 receptors, which are synthesized on T-cells after activation.
2. Anti-MHC antibodies are directed against the major histocompatibility complex (MHC) class II molecules present on antigen presenting cells. The MHC class II molecules on the cell surface present antigens for recognition by T-cells.
3. Manipulation of the T-helper cells, Th1 and Th2, responses is feasible by the cytokines produced by each of these subsets. Th1 and Th2 cells exert mutual inhibition through their cytokines (see Fig. 4.2).
4. The potential effects of IVIG administration are given in Table 4.2.
5. Induction of oral tolerance in auto-immune disease may be obtained by oral administration of competitive antigens, e.g. myelin basic protein in experimental encephalomyelitis.

Adapted from Amital, 1996 with permission.

INTERFERONS

Interferons (IFNs) are cytokines (glycoproteins) produced in response to virus infections. They have potent antiviral properties. There are two types of human interferon, Type I (α and β) and Type II (γ). Interferon-α (IFN-α) has best been studied. It produces significant clearing of hepatitis B virus in chronic carriers and induces marked biochemical and histological improvements in about half of

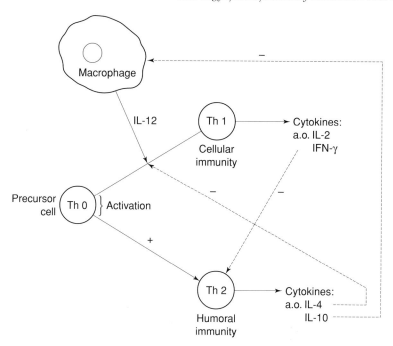

Figure 4.2 Cross regulation by T helper, Th1 and Th2, cells. Recent evidence indicates that Th cells vary in their ability to produce combinations of cytokines and to stimulate preferentially either cell-mediated immunity or antibody-mediated immunity. Th1 cells produce, amongst other cytokines, IL-2 and IFN-γ which stimulate cytotoxic cells and macrophages resulting in cell-mediated immunity). In contrast, Th2 cells produce, amongst other cytokines, IL-4 and IL-10, which stimulate B-cells and antibody production. These two subsets are thought to arise from a common precursor cell, Th-0. Macrophage-derived IL-12 stimulates the development of Th1 cells, whereas IL-4 (probably from mast cells or basophils) stimulates development of Th2 cells. Th1 and Th2 cells exert mutual inhibition through the cytokines they produce: IFN-γ inhibits proliferation of Th2 cells, whereas IL-4 inhibits the development of Th1 cells.

patients with chronic virus hepatitis C. The toxic effects of IFN-α are usually tolerable and are most commonly flu-like symptoms, such as fever, malaise, myalgias, anorexia and mental confusion. These effects are most pronounced during the first three months of therapy. More serious side effects include reversible bone marrow depression, proteinuria, liver dysfunction and cardiotoxicity. There are some reports on exacerbations of auto-immune diseases, including thyroiditis, which may be lethal (Durelli *et al.*, 1998). IFN-γ activates macrophages. Its action is most impressive in conditions in which macrophage function is defective, for instance in lepromatous lepra and chronic granulomatous disease.

Interferons in neurological disease
The use of interferons in MS stems from the idea that this disease may be caused by a virus. Although the explanation for the favourable effect of IFN-β in MS is not

Table 4.7 Cytokine manipulation of auto-immune conditions in animal experiments

Cytokine manipulation	Disease
Anti-TNFα antibodies	Collagen-induced arthritis, RA
Anti-IL-6 antibodies	RA
Anti-IFN-γ antibodies	(NZB×NZW) F mice; NOD mice
Anti-IL-10 antibodies	NZB/W mice; RA
Natural IL-1 inhibitors	BB diabetic mice
Anti-IL-2 receptor antibodies	NOD mice
Anti-IL-12 antibodies	NOD mice, EAE
IL-4	EAE
IL-10	EAE
IL-13	EAE
IL-2 conjugates	Adjuvant arthritis
212 bismuth	
pseudomonas toxin	
Soluble IL-1 receptor	RA
IL-1 receptor antagonists	RA

Abbreviations: BB and NZB/NZW, strains of experimental animals; EAE, experimental auto-immune encephalitis; IFN, interferon; IL, interleukin; NOD, non-obese diabetes; TNF, tumour necrosis factor; RA, rheumatoid arthritis. Adapted from Amital *et al* (1996), with permission.

known, it probably has nothing to do with its antiviral influences (IFN-β Multiple Sclerosis Study Group, 1993; Durelli *et al.*, 1994). Treatment of chronic inflammatory demyelinating polyneuropathy (CIDP) with IFN-α 2A may be effective in patients who failed to respond to steroids, IVIG, and plasma exchange, (Gorson *et al.*, 1998). Variable effects of IFN-α in patients with mixed cryoglobulinaemia, hepatitis virus infection, and polyneuropathy have been registered (La Civita *et al.*, 1996; Zuber and Gause, 1997).

MONOCLONAL ANTIBODIES (MOABs)

Recombinant DNA technology has enabled researchers to produce cytokines and cytokine receptors, as well as monoclonal antibodies against these proteins. Along with these antibodies, new therapeutic strategies have been developed. As the effects of MOABs in manipulating the immune response in the ICTDs are still far from clear, we shall restrict this review to some aspects of potential clinical interest.

Anti-CD4
These offer the chance to influence function and behaviour of CD4+ T-cells directly. Multicentre placebo-controlled studies in rheumatoid arthritis (RA) are underway (Kalden and Manger, 1997; Weinblatt *et al.*, 1995).

Anti-CD3
These interfere with the normal activation of T-cells, as well as contribute to the prevention of allograft rejection and the treatment of graft-versus-host-disease (Chatenoud, 1994).

Anti-CD5 and anti-CD7

These are directed against pan-T-cell antigens, such as CD5 and CD7, and against CD5 + B-cells. CD5 + B-cells comprise up to about 25% of the circulating B-cell population. This CD5+ B-cell subset is expanded in auto-immune conditions (Youinou *et al.*, 1993). In mice and in patients with RA and SLE, beneficial effects were noted from administration of anti-CD5. Positive results were also reported from treatment with anti-CD7 (Amital *et al.*, 1996).

Anti-T-cell receptor antibodies

These can be directed against different T-cell antigen receptors. In experimental auto-immune neuritis (an experimental model of Guillain-Barré syndrome), anti-α/β cell receptor treatment immediately after the induction of the disease prevented development of its clinical and electrophysiological signs and alleviated the disease in animals (Jung *et al.*, 1992).

In mice with experimental auto-immune encephalitis (EAE), favourable results were obtained with administration of a MOAB against the Vβ8 T-cell receptor. Preventive therapy with the combination of Vβ8 and Vβ13 antibodies gave a marked reduction in the incidence of EAE. Additionally, when these antibodies were given to mice after the first signs of EAE had developed, an impressive convalescence followed (Zaller *et al.*, 1990).

Anti-MHC class II antibodies

Antibodies directed against MHC class II histocompatibility antigens suppress the immune response against specific antigens that are under immunoregulatory gene control. Beneficial effects were reported in collagen-induced arthritis models, experimental MG, EAE and SLE (Amital *et al.*, 1996).

Anti-cytokine antibodies

Anti-TNF-α treatment in RA reduces serum concentrations of IL-1β, IL-6, soluble CD14 (monocytes and macrophages), and ICAM-1 (adhesion molecule, CD54) (Lorentz *et al.*, 1996). This may partly explain the anti-inflammatory effect of anti-TNF-α, as down regulation of cytokine-induced vascular adhesion molecules interferes with cell trafficking.

Anti-interleukin-1 and anti-inflammatory cytokines

Combined anti-IL-1 and anti-TNF-α therapy has proven to be more effective than monotherapy in collagen-induced arthritis models (Kalden and Manger, 1997).

Antibodies against adhesion molecules

Accumulation of leukocytes in inflammatory tissue is regulated by adhesion molecules. These molecules are expressed on endothelial cells after activation by cytokines. Following this interaction, endothelial cells are capable of activating further leukocytes by cytokines which are secreted locally. Inhibiting this step in the inflammation cascade might prevent the initiation of the inflammatory process. In EAE, a MOAB directed against the α4β1 integrin adhesive molecules (integrin is a member of a family of cell-surface adhesion molecules that binds mainly to the extracellular matrix) prevents the accumulation of leukocytes within the CNS by blocking their attachment to the α4β1 integrin. The development of EAE was delayed and reduced, and the attenuation of symptoms was noted (Yednock *et al.*, 1992).

BONE MARROW TRANSPLANTATION

Bone marrow transplantation is still in the experimental stage in auto-immune diseases, but there are a number of anecdotal reports about results in selected cases of RA, SLE, scleroderma (limited systemic sclerosis), MS, and severe juvenile chronic arthritis (Euler *et al.*, 1996; Fassas *et al.*, 1997; Wulffraat *et al.*, 1997). As it stands now, it seems likely that there will be a place for bone marrow transplantation for selected patients with intractable auto-immune disease.

DEHYDROEPIANDROSTERON (DHEA)

A putative role for sex hormones in both the aetiopathogenesis and therapy of auto-immune diseases has been suggested. Especially, this holds for diseases like SLE and Sjögren's syndrome. The effect of DHEA on the immune system of experimental animals is well known, but little is known yet about the results of DHEA administration in humans on auto-immune disease mechanisms and clinical manifestations. In patients with MS, a favourable effect on mood and psychic energy has been observed (Regelson and Kalimi, 1994). A double-blind placebo controlled study with 200 mg DHEA daily versus placebo for three months in 28 patients with mild to moderate SLE showed a decrease in clinical activity, but anti-DNA titre and complement levels did not change (van Vollenhove *et al.*, 1995). DHEA has been reported in several studies to achieve a sense of well-being with improvement in mood, fatigue, and psychic energy. Therefore, it might prove to be of value as adjunct therapy in SLE and Sjögren's syndrome (McKinley *et al.*, 1995).

OTHER APPROACHES TO TREATMENT

ORAL TOLERANCE

Attempts to induce tolerance to auto-antigens by oral administration of antigen have been undertaken first in animal experiments and subsequently in humans. Positive effects have been reported in RA, MS and uveitis (Thomson and Forrester, 1994). More research is needed before conclusions can be drawn.

DIETARY FISH OILS

It seems premature to recommend fish oil or other unsaturated fatty acids as treatment for auto-immune diseases. However, as unsaturated fatty acids may have beneficial effects on some aspects of these diseases, *e.g.* atherosclerosis in SLE, it is appropriate to recommend diets enriched with unsaturated fatty acids.

CONCLUSIONS

As the aetiology of most of the ICTDs is obscure and the pathogenetic mechanisms not well understood, we are forced to use agents that are still relatively non-specific in their immunosuppressive and anti-inflammatory properties. We may do harm by trading the problems of the disease for problems of the treatment! It should be stressed, however, that the serious side effects enumerated in this chapter have been registered largely in anti-tumour and transplantation therapy with doses much higher than customary in the auto-immune diseases. The complexity of the immune function in health and in disease has been enlightened during the past years. Greater insight into the multiple pathways of activation and the suppression of humoral and cellular processes involved have led clinicians and researchers to search for better strategies to modify disease processes in a more physiological manner. We have learnt that T-cell antigens, cytokines, MHC antigens and adhesion molecules normally keep the body in balance and health preserved. When out of balance, dysfunction of the body will result. Immuno-intervention by biological agents are becoming within our scope. These more physiological ways of intervention may have the advantage of restoring the immune balance, leaving those responses essential for host defence intact.

REFERENCES

Adachi JD, Bensen WG, Brown J *et al* (1997) Intermittent etidronate therapy to prevent corticosteroid-induced osteoporosis. *N Engl J Med* **37**, 382–387.

Adams EM and Plotz PH (1995) The treatment of myositis: How to approach resistant disease. *Rheum Dis Clin N Amer* **21**, 179–202.

Adorini L, Guery JC and Trembleau S (1996) Manipulation of the Th1/Th2 cell balance: An approach to treat human autoimmune diseases? *Autoimmunity* **23**, 53–69.

Alam SM, Kyriakides T, Lawden M *et al* (1993) Methylprednisolone in multiple sclerosis: A comparison of oral with intravenous therapy at equivalent high dose. *J Neurol Neurosurg Psychiat* **56**, 1219–1220.

Al-Janadi M, Smith CD and Karsh J (1989) Cyclophosphamide treatment of interstitial pulmonary fibrosis in polymyositis/dermatomyositis. *J Rheumatol* **16**, 1592–1596.

Al-Lozi MT, Pestronk A, Yee WC *et al* (1994) Rapidly evolving myopathy with myosin-deficient muscle fibres. *Ann Neurol* **35**, 273–279.

Alijotas J, Barquinero J, Ordi J *et al* (1990) Polymyositis and cyclosporin A (letter). *Ann Rheum Dis* **49**, 66.

American College of Rheumatology Task Force on Osteoporosis Guidelines (1996) Recommendations for the prevention and treatment of glucocorticoid-induced osteoporosis. *Arthritis Rheum* **39**, 1791–1801.

Amital H, Swissa M, Bar-Dayan Y *et al* (1996) New therapeutic avenues in autoimmunity. *Res Immunol* **147**, 361–376.

Andoh TF, Burdman EA and Bennett WM (1997) Nephrotoxicity of immunosuppressive drugs: Experimental and clinical observations. *Sem Nephrol* **17**, 34–45.

Batchelor TT, Taylor LP, Thaler HT *et al* (1997) Steroid myopathy in cancer patients. *Neurology* **48**, 1234–1238.

Block JA (1998) Hydroxychloroquine and retinal safety. *Lancet* **351**, 771.

Boumpas DT (1996) A novel action of glucocorticoids-NF-kappa B inhibition (editorial). *Brit J Rheumatol* **35**, 709–710.

Bowyer SL, LaMothe MP and Hollister JR (1985) Steroid myopathy: Incidence and detection in a population with asthma. *J Allergy Clin Immunol* **6**, 234–242.

Buch TW, Worthington JW, Combs JJ *et al* (1980) Azathioprine with prednisone for polymyositis. *Ann Intern Med* **92**, 365–369.

Calabresi P and Chabner BA (1990) Antineoplastic agents. In: Goodman, Gilman A, Rall TW, Niew AS *et al* (eds) *The Pharmacological Basis of Therapeutics*, pp 1209. New York: McGraw-Hill.

Cantu TG, Hoehn-Sarie EW, Burgess KM *et al* (1995) Acute renal failure associated with immunoglobulin therapy. *Am J Kidney Dis* **25**, 228–234.

Chatenoud L (1994) Use of CD3-antibodies in transplantation and autoimmune diseases. *Transplant Proc* **26**, 3191–3193.

Cheson BD, Vena DA, Foss FM *et al* (1994) Neurotoxicity of purine analogs: A review. *J Clin Oncol* **12**, 2216–2228.

Chou SM (1992) Pathology of the neuromuscular junction. In: Mastaglia FL and Lord Walton of Detchant (eds) *Skeletal Muscle Pathology*, 2 ed, pp 599–637. Edinburgh: Churchill Livingstone.

Chrousos GP (1995) The hypothalamic-pituitary-adrenal axis and immune-mediated inflammation. *N Engl J Med* **332**, 1351–1362.

Chrousos GA, Kattah JC, Beck RW *et al.* (1993) Side effects of glucocorticoid treatment. Experience of the Optic Neuritis Treatment Trial. *JAMA* **269**, 2110–2112.

Clements PJ and Davis J (1986) Cytotoxic drugs: Their clinical application to the rheumatic diseases. *Semin Arthritis Rheum* **15**, 231–254.

Conaghan PG, Lehman T and Brooks P (1997) Disease-modifying anti-rheumatic drugs. *Curr Opin Rheumatol* **9**, 183–190.

Cosi V, Lombardi M, Erbetta A *et al.* (1993) Azathioprine as a single immunosuppressive drug in the treatment of myasthenia gravis. *Acta Neurol* **15**, 123–131.

Cronstein BN (1995) The antirheumatic agents sulphasalazine and methotrexate share an anti-inflammatory mechanism. *Brit J Rheumatol* **34** (suppl 2), 30–32.

Dalakas (1994) High-dose intravenous immunoglobulin and serum viscosity: Risk of precipitating thromboembolic events. *Neurology* **44**, 223–226.

Dalakas MC, Illa I, Dambrosia JM *et al* (1993) A controlled trial of high dose immune globulin infusions as treatment for dermatomyositis. *N Engl J Med* **329**, 1993–2000.

Dekhuijzen PNR and DeCramer M (1992) Steroid-induced myopathy and its significance to respiratory disease: A known disease rediscovered. *Eur Respir J* **5**, 997–1003.

Delattre JY and Posner JB (1989) Neurological complications of chemotherapy and radiation therapy. In: Aminoff J (ed) *Neurology and General Medicine*, pp 365–387. New York: Churchill Livingstone.

Dequeker J (1998) Intermittent therapy with etidronate and calcium helps prevent osteoporosis secondary to steroids. *Clin Exp Rheumatol* **16**, 117–118.

Diamond T, McGuigan L, Barballo S *et al* (1995) Cyclical etidronate plus ergocalciferol prevents glucocorticoid-induced bone loss in postmenopausal women. *Am J Med* **98**, 450–463.

Dropcho EJ, Soong SJ (1991) Steroid-induced weakness in patients with primary brain tumors. *Neurology* **41**, 1235–1239.

Durelli L, Bongioanni MR, Cavallo R *et al* (1994) Chronic systemic high-dose recombinant interferon alpha 2a reduces exacerbation rate, MRI signs of disease activity and lymphocyte interferon gamma production in relapsing-remitting multiple sclerosis. *Neurology* **44**, 406–413.

Durelli L, Bongioanni MR, Ferrero B *et al* (1998) Interferon treatment for multiple sclerosis: Autoimmune complications may be lethal (letter). *Neurology* **50**, 570.

Dwyer JM (1992) Manipulating the immune system with immune globulin. *N Engl J Med* **326**, 107–116.

Eastell R (1995) Management of corticosteroid induced osteoporosis. *J Intern Med* **237**, 439–447.

Eastell R (1998) Drug therapy: Treatment of postmenopausal osteoporosis. *N Engl J Med* **338**, 736–746.

Efros MD, Ahmed T, Coombe N *et al.* (1994) Urologic complications of high-dose chemotherapy and bone marrow transplantation. *Urology* **43**, 355–360.

Euler HH, Schroeder JO, Harten P *et al.* (1994) Treatment-free remission in severe systemic lupus erythematosus following synchronization of plasmapheresis with subsequent pulse cyclophosphamide. *Arthritis Rheum* **37**, 1784–1794.

Euler HH, Marmont AM, Bacigalupo A *et al* (1996) Early recurrence or persistence of autoimmune disease after unmanipulated autologous stem cell transplantation. *Blood* **88**, 3621–3625.

Fassas A, Anagnostopoulos A, Kazis A *et al* (1997) Peripheral blood stem-cell transplantation for treatment of progressive multiple sclerosis: First results of a pilot study. *Bone Marrow Transplantation* **20**, 631–638.

Feutrin G and Mihatsch MJ (1992) Risk factors for cyclosporine-induced nephropathy in patients with autoimmune diseases. *N Engl J Med* **326**, 1654–1660.

Frei U, Bode V, Repp H *et al* (1993) Malignancies under cyclosporine after kidney transplantation: Analysis of a 10 year period. *Transplant Proc* **25**, 1394–1396.

Fruet P, Sheela R and Pelletier L (1995) Th1 and Th2 cells in autoimmunity. *Clin Exp Immunol* **101** (Suppl), 9–12.

Furst DE (1995) Practical clinical pharmacology and drug interactions of low dose methotrexate therapy in rheumatoid arthritis. *Brit J Rheumatol* **34** (suppl 2), 20–25.

Gay CT, Bodensteiner JB, Nitsche R *et al* (1994) Reversible treatment related leukoencephalopathy. *J Child Neurol* **4**, 208–212.

Gelder M, Gath D, Mayou R *et al* (1996) Oxford Textbook of Psychiatry, 3 ed. Oxford: Oxford University Press.

George WE, Wilmot M, Greenhouse A *et al* (1983) Medical management of steroid-induced epidural lipomatosis. *N Engl J Med* **308**, 316–319.

Gorson KC, Ropper AH, Clark BD *et al* (1998) Treatment of chronic inflammatory demyelinating polyneuropathy with interferon α 2A. *Neurology* **50**, 84–87.

Govert JA, Patton S and Fine RL (1992) Pancytopenia from using trimethoprim and methotrexate (letter). *Ann Intern Med* **117**, 877–878.

Griggs RC, Askanas V, DiMauro S *et al*. (1995) Inclusion body myositis and myopathies. *Ann Neurol* **38**, 705–713.

Guillevin L, Lhote F, Cohen P *et al* (1992) Corticosteroids plus pulse cyclophosphamide and plasma exchanges versus corticosteroids plus pulse cyclophosphamide alone in the treatment of polyarteritis nodosa and Churg Strauss syndrome patients with factors predicting poor outcome. A prospective randomized trial in 62 patients. *Arthritis Rheum* **38**, 1638–1645.

Hahn AF, Bolton CF, Zochodne D (1996) Intravenous immunoglobulin treatment in chronic inflammatory demyelinating polyneuropathy. A double-blind, placebo-controlled, cross-over study. *Brain* **119**, 1067–1077.

Hawkey CJ, Karrash JA, Szczepanski L, Walker DG *et al*. (1998) Omeprazole compared with misoprostol for ulcers associated with non-steroidal anti-inflammatory drugs. *N Engl J Med* **338**, 727–734.

Hilliquin P, Renoux M, Perrot S *et al* (1996) Occurrence of pulmonary complications during methotrexate therapy in rheumatoid arthritis. *Clin Rheumatol* **35**, 446–452.

Hirano F, Tanaka H, Nomura Y *et al* (1993) Successful treatment of refractory polymyositis with pulse intravenous cyclophosphamide and low-dose weekly oral methotrexate therapy. *Intern Med* **32**, 749–752.

Hoffman GS, Leavitt RY, Fleisher TA *et al* (1990) Treatment of Wegener's granulomatosis with intermittent high-dose intravenous cyclophosphamide. *Am J Med* **89**, 403–410.

Hohlfeld R and Toyka KV (1993) Therapies. In: De Baets MH and Oosterhuis HJGH (eds) *Myasthenia Gravis*, pp 235–261. Boca Raton: CRC Press.

Hoogenraad TU (1996) *Wilson's Disease*, pp 141–148. London: WB Saunders Co Ltd.

IFNB Multiple Sclerosis Study Group (1993) Interferon beta 1b is effective in relapsing intermitting multiple sclerosis. 1. Clinical results of a multicenter randomized double blind placebo-controlled trial. *Neurology* **43**, 655–661.

Joffe MM, Love LA, Leff RL *et al* (1993) Drug therapy of the idiopathic inflammatory myopathies: Predictors of response to prednisone, azathioprine, and methotrexate and a comparison of their efficacy. *Am J Med* **94**, 379–387.

Jongen JLM, van Doorn PA and van der Meché FGA (1998) High-dose intravenous immunoglubulin therapy for myasthenia gravis. *J Neurol* **245**, 26–31.

Jongen PJ, ter Laak HJ, van de Putte LBA (1995) Inclusion body myositis responding to long term chlorambucil treatment (letter). *J Rheumatol* **22**, 576–578.

Jundt JW, Browne BA, Fiocco GP *et al* (1993) A comparison of low dose methotrexate bioavailability: Oral solution, oral tablet, subcutaneous and intramuscular dosing. *J Rheumatol* **20**, 1845–1849.

Jung S, Kramer S, Schluesner HJ *et al* (1992) Prevention and therapy of experimental autoimmune neuritis by an antibody against T-cell receptors α/β. *J Immunol* **148**, 3768–3775.

Kahan BD (1996) The three fates of immunosuppression in the next millenium: Selectivity, synergy and specificity. *Transpl Int* **9**, 527–534.

Kakulas BA and Mastaglia FL (1992) Drug-induced, toxic and nutritional myopathies. In: Mastaglia FL and Detchant Lord Walton (eds) *Skeletal Muscle Pathology*, 2ed, pp 511–540. Edinburgh: Churchill Livingstone.

Kalden JR and Manger B (1997) Biological agents in the treatment of inflammatory rheumatic diseases. *Curr Opin Rheumatol* **9**, 206–212.

Kaldor JM, Day NE, Petterson F *et al* (1990) Leukemia following chemotherapy for ovarian cancer. *N Engl J Med* **322**, 1–13.

Kallenberg CGM (1998) Immunologie in de medische praktijk. IX. Systemische vasculitis. *Ned Tijdschr Geneesk* **142**, 118–123.

Kaplan SR and Calabresi P (1973) Immunosuppressive agents. (Second of two parts) *N Engl J Med* **289**, 1234–1238.

Kater L, Baart de la Faille N and Talal N (1995) Remarks on the use of therapeutic agents and their possible actions. In: Kater L and Baart de la Faille H (eds) *Multisystemic Autoimmune Diseases: An integrated Approach*, pp 307–323. Amsterdam: Elsevier.

Kelly WN, Harris Jr ED, Ruddy S, Sledge CB (eds) (1997) *Textbook of Rheumatology*, 5th ed., Philadelphia: W.B. Saunders Co.

Kinlen LJ, Sheil AG, Peto J *et al* (1979) Collaborative United Kingdom–Australian study of cancer in patients treated with immunosuppressive drugs. *Brit Med J* **2**, 1461–1466.

Kinto T, Hatanaka H, Miyata S *et al* (1987) FK 506, a novel immunosuppressant isolated from a streptomyces II. Immunosuppressive effects of FK 506 in vitro. *J Antibiot (Tokyo)* **40**, 1256–1265.

Klippel JH, Dieppe P (1998) *Rheumatology*, 3rd ed., St. Louis: Mosby

Knysak DJ, McLean JA, Solomon WR *et al* (1994) Immediate hypersensitivity reaction to cyclophosphamide. *Arthritis Rheum* **37**, 1101–1104.

Koskinen S, Tolo H, Hirvonen M *et al* (1995) Long-term follow-up of anti-IgA antibodies in healthy IgA-deficient adults. *J Clin Immunol* **15**, 194–198.

Kremer JM, Alarcon GS, Lightfoot RW *et al* (1994) Methotrexate for rheumatoid arthritis. Suggested guidelines for monitoring liver toxicity. *Arthritis Rheum* **37**, 316–328.

Kroemer G, Hirsch F, Gonzalez-Garcia A *et al* (1996) Differential involvement of Th1 and Th2 cytokines in autoimmune diseases. *Autoimmunity* **24**, 25–33.

La Civita L, Zignego AL, Lombardini F *et al* (1996) Exacerbation of peripheral neuropathy during alpha-interferon therapy in a patient with mixed cryoglobulinaemia and hepatitis B virus infection. *J Rheumatol* **23**, 1641–1643.

Lacomis D, Guiliani MJ, Van Cott A *et al* (1996) Acute myopathy of the intensive care: Clinical electromyographic and pathologic aspects. *Ann Neurol* **40**, 645–654.

Lacki JK, Samborski W and Mackieqicz SH (1993) Transient increase of aminotransferases in RA patients treated with methotrexate. *Z Rheumatol* **52**, 232–235.

Langford CA and Sneller MC (1997) New developments in the treatment of Wegener's granulomatosis, polyarteritis nodosa, microscopic polyangiitis and Churg-Strauss syndrome. *Curr Opin Rheumatol* **9**, 26–30.

Leff RL, Miller FW, Hicks J *et al* (1993) The treatment of inclusion body myositis (IBM): a retrospective review and a randomized prospective trial of immunosuppressive therapy. *Medicine* **72**, 225–235.

Lems WF, Jacobs JWG, Bijlsma JWJ *et al* (1997) Is addition of sodium fluoride to cyclical etidronate beneficial in the treatment of corticosteroid induced osteoporosis? *Ann Rheum Dis* **56**, 357–363.

Levy GD, Munz SJ, Paschal J *et al* (1997) Incidence of hydroxychloroquine retinopathy in 1207 patients in a large multicenter outpatient practice. *Arthritis Rheum* **40**, 1482–1486.

Lorentz HM, Antoni C, Valerius T *et al* (1996) In vivo blockade of TNF-alpha by intravenous infusion of a chimeric monoclonal TNF-alpha antibody in patients with rheumatoid arthritis: Short term cellular and molecular effects. *J Immunol* **156**, 1646–1653.

Lukert BP and Raisz LG (1990) Glucocorticoid-induced osteoporosis: pathogenesis and management. *Ann Intern Med* **112**, 352–364.

Machkhas H, Harati Y and Rolak LA (1997) Clinical pharmacology of immunosuppressants: Guidelines for neuroimmunotherapy. In Rolak LA and Harati Y (eds) *Neuro-Immunology for the Clinician*, pp 77–104. Boston: Butterworth-Heinemann.

Mandell BF (1996) Intravenous gammaglobulin therapy: The nuts and bolts. *J Clin Rheumatol* **2**, 317–324.

Martin F, Lauwerys B, Lefebvre C *et al.* (1997) Side-effects of intravenous cyclophosphamide pulse therapy. *Lupus* **6**, 254–257.

Mastaglia FL, Phillips BA and Zilko P (1997) Treatment of inflammatory myopathies. *J Neurol Neurosurg Psychiat* **20**, 651–664.

Matsubara S, Sawa Y, Takamori H *et al.* (1994) Pulsed intravenous methylprednisolone combined with oral steroids as the initial treatment of inflammatory myopathies. *J Neurol Neurosurg Psychiat* **57**, 1008–1009.

Mayer AD, Dmitrewski J, Squiffet JP *et al* (1997) Multicenter randomized trial comparing tacrolimus (FK 506) and cyclosporine in the prevention of renal allograft rejection. *Transplantation* **64**, 436–443.

McKinley PS, Ouelette SC and Winkel GH (1995) The contributions of disease activity, sleep patterns and depression to fatigue in systemic lupus erythematosus. *Arthritis Rheum* **38**, 826–834.

Milligan NM, Newcombe R and Compston DA (1987) A double-blind controlled trial of high dose methylprednisolone in patients with multiple sclerosis. *J Neurol Neurosurg Psychiat* **50**, 511–516.

Miller LC, Heckmatt JZ and Dubowitz V (1983) Drug treatment of juvenile dermatomyositis. *Arch Dis Child* **58**, 445–450.

Miller FW, Leitman SF, Cronin ME *et al* (1991) Controlled trial of plasma exchanges and leukapheresis in polymyositis and dermatomyositis. *N Engl J Med* **326**, 1380–1384.

Miller PD, Bonnick CK and Rosen CJ (1996) Clinical utility of bone mass measurement in adults: Consensus of an international panel. *Semin Arthritis Rheum* **25**, 361–372.

Murgia MG, Jordan S and Kahan BD (1996) The side effect profile of sirolimus: A phase I study in quiescent cyclosporine-prednisone-treated renal transplant patients. *Kidney Int* **49**, 209–216.

Morand E (1997) Corticosteroids in the treatment of rheumatologic diseases. *Curr Opin Rheumatol* **9**, 200–205.

Newman ED and Scott DW (1995) The use of low-dose methotrexate in the treatment of polymyositis and dermatomyositis. *J Clin Rheumatol* **1**, 99–102.

Ramirez F, Fowell DJ, Puklavec M *et al* (1996) Glucocorticoids promote a Th2 cytokine response by CD4+ T-cells in vitro. *J Immunol* **156**, 2406–2412.

Regelson W and Kalimi M (1994) Dehydroepiandrosteron (DHEA). The multifunctional steroid. II. Effects on the CNS, cell proliferation, metabolic and vascular, clinical and other effects. Mechanism of action? *Ann NY Acad Sci* **719**, 564–575.

Rich MM, Teener JW, Raps EC *et al* (1996) Muscle is electrically inexcitable in acute quadriplegic myopathy. *Neurology* **46**, 731.

Ritters B, Grabensee B and Heering P (1994) Malignancy under immunosuppression therapy including cyclosporine. *Transplant Proc* **26**, 2656–2657.

Romagnani S (1995) Biology of human TH1 and TH2 cells *J Clin Immunol* **15**, 121–129.

Rubin CM, Nesbit ME Jr, Kim TH *et al* (1992) Chromosomal abnormalities in skin following total lymphoid irradiation. *Genes Chromosome Cancer* **4**, 141–145.

Russel G, Graveley R, Seid J *et al* (1992) Mechanisms of action of cyclosporine and effects on connective tissue diseases. *Semin Arthr Rheum* **21**, 16–22.

Sandoval DM, Alarcon GS and Morgan SL (1995) Adverse events in methotrexate-treated rheumatoid arthritis patients. *Brit J Rheumatol* **34** (suppl 2) 49–56.

Schnabel A, Dahlhoff K, Bauerfeind S *et al* (1996) Sustained cough in methotrexate therapy for rheumatoid arthritis. *Clin Rheumatol* **15**, 277–282.

Sekul EA, Cupler EJ and Dalakas MC (1994) Aseptic meningitis associated with high dose intravenous immunoglobulin therapy: Frequency and risk factors. *Ann Intern Med* **121**, 259–262.

Silverstein FE, Graham DY, Senior JR *et al.* (1995) Misoprostal reduces serious gastrointestinal complications in patients with rheumatoid arthritis receiving non-steroidal anti-inflammatory drugs. Amized double blind placebo controlled trial. *Ann Intern Med* **123**, 241–249.

Sinoway PA and Callen JP (1993) Chlorambucil. An effective corticosteroid-sparing agent for patients with recalcitrant dermatomyositis. *Arthritis Rheum* **36**, 319–324.

Sipe JC, Romine JS, Koziol JA *et al* (1994) Cladibrine in treatment of chronic progressive multiple sclerosis. *Lancet* **344**, 9–13.

Snijder LS, Heigh RI and Anderson ML (1993) Cyclophosphamide induced hepatotoxicity in a patient with Wegener's granulomatosis. *Mayo Clin Proc* **68**, 1203–1204.

Stillwell THJ, Benson RC, DeRemee RA, McDonald THJ *et al* (1988) Cyclophosphamide-induced bladder toxicity in Wegener's granulomatosis. *Arthritis Rheum* **31**, 465–470.

Strober S and Farinas MC (1989) Cellular mechanisms in immune tolerance and treatment of autoimmune disease: Studies using total lymphoid irradiation. In: Bach JF (ed) *Immunointervention in Autoimmune Diseases*, pp 197–206. London: Academic Press.

Talar-Williams G, Hijazi TM, Schnaubec A *et al.* (1996) Cyclophosphamide induced cystitis and bladder cancer in patients with Wegener's granulomatosis. *Ann Int Med* **124**, 477–484.

Ten Berghe RHJM (1997) New immunosuppressive drugs: A welcome addition? *Neth J Med* **51**, A13–A14.

Thomas E, Leroux JL, Hellier JP *et al* (1993) Seizure and methotrexate therapy (letter.) *J Rheumatol* **20**, 1632.

Thomson AW and Forrester JV (1994) Therapeutic advances in immunosuppression. *Clin Exp Immunol* **98**, 351–357.

Thomson AW and Nield GH (1992) Cyclosporine: Use outside transplantation. *Brit Med J* **302**, 4–5.

Tindall RSA, Philips TH, Rollins J *et al* (1993) A clinical therapeutic trial of cyclosporine in myasthenia gravis. *Ann New York Acad Sci* **581**, 539–551.

Travis LB, Curtis RE, Glimelius B *et al* (1995) Bladder and kidney cancer following cyclophosphamide therapy for non-Hodgkin's lymphoma. *J Natl Cancer Inst* **87**, 524–530.

Troiano R, Halstein M, Ruderman M *et al* (1984) Effect of high dose intravenous steroid administration on contrast-enhanced computed tomographic scan lesion in multiple sclerosis. *Ann Neurol* **15**, 257–263.

Turner-Stokes L and Turner-Warwick M (1982) Intrathoracic manifestations of SLE. *Clin Rheum Dis* **8**, 229–242.

Usman AR and Yunus MB (1996) Non-Hodgkin lymphoma in patients with rheumatoid arthritis treated with low dose methotrexate. *J Rheumatol* **234**, 1095–1097.

Van den Berg LH, Kerkhoff H, Oey PL *et al* (1995) Treatment of multifocal motor neuropathy with high dose intravenous immunoglobulins: A double blind placebo controlled study. *J Neurol Neurosurg Psychiat* **59**, 248–252.

Van der Meché FGA, van Doorn PA (1997) The current place of high dose immunoglobulins in the treatment of neuromuscular disorders. *Muscle Nerve* **20**, 136–147.

Van der Meché FGA, Schmitz PI and Dutch Guillan-Barré Study Group (1992) A randomized trial comparing intravenous immune globulin and plasma exchange in Guillain-Barré syndrome. *N Engl J Med* **326**, 1123–1129.

Van der Wouden F (1998) Mycophenolate mofetil – a comparison with cyclophosphamide (CPH). *Third Int Conf on New Trends in Clinical and Experimental Immunosuppression*, Abstract, 100. Geneva, Switzerland.

van Vollenhoven RF, Engleman EG and McGuire JL (1995) Dehydroepiandrosterone in systemic lupus erythematosus. *Arthritis Rheum* **38**, 1826–1831.

Villalba L and Adams EM (1996) Update on refractory dermatomyositis and polymyositis. *Curr Opin Rheumatol* **8**, 544–551.

Viraben R, Brousse P and Lamant L (1996) Reversible cutaneous lymphoma occurring during methotrexate therapy. *Brit J Dermatol* **135**, 116–118.

Vita S de, Neri S and Bombardieri S (1991) Cyclophosphamide pulses in the treatment of rheumatic disease: An update. *Clin Exp Rheumatol* **9**, 179–193.

Vose JM, Reed EC, Pippert GC *et al* (1993) Mesna compared with continuous bladder irrigation as uroprotection during high dose chemotherapy and transplantation: A randomized trial. *J Clin Oncol* **11**, 1306–1310.

Walker AE and Adamkiewitcz JJ (1964) Pseudotumor cerebri associated with prolonged corticosteroid therapy: Reports of four cases. *JAMA* **188**, 779–784.

Walker RW and Brochstein JA (1988) Neurologic complications of immunosuppressive agents. *Neurol Clin* **6**, 261–278.

Wallace DJ, Hahn BH (eds) (1997) *Dubois' Lupus Erythematosus*, Baltimore: Williams and Williams.

Weinblatt ME, Maddison PJ, Bulpitt KJ *et al* (1995) Campath-1H humanized monoclonal antibody in refractory rheumatoid arthritis: An intravenous dose-escalation study. *Arthritis Rheum* **38**, 1589–1594.

Weiner P, Azgad Y and Weiner M (1993) The effect of corticosteroids on inspiratory muscle performance in humans. *Chest* **104**, 1788–1791.

Wernicke R, Smith DL (1989) Central nervous system low toxicity associated with weekly low dose methotrexate treatment. *Arthritis Rheum* **32**, 770–775.

Williamson RA and Karp LE (1981) Azathioprine teratogenicity: Review of the literature and a case report. *Obstet Gynecol* **58**, 247–250.

Worthley SG and McNeil JD (1995) Leukoencephalopathy in a patient taking low-dose oral methotrexate therapy for rheumatoid arthritis. *J Rheumatol* **22**, 335–337.

Wulffraat NW, van Royen A, Slaper I *et al.* (1997) Autologous bone marrow transplantation in a case of refractory systemic juvenile chronic arthritis. *Arthritis Rheum* **40**, (Supplement) S46.

Yednock TA, Cannon C, Fritz LC *et al* (1992) Prevention of experimental autoimmune encephalo-pathy by antibodies against α4β1 integrin. *Nature* **356**, 63–66.

Youinou P, Buskila D, MacKenzie LE *et al* (1993) CD5 positive B-cells and disease. In: Shoefeld Y and Isenberg DA (eds) *Natural Autoantibodies*, pp 143–165. Boca Raton: CRC Press.

Zaller DM, Osman G, Kanagawa O *et al* (1990) Prevention and treatment of murine experimental allergic encephalomyelitis with T-cell receptor Vβ-specific antibodies. *J Exp Med* **171**, 1943–1955.

Zuber M and Gause A (1997) Peripheral neuropathy during interferon-α therapy in patients with cryoglobulinaemia and hepatitis virus infection. *J Rheumatol* (letter) **24**, 2488.

5

Vasculitis

INTRODUCTION

A bewildering number of disorders have one pathological feature in common: inflammation with damage of blood vessels. The term *inflammation* implies that mononuclear or polynuclear white blood cells are present in and near the walls of blood vessels. A perivascular inflammatory cell infiltrate should not be considered proof of vasculitis, though some vessels in biopsies from patients with proven vasculitis are surrounded only by inflammatory cells. Vasculitis may cause stenosis of vessel lumina, occlusion by secondary thrombosis, (micro)aneurysmata, rupture and haemorrhage of blood vessels, and dissection of blood vessel walls. Before discussing the neurology of these diseases, a choice has to be made between one of the current classification systems of the vasculitides, none of which is likely to survive for very long. For an analysis of the problematic nature of the present systems, the reader is referred to the literature (Lie, 1994). Here, we just link up to the system that is most recent and most 'en vogue'.

Table 5.1 shows that a distinction can be made between the primary and secondary vasculitides. The *primary vasculitides* are arranged according to the proposal of the Chapel Hill Consensus Conference (Jennette *et al.*, 1994). A few other relevant diseases are grouped under the heading 'miscellaneous'. They are also 'primary', but for historical and other reasons are usually not included under this heading. For the purpose of this chapter, the isolated vasculitides of the central and peripheral nervous systems (CNS and PNS) have been grouped together. The neurological aspects of each of these diseases will be reviewed against a description of their general features. A full discussion of the secondary vasculitides is not within the scope of this book. However, we shall indicate which of these diseases give rise to prominent neurological manifestations and provide references to relevant reviews. For the vasculitides secondary to inflammatory connective tissue diseases (ICTDs), we refer to other chapters in this monograph. A review of the neurological aspects of systemic vasculitides was published by Cohen Tervaert and Kallenberg in 1993.

Table 5.1 Classification of vasculitides

Primary Vasculitides	
Affecting large vessels	Takayasu's disease
	Giant cell (temporal) arteritis
Affecting medium-sized vessels	Polyarteritis nodosa (classic)
	Kawasaki disease
Affecting small vessels	Microscopic polyangiitis
	Churg-Strauss syndrome
	Wegener's granulomatosis
	Henoch-Schönlein purpura
	Essential cryoglobulinaemic vasculitis
	Cutaneous leukocytoclastic vasculitis
Miscellaneous	Behçet's disease
	Degos' disease
	Cogan syndrome
Nervous System Vasculitis	Primary angiitis of the CNS
	Benign angiitis of the CNS
	Vasculitis of the PNS
Secondary Vasculitides	Secondary to connective tissue disease
	Infection related
	Malignancy related
	Drug related
	Hypocomplementaemic urticarial
	Post-organ transplant

Adapted from Jennette *et al.* (1994), with permission.

CLINICAL DIFFERENCES BETWEEN THE VASCULITIDES

The value of clinical indices for the differential diagnosis of the vasculitides is not to be underestimated. A prerequisite for the diagnosis of these diseases is nearly always the histological demonstration of a vasculitis. Once this has been established, a decision on the type of vasculitic disease is usually taken on the basis of clinical characteristics. Serum antibody profiles play a role in the diagnostic process, but at present they are of secondary importance in most diseases. Clinical features differ depending on age, gender, and the affected organs (Table 5.2). The table shows a few striking points. In general, the vasculitides affect the skin more frequently than any other organ. As far as incidence is concerned, the CNS is relatively spared, but once it is involved the consequences are often serious. Takayasu's disease and giant cell arteritis (GCA) are apparently related diseases. They differ distinctly from all other vasculitides in gender and organ preference.

THE PRIMARY VASCULITIDES

TAKAYASU'S DISEASE

Definition and epidemiology
Takayasu's disease or *Takayasu's arteritis* (Tk.A) is a chronic granulomatous vasculitis of unknown origin. Predominantly, it affects large arteries: the aorta, the main

Table 5.2 The primary vasculitides and related disorders: Clinical differences in age, gender and main affected organs

Disease	Pref Ages	Sex	Hd	Eyes	Skin	Joints	Heart	Re sy		Kidn		GI sy	PNS	CNS
								U	L	H	G			
Tk	≤40	M<F	+	+										
GCA	≥50	M<F	+	+										
PAN	All	M≥F			+	+				+			+	
Ka	≤5	M=F			+		+							
MPA	All	M>F			+				+	+				
CSS	All	M>F			+		+		+					+
WG	>20	M>F		+	+			+	+	+				+
HSP	J&C	M=F			+	+					+	+		
EC	>40	M=F			+						+	+		
CLV	All	M=F			+									
Beh	>YA	M=F		+	+									
Dego	All	M=F			+									
Cog	>YA	M=F	+*											

Vertical abbreviations: Tk, Takayasu's disease; GCA, giant cell arteritis; PAN, polyarteritis nodosa; Ka, Kawasaki disease; MPA, microscopic polyangiitis; CSS, Churg–Strauss syndrome; WG, Wegener's granulomatosis; HSP, Henoch–Schönlein purpura; EC, essential cryoglobulinaemia; CLV, cutaneous leukocytoclastic vasculitis; Beh, Behçet's disease; Dego, Degos' disease; Cog, Cogan syndrome; M, males; F, females; J&C, juveniles and children; >YA, preferentially young adults.

Horizontal Abbreviations: Pref, preferred; Hd, headache; Skin, skin and mucous membrane; Re sy U, respiratory system upper; Re sy L, respiratory system lower; Kidn H, renal vascular disease and hypertension; Kidn G, glomerulonephritis; GI sy, gastrointestinal system including liver; PNS, peripheral nervous system; CNS, central nervous system

*Bilateral interstitial keratitis and vestibuloauditory dysfunction

branches of the aorta, and the coronary and pulmonary arteries. There are considerable regional differences in epidemiological and clinical aspects of the disease (Numano, 1997). Tk.A is 'common' in Japan, South-East Asia and Africa, and rare in Europe and the USA. The estimated annual incidence in Olmsted County in Minnesota is 2.6 per million (Hall *et al.*, 1985). In Japan, Tk.A is a disease predominantly of females of childbearing age, with a peak incidence in the third decade. In India and Israel, men and women are affected equally at a mean age of 41 years (see Kerr, 1995). According to Japanese authors, the disease is linked with increased frequency to HLA-Bw52, Dw12, DR2 and DQw1, but this has not been confirmed in Western countries. Familial Tk.A has been reported in Japan. In Japan, Tk.A presents mostly as an aortic arch syndrome and in South-East Asia and Mexico as a disorder of the descending aorta.

Pathogenesis and pathology

Tk.A is considered an immune-mediated disease on the basis of 'anecdotal and sporadic' reports and on case reports that suggest frequent association with other autoimmune diseases (Kerr, 1994). Serum levels of gammaglobulins and circulating immune complexes are high, and rheumatoid factor (RF) is often positive. Serum anti-endothelial antibody titres are high in approximately 90% of patients (17/18 cases) (Sima *et al.*, 1994). The histopathology in the active stage of Tk.A is characterized by a granulomatous panarteritis with a mixed cellular infiltrate, as in GCA, and cannot be distinguished from GCA by histological criteria. In the healed end-stages, there is fibrosis and constriction with scant or no inflammatory infiltrate anymore (Lie, 1995).

Clinical features
Patients still may be asymptomatic when unequal or absent pulses are discovered by chance, or alternatively, they may suddenly and unexpectedly present with heart failure, stroke, or aneurysmal bleeding. A minority of patients (see Kerr *et al.*, 1994) complain initially about fatigue, fever, weight loss or arthralgia and subsequently, in a second phase of the disease, about symptoms of vessel inflammation, such as vessel pain and tenderness at palpation. The third and last phase is characterized by unequal or absent pulses; unequal blood pressure; limb claudicatio in upper limbs, and less often in the lower; neurological manifestations (see below); and evidence of ischaemia of other organs. Hypertension (due to renal arterial stenosis), angina pectoris, heart failure and cardiomegaly may all be present. As well, although more rare, gastrointestinal symptoms like nausea, diarrhoea and abdominal pain may be present. Erythema nodosa occurs in a small minority of patients (Hall *et al.*, 1985; Kerr *et al.*, 1994). Several patients have been reported with the combination of either sarcoidosis and Tk.A (Rose *et al.*, 1990; Kerr *et al.*, 1994) or inflammatory bowel disease and Tk.A (Achar and Al-Nakib, 1986; Kerr *et al.*, 1994).

Diagnosis
Tk.A is diagnosed on the basis of its clinical presentation, four limb blood pressure readings, and arteriography or imaging by non-invasive techniques of large blood-vessels (Kerr *et al.*, 1994). The affected arteries show irregularities of the vessel walls, mural thrombi, stenosis or obstruction, post-stenotic dilatations, and aneurysms (Fig. 5.1). Long stenotic lesions are a feature of the disease and were detected by Kerr *et al.* (1994) in nearly all of their 60 cases. Calcifications in vessel walls are rare and occur mostly in the aorta abdominalis. Dissection was not observed in any of the large series reviewed here. When arteritis has been established by biopsy investigation, classification as Tk.A is possible by the criteria provided by the American College of Rheumatology in 1990 (Table 5.3); these are meant for epidemiological investigations and other research purposes and not for the diagnosis of the individual case.

The differential diagnosis of Tk.A with GCA will be discussed in the next section.

Therapy and outcome
Corticosteroids, cyclophosphamide and methotrexate have been evaluated in uncontrolled open trials and are recommended for treatment of patients in acute or active stages (Kerr, 1995; see Chapter 4 for doses and side effects). In view of dose related serious side effects, cyclophosphamide should be prescribed only in life or organ threatening situations. Antiplatelet agents (primarily acetylsalicylic acid) are advised in patients with a hypercoagulable state (see Chapter 2, *Secondary Prevention of Ischaemic Stroke*). Surgical interventions are often required for abolishment of stenotic lesions, by-passes, and removal of aneurysms. These operations should be performed preferably when the disease is inactive, but unfortunately there are no adequate criteria for disease activity. For lack of anything better, the erythrocyte sedimentation rate (ESR) is used. However, surgical specimens often show histological evidence of disease activity in patients with normal ESR. Relapse

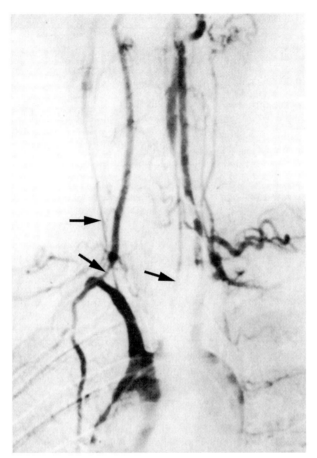

Figure 5.1 Takayasu's arteritis. Angiography. Long segments of critical stenoses of the two common carotid arteries, the subclavian artery and the proximal right vertebral artery (with permission from Kerr *et al.*, 1994).

rates are as high as 45% and long treatment courses are therefore advocated. The prognosis *quoad vitam* in well-treated and controlled patients is favourable nevertheless. Survival rates of 5–10 years have been documented in 80–97% of patients (see Kerr, 1994). Sudden death is rare and is commonly due to myocardial infarction, stroke or aneurysmal bleeding (Kerr *et al.*, 1994; Kerr, 1995).

Neurology
The neurological symptoms depend on the degree of involvement of the aorta, and the innominate, carotid and vertebral arteries. Patients complain about tenderness in the neck due to carotodynia, headache, dizziness and syncope. They may present with seizures, visual disturbances, transient ischaemic attacks (TIAs) and stroke.

Headache and dizziness. These are common symptoms in Tk.A. In different series, headache was present in 57% (Lupi-Herrera *et al.*, 1977), 31% (Hall *et al.*, 1985) and

Table 5.3 1990 criteria for the classification of Takayasu's arteritis

Criterion	Definition
Age at disease onset ≤ 40 years	Development of symptoms or findings related to Takayasu arteritis at age ≤ 40 years
Claudicatio of extremities	Development and worsening of fatigue and discomfort in muscles of 1 or more extremities while in use, especially the upper extremities
Decreased brachial artery pulse	Decreased pulsation of 1 or both brachial arteries
BP difference >10 mm Hg	Difference of > 10 mm Hg in systolic blood pressure between arms
Bruit over subclavian arteries or aorta	Bruit audible on auscultation over 1 or both subclavian arteries or abdominal aorta
Arteriogram abnormality	Arteriographic narrowing or occlusion of the entire aorta, its primary branches, or large arteries in the proximal upper or lower extremities, not due to arteriosclerosis, fibromuscular dysplasia or similar causes; changes usually focal or segmental

For purposes of classification, a patient shall be said to have Takayasu's arteritis if at least 3 of these 6 criteria are present. The presence of any 3 or more criteria yields a sensitivity of 90.5% and a specificity of 97.8%. Abbreviation: BP, blood pressure (systolic, difference between arms).
From Arend *et al.* (1990), with permission.

42% (Kerr *et al.*, 1994) of patients. Hall *et al.* (1985) stressed that dizziness (present in 39% of their cases) had a postural aspect. One of their patients experienced dizziness to such a degree that sitting upright prompted syncope. Syncope was a feature of 13% (*n*=14) of the patients of Lupi-Herrera *et al.* (1977). Light-headedness or dizziness occurred in one third of the patients of Kerr *et al.* (1994), and was a symptom of 57% of patients with vertebral artery stenosis and of 23% of patients without vertebral artery disease.

Visual disturbances. Visual disorders are not uncommon and are due to hypertensive ophthalmopathy, hypoperfusion of the retina, ischaemia of the optic nerves, ischaemia of the oculomotor nerves, and occasionally occipital infarcts, though this is rare. Though diplopia occurred in three patients of Hall *et al.* (1985), it is exceptional and has not been reported in other series. Monocular blindness is rare as well, occurring in only one of 32 patients of Hall *et al.* (1985), in one of 88 patients of Subramanyan *et al.* (1989), and in one of 60 patients of Kerr *et al.* (1994). Visual loss of one or both eyes has been described in case histories by Edwards *et al.* (1989), Bodker *et al.* (1993) and Rodriguez-Pla *et al.* (1996).

Vascular disorders in the CNS. Tk.A carries an increased risk of focal cerebral lesions. Lupi-Herrera *et al.* (1977) had eight cases of hemiplegia in their series (7%); Hall *et*

al. (1985) had one case among 35 patients with right-sided hemiplegia and aphasia; and Subramanyan *et al.* (1989) reported hemiplegia in six of 88 consecutive cases of Tk.A and subarachnoid haemorrhage in one. In the study of Kerr *et al.* (1994), ten out of 60 patients had TIAs or stroke. In most series, there is an occasional case of hypertensive encephalopathy. Spinal cord lesions are very rare: only Lupi-Herrera *et al.* (1977) had a case of paraplegia in their series.

Management of patients with neurological manifestations
Apart from symptomatic measures, therapy does not change by the presence of neurological signs (see this Chapter, *Therapy and Outcome of Tk.A* and Chapter 2, *Ischaemic Stroke* and *Intracranial Haemorrhage*).

GIANT CELL ARTERITIS (GCA)

Definition and epidemiology
GCA, also known as *temporal arteritis* (TA) or *cranial arteritis*, is a disease of middle and old age (mean age 70 and age range 50–90) and is the most common form of primary arteritis. It affects predominantly branches of the aortic arch (aa. temporalis superficialis, vertebralis, ophthalmica, and ciliaris posterior, and less often the aa. carotis externa and interna and centralis retinae) and the aorta itself. The upper limb arteries and other arteries and venae, including the lower limb arteries, may be involved as well (Hunder, 1997; Evans and Hunder, 1997; Evans *et al.*, 1995; Lie, 1995; Lie and Togaguwa, 1995). Intracranial arteries are usually spared.

The incidence of GCA is highest in Scandinavian countries ($29/10^5$ in residents older than 50 years in South Norway) (Gran and Myklebust, 1997, see Cotch and Rao, 1996). Women are affected twice as often as men (Salvarini *et al.*, 1995). There is an as yet unexplained association of GCA with polymyalgia rheumatica (PMR) (see Chapter 12); in a recent prospective study, 20–30% of patients with PMR also had GCA (Gran and Myklebust, 1997). Hereditary predisposition is likely to play a role in the aetiology of the disease. Siblings are at an increased risk for the disease (Bengtsson and Malmvall, 1982), and HLA-DR4 is associated both with GCA and PMR more often than explainable by chance (Weyand *et al.*, 1994).

Pathogenesis and pathology
Immunological reactions are probably decisive in the mechanism that underlies the disease. Serum levels of adhesion molecules and immune complexes are increased (Hunder, 1997). The majority of the circulating monocytes are activated both in GCA and PMR and secrete cytokines that promote inflammatory responses (Weyand and Goronzy, 1995). Findings in a retrospective, matched case-control study suggest that onset of GCA is related to infections – predominantly urinary – by *E. coli*, *Proteus* and *Klebsiella* (Russo *et al.*, 1995). In a case of corticosteroid resistant GCA, evidence for *Borrelia burgdorferi* infection was found in the cerebrospinal fluid (CSF); signs of GCA vanished rapidly after initiation of antibiotic treatment (Fontana *et al.*, 1997).

The pathology of GCA at an early stage is characterized by thickening of the intima and by lymphocyte infiltration, predominantly T-helper cells, more in the adventitia than in the media or intima. The inflammatory cells are suggested to derive predominantly from the microvasculature in the adventitia, and to target antigens in the outer part of the intima or the internal elastic membrane (Nordborg and Nordborg, 1998). At a more advanced stage, there may be fibrinoid necrosis of the intima and then the vessel wall is infiltrated by lymphocytes, plasma cells and some eosinophils. In approximately 70% of the biopsies (Myklebust and Gran, 1996), granuloma's with multinucleated histiocytes and foreign body giant cells are present, usually in the peripheral half of the intima, centring on a disrupted internal elastic lamina. At the end–stage, the inflammatory infiltrate has disappeared and fibrosis and constriction are the only remains. GCA cannot be distinguished from Tk.A by the histological changes (Lie, 1995).

Clinical features

With few exceptions (Nordborg and Bengtsson, 1990), symptoms and signs of GCA appear only in patients older than 50 years of age. While onset is usually abrupt, it may be insidious in some patients (Myklebust and Gran, 1996). Local signs of vasculitis become manifest against the background of systemic symptoms, for example fatigue, loss of appetite and weight, and a raised body temperature, even up to 39°C. The cranial symptoms are the most characteristic for the disease and comprise headache, loss of vision, diplopia, pain in the jaw when eating (jaw claudicatio), and ischaemia of the tongue or skin of the head. TIAs and stroke are rare. Impaired blood supply to the cochlear and vestibular vessels may cause deafness and vertigo (see *The Neurology*, below).

Extracranial changes are less prominent than cranial abnormalities or entirely absent, though they may dominate the clinical picture in some cases. There may be bruits over large arteries; absent, diminished or unequal pulses in the upper limbs or even in the lower limbs; ischaemic or gangrenous digits; and myocardial infarction due to coronary arteritis. Aortic aneurysms are 17 times more frequent during, or more usually following, GCA than in controls (Cotch and Rao, 1996). Aortic dissection due to GCA is not that rare and causes manifestations usually at a late stage (Liu *et al.*, 1995).

Diagnosis

The golden standard for the diagnosis of GCA is histological confirmation by a temporal artery biopsy. In some cases, temporal artery pathology can be predicted clinically when the vessel is swollen, when pulsations are decreased, or when they cannot be felt. However, biopsy is justified also when these changes are not obvious. Colour duplex ultrasonography has proven to demonstrate reliably obstruction of lumina of temporal arteries and oedema of the temporal artery wall. The lack of abnormal findings at colour duplex ultrasonography is, however, not sufficient reason to renounce biopsy investigation. At present, it is likely that colour duplex ultrasonography will be a valuable method for screening purposes, for instance in patients with PMR (Schmidt *et al.*, 1997).

As vascular inflammation by GCA is patchy, biopsies should be long to increase the chance that they contain an inflamed portion or remnants of inflammation. The biopsy material should be divided in small portions before embedding or freezing and sections should be made of each portion to confirm or exclude evidence of inflammation definitely. A negative biopsy does not, however, rule out GCA. ESR (Westergren method) or C-reactive protein are raised high nearly always, but exceptions do occur (Myklebust and Gran, 1996). Elevated liver function tests are found in 25% of patients, and invariably return to normal when therapy has started.

The 1990 criteria of the American College of Rheumatology for GCA concern patients in whom vasculitis has been established (Hunder *et al.*, 1990). They are meant primarily for research purposes and not as much for the diagnosis of individual patients (Table 5.4).

The overlap between Tk.A and GCA in epidemiological (predominantly women), clinical (headache and visual aberrations), arteriographic (stenotic lesions, obstruction, aneurysms of the aorta and its branches), and histological (granulomatous inflammation) features has given rise to suggestions that these disorders are slightly different manifestations of the same disease. Michell and Hunder (1996) used the prospectively gathered, large data set of the American College of Rheumatology Vasculitis Criteria Databank to investigate this subject in more detail (Table 5.5). There are a number of very striking differences between the two diseases, the most obvious being the divergence in preferred age, differences in blood pressure between the arms, and involvement of the abdominal aorta.

Treatment and outcome
Corticosteroid medication generally has a favourable effect and prevents or improves eye complications and other neurological changes. Treatment should be started without delay with prednisolone, 40–60 mg/day for one week (see Nordborg *et al.*, 1995). This dose may be reduced slowly during the weeks thereafter. A daily dose of 2.5–7.5 mg should be maintained until patients are without symptoms for six months. When medication is stopped relapse follows in up to 50% of patients, and corticosteroid medication should be resumed then (10–15 mg/day). Controlled intervention studies have not been performed.

Table 5.4 The American College of Rheumatology 1990 criteria for the classification of giant cell arteritis

Criterion	Definition
Age at disease onset ≥ 50 years	Development of symptoms or findings beginning at age 50 or older
New headache	New onset of or new type of localized pain in the head
Temporal artery abnormality	Temporal artery tenderness to palpation or decreased pulsation unrelated to arteriosclerosis of cervical arteries
Elevated erythrocyte sedimentation rate	Erythrocyte sedimentation rate ≥ 50 mm/h by the Westergren method
Abnormal artery biopsy	Biopsy specimen with artery showing vasculitis characterized by a predominance of mononuclear cell infiltration or granulomatous inflammation usually with multinucleated giant cells.

For purpose of classification a patient shall be said to have giant cell (temporal) arteritis if at least 3 of these 5 criteria are present. The presence of any 3 or more criteria yields a sensitivity of 93.5% and a specificity of 91.2%.
From Hunder *et al.* (1990), with permission.

Table 5.5 Differences between Takayasu's arteritis and giant cell arteritis from data on the two diseases by the American College of Rheumatology Vasculitis Criteria Databank (see Michell and Hunder, 1996).

	Takayasu's disease	*Giant cell arteritis*
Mean age at onset	26 yrs	69 yrs
Frequent, characteristic, clinical features	Signs of vascular insufficiency of the upper limbs and less frequently the lower limbs Bruits and decreased pulsations of the aorta and the proximal branches of the aorta	Jaw claudicatio, proximal aching, musculoskeletal stiffness Temporal artery abnormality Scalp tenderness Vascular upper limb insufficiency in 15%
Systolic BP difference in arms	74%	4%
Thoracic part of aorta	Affected in nearly 100%	Affected in 54%
Abdominal part of aorta	Affected in 76%	Affected in 14%
ESR mean ± S.D.	65 ± 39 mm	90 ± 33 mm

Neurology

Headache. Headache is prominent in 80–90% of patients (Hunder, 1997; Myklebust and Gran, 1996; Nordborg *et al.*, 1995). This type of headache is new for the patient; it is chronic or paroxysmal, sometimes mainly temporal but more often diffuse, and burning in some cases. Touching the head may be painful. The temporal arteries and less often the carotid artery may be tender (Gonzalez-Gay and Garcia-Porrua, 1998).

Visual loss. Visual loss is the most notorious manifestation of GCA. In a large, retrospective study in a tertiary referral centre (the Mayo Clinic), 35 of 166 patients (21%) had neuro-ophthalmologic symptoms compared to seven of 37 patients (18%) in a recent prospective Norwegian study (Caselli *et al.*, 1988a; Myklebust and Gran, 1996). Most patients in the American study had either transient (17 patients) or permanent loss of vision (14 patients), either in one eye (12 patients) or both (2 patients). For the Norwegian study, these figures were six cases with transient, usually very slight, visual loss and one case with bilateral permanent visual loss. Scintillating scotoma's or amaurosis fugax precede permanent visual loss in a minority (approximately 20%) and may serve as a warning. Visual loss in GCA is due to ischaemia of the optic tract or nerve and is caused by arteritis and obstruction of blood flow in the ophthalmological or posterior ciliary arteries. Probably a very rare cause of visual loss is (are) occipital infarction(s) due to obstruction of the top of the basilar artery (Caselli *et al.*, 1988a). Bright-light amaurosis fugax is a curious phenomenon that occurs in some patients. It lasts for up to several minutes, for example immediately after dilated fundoscopic examination, and is attributed to delayed regeneration of retinal pigment secondary to insufficient oxygen/blood flow (Galetta *et al.*, 1997a; Furlan *et al.*, 1979). Posture related changes in vision have been documented in patients with presumably marginal artery blood flow (Galetta *et al.*, 1997a) (compare with posture related dizziness in Tk.A). Visual loss cannot always be prevented by corticosteroid treatment (Aiello *et al.*, 1993; Galetta *et al.*, 1997b).

Diplopia. Diplopia is much less frequent than loss of vision (two out of 166 patients in the study from the Mayo Clinic and none in the Norwegian study), but exceptionally can be one of the presenting signs of GCA. It may be due to palsy of one of the oculomotor nerves (Mehler and Rabinowich, 1988; Bondeson and Asman, 1997); very rarely to internuclear ophthalmoplegia (INO) (see Chapter 7, *Internuclear Ophthalmoplegia* (Thomson *et al.*, 1989); to a pontine one and a half syndrome (Galetta *et al.*, 1997a); or perhaps also to ischaemic necrosis of extraocular muscle (Barricks *et al.*, 1977).

TIAs, stroke and spinal infarctions. Twelve of 166 patients (7%) in the Mayo Clinic study had TIAs or stroke that were, in time, related to GCA. These events were located in the vertebrobasilar region slightly more often than expected from figures about such events from all causes. Of course, in view of the age category to which patients with GCA belong it is not certain that all these events were caused by vasculitis, but it is also unlikely that all of them had other causes. Three patients developed abrupt cognitive decline during corticosteroid taper, one several months after GCA had been diagnosed, and appeared to have multiple infarcts. They improved in part when high-dose corticosteroid treatment was resumed (Caselli, 1990). One patient in the Mayo Clinic series developed signs of myelopathy first, and cranial symptoms suggestive for GCA subsequently. The diagnosis was then confirmed by temporal artery biopsy. Myelopathy due to spinal cord infarction has been described in several case reports and anterior spinal arteritis has been demonstrated (Galetta *et al.*, 1997b).

Other cranial symptoms. Four patients in the Mayo Clinic series had transient numbness of the tongue. There are case reports on simultaneous, unilateral involvement of the IXth and Xth cranial nerves (Vernet's syndrome) suggested to be due to vasculitis of the ascending pharyngeal artery (Cherin *et al.*, 1992; Gout *et al.*, 1998).

Peripheral neuropathy. Neuropathy in GCA has been reported and should be considered against the incidence of such changes in the general population. The prevalence of carpal tunnel syndrome in women between 25–74 years is 9.2% (de Krom *et al.*, 1992), and the incidence of generally mild polyneuropathy is probably somewhat lower than 3–4% in subjects older than 55 years (The Italian General Practitioner Study Group, 1995). The incidence of cervical radiculopathy is approximately $107/10^6$ (Hoffman *et al.*, 1993). In a retrospective review of 166 biopsy-proven cases of GCA (128 women), two had carpal tunnel syndrome, one had ulnar neuropathy, 10 had mild polyneuropathy, and one had moderately severe polyneuropathy (Caselli *et al.*, 1988b). This may still be in the expected range for the age category of patients with GCA, but there were also nine patients with multiple mononeuropathies, three of which were severe, acute in onset, and related in time to the onset of GCA. Two of these patients had lower limb claudicatio and multiple mononeuropathies in these limbs. In one of them, lower limb vasculitis with ischaemic necrosis of peripheral nerves was observed histologically in limbs be amputated because of gangrene. Inflammation of vasa nervorum was not reported (Caselli *et al.*, 1988b). There are only few case reports on peripheral neuropathy in GCA and they are not very recent (Feigal *et al.*, 1985; Massey and Weed, 1978). In a review on nerve biopsies from disabling neuropathy in the elderly, vasculitic neuropathy was mentioned in two cases of 'cranial arteritis' (Chia *et al.*, 1996). GCA should be in the differential diagnosis when patients above 50 years of age present with mononeuritis multiplex or polyneuropathy of unknown origin. There is a case report on bilateral brachial plexopathy due to GCA (Silva *et al.*, 1998).

Management of patients with neurological or ophthalmological manifestations
Early diagnosis and onset of corticosteroid treatment as a rule prevents neurological and ophthalmological manifestations. In therapy resistant cases, one should consider the possibility of an underlying infection (Fontana *et al.*, 1997; Russo *et al.*, 1995). When neurological and ophthalmological complications have developed, additional symptomatic treatment is required.

POLYARTERITIS NODOSA (PAN)

Definition
Polyarteritis nodosa (PAN) was initially the diagnostic label for all forms of systemic necrotizing vasculitis. This changed when smaller entities were delineated, like Churg-Strauss syndrome (CSS), microscopic polyangiitis (MPA), and Kawasaki disease (previously designated infantile PAN). The 1990 classification criteria of the American College of Rheumatology for PAN (Lightfoot *et al.*, 1990) still include MPA but not CSS. The recent guidelines of the Chapel Hill conference maintain the PAN label only for cases of systemic necrotizing vasculitis of medium-sized and small arteries (no vessels smaller than arteries are involved) and classify CSS and MPA as disorders of predominantly small vessels (Jennette *et al.*, 1994; Jennette and Falk, 1997) (see Table 5.1). Not everyone agrees that there exists a vasculitis of medium-sized and small arteries only, as, according to the opponents, smaller vessels (the arterioles, capillaries and venules) are never entirely spared (Lie *et al.*, 1994; Guillevin *et al.*, 1996).

Epidemiology
PAN has never been a common disease and since the recent changes in definition it has become very rare. In a well-defined area in the UK with a stable population, vasculitis (not including GCA, isolated cutaneous vasculitis, and patients < 16 years) was diagnosed during a six year period in 126 patients. According to the criteria of the Chapel Hill conference, the annual incidence for MPA was $3.6/10^6$. Not a single patient met the Chapel Hill criteria for PAN. The investigators wondered whether PAN had been classified out of existence (Watts *et al.*, 1995 and 1996). In a retrospective review of 66 cases of necrotizing vasculitis by authors from the group of Moutsopoulos (Boki *et al.*, 1997), seven patients had so called 'classic PAN' according to the Chapel Hill criteria, nine had MPA, seven had CSS, 37 had Wegener's granulomatosis (WG), and six could not be classified.

Pathology and pathogenesis

The vascular lesions are patchy and often asymmetrical, with or without fibrinoid necrosis of the intima. They contain a mixed cellular infiltrate of predominantly macrophages and lymphocytes (mainly CD4+) and a variable percentage (0–45%) of polymorph nuclears (Lie, 1995). Vasculitis in PAN is usually attributed to deposition of immune complexes in arterial walls and a subsequent inflammatory reaction. The antigens for these immune complexes are conceived to be derived from infectious agents. Compatible with this hypothesis is that PAN is associated with hepatitis B virus (HBV) in 10–54% of cases (Scott *et al.*, 1982; Guillevin *et al.*, 1995; Boki *et al.*, 1997; see Christian, 1991 and Somer and Finegold, 1995), and that some patients have circulating immune complexes containing HBV surface antigens. PAN may also be associated with hepatitis C virus (HCV), and essential mixed cryoglobulinaemia (see this Chapter, *Essential Cryoglobulinaemia*), parvovirus B19, human immunodeficiency virus (HIV), and streptococcal and other bacterial infections (see Somer and Finegold, 1995). PAN also has been related to immunization against HBV, HCV, and influenza virus. Interestingly, PAN is occasionally associated with hairy cell leukaemia (see Fortin, 1996; Lie, 1996; Wooten and Jasmin, 1996) and other disorders (Table 5.6). Few data concerning a possible genetic predisposition are available. Familial occurrence has been documented (Mason *et al.*, 1994). It will be clear that the PAN that is described in association with infections, immunizations or malignancies is not very likely to have been screened in all cases for compatibility with the Chapel Hill criteria.

Clinical features

The clinical features are quite variable. Onset is usually with malaise, weight loss, fever and often cutaneous manifestations (Boki *et al.*, 1997). The most common disorders of patients with PAN comprise peripheral neuropathy; usually mononeuritis multiplex (50–70% of cases); skin lesions (purpura, ulcera, subcutaneous nodules, livedo reticularis, distal gangrene), arthralgia and myalgia; and vascular nephropathy with hypertension. Progressive glomerulonephritis is not a feature of PAN and pulmonary disorders are not frequent or prominent. Bowel ischaemia may cause abdominal pain, haemorrhage and perforation. Some patients have vasculitis of the appendix or gall bladder, infarctions or haemorrhage in the liver, and cardiac manifestations due to malignant hypertension or vasculitis of coronary

Table 5.6 Pan-associated diseases

Infections		Immunizations against	Malignancies	Other
Viral	*Bacterial*			
HBV*	Streptoc[+]	Influenza[+]	Hairy cell leukaemia[+]	Kawasaki disease[+]
HCV*	Psdmona[+]	HBV[+]	Gastric adenoma[+]	Whipple's disease[+]
Parvov[+]	Yersinia[+]	HCV[+]		
HIV*	Klebsiella[+]			

Abbreviations: HBV, hepatitis B virus; HCV, hepatitis C virus; Parvov, Parvovirus B19; HIV, human immunodeficiency virus; Streptoc, streptococcus; Psdmonas, Pseudomonas. *Frequent or not rare; [+]rare. For references concerning associations of PAN with infections, malignancies and Kawasaki disease, see the appropriate sections in this chapter. For Wipple's disease, see Middlekauf *et al.*, 1987.

arteries. Orchitis, breast and uterine disease, ocular manifestations and CNS disorders are less frequent. The clinical features of HBV-related PAN, according to Guillevin and collaborators, do not differ significantly from other cases of PAN (Guillevin *et al.*, 1995; Lhote and Guillevin, 1995).

There are several limited forms of PAN or necrotising vasculitis, as for instance, of the skin (cutaneous PAN) or the PNS (Dyck *et al.*, 1987; Cohen Tervaert and Kallenberg, 1993). Several authors tend to consider 'non-systemic vasculitic neuropathy', however, as its own entity, differing from idiopathic PAN (Davies *et al.*, 1996).

Diagnosis
The three main diagnostic criteria for PAN are: (1) evidence of a systemic (generalized) disorder; (2) a necrotizing vasculitis of medium-sized and small arteries in a biopsy of an affected organ; and (3) vascular changes of medium-sized and small arteries visualized by arteriography or another comparable method and accepted as due to vasculitis. These would be multiple small aneurysms, stenosis and post-stenotic dilations and obstruction not due to arteriosclerosis, fibromuscular dysplasia or other non-inflammatory changes (Lightfoot *et al.*, 1990) (Fig. 5.2). When the first two criteria are met, imaging of the vascular system is not required. Due to the patchy nature of the vascular lesions, biopsies of affected organs may be uninformative. In these cases, a second biopsy or imaging of the visceral system should be considered. ESR is commonly increased, serum complement levels may be decreased, and antineutrophil cytoplasmic antibody (ANCA) (not specified) was found positive in a minority of patients (< 20% according to Guillevin *et al.*, 1993b; 6.6% according to Guillevin *et al.*, 1996). ANCA was absent in 23/24 HBV-related cases of PAN (Guillevin *et al.*, 1995) (see Chapter 3 for a discussion of antineutrophil cytoplasmic antibodies). The American College of Rheumatology criteria allow classification of patients with established vasculitis for research purposes and do not distinguish PAN from MPA (Lightfoot *et al.*, 1990) (Table 5.7). When PAN is diagnosed, one should always search for an associated disorder (see Table 5.6).

Treatment and outcome
There is no consensus on the preferred treatment of PAN. We prefer to start with intravenous pulse doses of methylprednisolone, 1000 mg (15 mg/kg) repeated twice with intervals of 24 h, followed by oral prednisone 1 mg/kg until remission is obtained or for 5 weeks, and then to taper slowly. In view of its toxicity, cyclophosphamide should be reserved for life or organ threatening emergency situations. According to Guillevin *et al.* (1992), steroids in combination with plasma exchanges offer no advantage in comparison to steroids only. Savage *et al.* (1997) propose treatment with prednisolone, 1 mg/kg, and oral cyclophosphamide, 2 mg/kg until remission is obtained. Cyclophosphamide should then be replaced by a less toxic agent, for instance by azathioprine 2 mg/kg daily. Patients of 60 years and older should be given a reduced dose of cyclophosphamide. Plasma exchange and antiviral agents (vidarabine or interferon alpha) are advocated for HBV-related PAN (Guillevin *et al.*, 1993a and 1994) (see Chapter 4 for a discussion of toxic effects of cyclophosphamide and interferon alpha).

Abu-Shakra *et al.* (1994) studied the records of all patients with PAN (presumably including MPA cases) seen in one vasculitic clinic in a 14 year period (1979–1993). Two of 12 patients died within months after they had been diagnosed. Ten patients

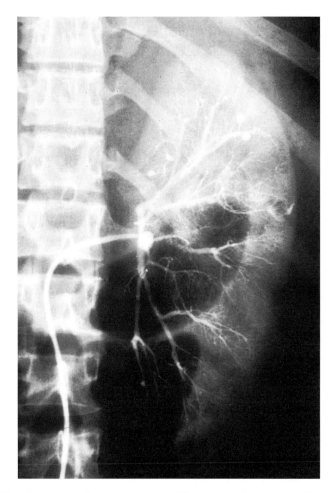

Figure 5.2 Renal angiography of a patient with polyarteritis nodosa showing multiple aneurysmata.

went in remission, of which one obtained prolonged remission (more than one year). These ten patients had 20 relapses in 650 patient-months, which is considerably more than in Churg-Strauss syndrome (CSS) (see this Chapter, section on CSS). These results show that, at present, PAN is not the fatal disease that it previously was reputed to be. Patients should remain under observation for a prolonged period in view of the high relapse rate.

Neurology

Peripheral neuropathy. This may present as mononeuritis or mononeuritis multiplex and can progress towards distal symmetric polyneuropathy, or also it may present from onset as a symmetric polyneuropathy. Nerves in the distal parts of the lower limbs are more often affected than nerves in the distal parts of the upper limbs.

Table 5.7 1990 criteria for the classification of polyarteritis nodosa (traditional format)

Criterion	Definition
Weight loss ≥ 4 kg	Loss of 4 kg or more of body weight since illness began, not due to dieting or other factors
Livedo reticularis	Mottled reticular pattern over the skin or portions of the extremities or torso
Testicular pain or tenderness	Pain or tenderness of the testicles, not due to infection, trauma or other causes
Myalgia, weakness, or leg tenderness	Diffuse myalgias (excluding shoulder and hip girdle), or weakness or tenderness of leg muscles
Mononeuropathy or polyneuropathy	Development of mononeuropathy, multiple neuropathies, or polyneuropathy
Diastolic BP ≥ 90 mm Hg	Development of hypertension with the diastolic BP higher than 90 mm Hg
Elevated BUN or creatinine	Elevation of BUN ≥ 40 mg/dl or creatinine > 1.5 ml/dl, not due to dehydration or obstruction
Hepatitis B virus	Presence of hepatitis B surface antigen or antibody in serum
Arteriographic abnormality	Arteriogram showing aneurysms or occlusions of the visceral arteries, not due to arteriosclerosis, fibromuscular dysplasia, or other non-inflammatory causes
Biopsy of small or medium-sized artery containing PMN	Histologic changes showing the presence of granulocytes or granulocytes and mononuclear leukocytes in the artery wall

For classification purposes, a patient shall be said to have polyarteritis nodosa if at least 3 of these 10 criteria are present. The presence of any 3 or more criteria yields a sensitivity of 82.2% and a specificity of 86.6%. Abbreviations: BP, blood pressure; BUN, blood urea nitrogen; PMN, polymorphonuclear neutrophils
From Lightfoot *et al.* (1990), with permission.

Neuropathy is commonly mixed sensomotor and often painful, but may present, according to Lhote and Guillevin (1995) and Cohen *et al.* (1980), as a sensory neuropathy in some cases. The prognosis of vasculitic (ischaemic) neuropathies is relatively favourable in general. When patients come in remission, motor and sensory symptoms and signs improve considerably in general, though slowly, demonstrating the regenerative power of the PNS (Moore and Fauci, 1981; see Chapter 2, *Mononeuritis Multiplex*).

CNS involvement. Data published on the frequency of CNS disorders vary widely, from more than 50% of cases to less than 1% (see Lhote and Guillevin, 1995, table on page 919). The reason for this striking variation is due at least in part to the inclusion, in reviews, of old data from the time that corticosteroids and cytostatic agents were not – or perhaps not adequately – applied (Frohnert and Shep, 1967; Sack *et al.*, 1975; Leib *et al.*, 1979). One should also take into account that in some series data are included of Churg-Strauss syndrome (Fortin *et al.*, 1995; Lhote and Guillevin, 1995) and that it is only since 1994 that MPA has been kept separated from PAN in series of patients with 'systemic necrotizing vasculitis' or 'PAN'. Below, data from two well known and often referred to publications from the early eighties are highlighted.

The study of Moore and Fauci (1981): This combined retrospective and prospective study of 25 patients with *systemic vasculitis* (which is classic polyarteritis nodosa, CSS, and polyangiitis overlap syndrome) revealed that 10 patients developed abnormalities of the brain, brainstem or cerebellum. In eight of these cases, the abnormalities developed late after onset of the disease (between 8 months and 3 years). With one exception, these 10 patients were all younger than 60 at onset of CNS manifestations. Most were younger than 40 and the youngest was 8. It is thus unlikely that the CNS manifestations can be explained by age-related disorders. Four patients were treated with corticosteroids at the time of the event, but doses were not specified and it was not stated whether the CNS manifestations occurred during relapse of PAN activity. Two kinds of neurological syndromes were distinguished: diffuse disorders and focal syndromes. In six patients, the neurological syndrome was considered diffuse because they had altered mental states (confusion, hallucinations, memory disorder, dementia, stupor, and coma) (see Chapter 2 for mechanisms underlying coma). Four of these patients had seizures and one (a 55-year-old man with dementia) had parietal lobe deficits. In four other cases, the neurological syndrome was predominantly focal, although evidence of dementia was present in one case. Mental alteration proved transient in general, with the exception of dementia.

CT in patients with focal syndromes revealed changes compatible with multiple infarcts in one case, with mild diffuse atrophy in a second case, and with occipital lobe haematoma in a third case. In two cases, angiography did not show any evidence of vasculitis. Three patients died, apparently due to their neurological disorder. Vasculitis was not found at post-mortem investigation; the brain was, however, not examined!

In retrospect, it is conceivable that the focal neurological manifestations resulted from damage, or previous damage, to vessels in the brain by the inflammatory process (vessel occlusions, rupture of aneurysms). Coma could have been due to a vascular lesion in the brainstem; dementia could have been due to small vessel vasculitis or multiple brain infarcts; and confusion and hallucinations could have been due to small vessel vasculitis, corticosteroid psychosis, or perhaps hypertensive encephalopathy.

The study by Cohen *et al.* (1980): The authors performed a retrospective investigation of 53 cases of 'polyarteritis' observed in the Mayo Clinics between 1970 and 1975. Patients were seen within months after onset and were followed for at least two years. At onset of the disease, they varied in age from 17–78 years. CSS and other forms of vasculitides were excluded but not MPA. When first seen, two patients had seizures previously, two had abducens nerve palsy, one had transient Horner's syndrome and 32 had peripheral neuropathy. Patients were treated with corticosteroids (36 patients), corticosteroids and cyclophosphamide (14) or not at all (three). Twenty-two patients (41%) died during the follow-up period: seven due to 'vasculitis' or uraemia within four months after onset, two due to 'vasculitis' after two and two and a half years, and five between seven and 63 months after onset by a 'cerebrovascular accident'. In patients with a cerebral cause of death, vasculitis was inactive at the time of death in three and in two information on vasculitis activity was not available. This study confirms that there is a considerable risk of serious CNS complications long after onset of PAN. Patients that died from uraemia would probably now have been classified as MPA.

The experience of the French Study Group for Polyarteritis Nodosa: Since the early eighties, this group has run a nationwide investigation in France on the effects of different interventions in patients with PAN (including MPA) and CSS. Without providing many details, CNS involvement is stated by this group now to be 'rare' (Lhote and Guillevin, 1995). Two of 41 cases of HBV-related cases of PAN diagnosed during an 11-year period and with a mean duration of follow-up of 69.6 months, had unspecified CNS manifestations. In one of these patients, signs of optic neuropathy persisted after recovery (Guillevin *et al.*, 1995). One other patient died due to 'bleeding' from an intracranial congenital anomaly.

Neuroimaging of CNS lesions: The causes for CNS manifestations in PAN are likely to be heterogeneous. In a recent study of the neuroradiology of five patients, three had encephalopathy and seizures (the diffuse type of neurological abnormality of Moore and Fauci, 1981) and two had hemiparesis and seizures (the focal type). Multiple cortical and subcortical infarcts were found in four patients and a single parietal infarct in one patient with hemiparesis. Vascular changes consistent with cerebral arteritis were demonstrated by arteriography in one of the encephalopathy patients, and cerebral arteritis was considered likely for clinical reasons in a second case. Cardiogenic embolism was the most probable cause of the parietal infarct in one of the two patients with a focal type of lesion (Provenzale and Allen, 1996a).

Prevention and management of neurological manifestations
The experience of the French Study Group for Polyarteritis Nodosa suggests that CNS complications may be prevented largely by vigorous treatment (see this Chapter, *Treatment of PAN*). PAN carries a high risk on relapses (Abu-Shakra *et al.*, 1994), and therefore patients should remain under observation for at least a year in order to be able to resume treatment as soon as relapses occur. Peripheral nerve disorders react favourably to treatment, but a study of the final handicap after recovery has not been performed yet.

KAWASAKI DISEASE

This disease affects mainly children less than five years of age. It was first diagnosed in Japan and subsequently recognized worldwide (see Jacobs, 1996; Dillon and Ansell, 1995). The incidence in Japan ($150/10^5$) is much higher than in the USA ($10.3/10^5$) and other countries (in the UK $2.9/10^5$). Kawasaki disease occurs in outbreaks and with seasonal variations, which are reasons why a relation with infections has been suggested (see Somer and Finegold, 1995 for lack of confirmation). Clinical symptoms at onset are fever for more than five days, redness of palms and soles with indurative oedema, polymorph exanthema, reddening of lips and a strawberry tongue, conjunctival injection and cervical lymphadenopathy. Additional clinical features are anterior uveitis, sterile pyuria, arthritis or arthralgia, and aseptic meningitis (Loh and Janner, 1996). Microscopy of cervical lymph node biopsies reveals necrotizing arteritis with foci of fibrinoid material containing nuclear debris. Kawasaki disease is notorious for its cardiovascular complications and its high incidence of coronary artery aneurysms (in 20–30% of patients). Among the associated changes of other organs are seizures and pleocytosis in the CSF. Some cases present as Kawasaki disease and progress subsequently to a PAN-like disorder (Bowyer *et al.*, 1994). Presentation with PAN and development of coronary artery aneurysmata thereafter occurs also (Engel *et al.*, 1995). Treatment includes prescription of antiplatelet agents, administration of intravenous gamma-globulins and coronary recanalization surgery. Treatment with corticosteroids is, in view of the proposed infectious cause, disputed and considered contraindicated by some authors. Outcome is favourably with a low figure for mortality (< 1%).

MICROSCOPIC POLYANGIITIS (MPA)

Introduction and epidemiology
A microscopic form of *periarteritis*, as MPA was called previously, with 'haemorrhagic extracapillary glomerulonephritis' was first described in 1923 by Wohlwil (Mercado, 1997). It was not until the Chapel Hill conference in 1994 (Jennette *et al.*, 1994) that MPA was classified definitely as a separate entity, distinct from PAN. It has an annual incidence in a small region in the UK of $3.6/10^6$ and affects males slightly more frequently than females.

Differences between MPA and PAN
As it stands now, MPA differs in clinical, histological and biochemical aspects from PAN.

1. MPA has as a main clinical manifestation – a segmental, necrotizing, rapidly progressive glomerulonephritis, which is present in nearly all (90% or more) cases (Jennette and Falk, 1997). It causes progressive renal failure but no or no excessive hypertension.
2. Lung disease with dyspnoea and haemoptysis is not rare in MPA, in contrast to PAN, and is due to alveolar capillaritis and haemorrhage. It is a potentially life-threatening complication.
3. Vasculitis in MPA affects arteriolae, capillaries and venulae and may affect small arteries. The vessel inflammation is PAN-like, but pauci-immune at least in the kidney, where it has been studied extensively.
4. Serum ANCAs are present in most cases and are usually of the perinuclear ANCA (pANCA) type, which means fluorescence at indirect immunofluorescent examination near the nuclei, indicating that the antibodies are directed against myeloperoxidase (MPO) or other antigens (see Chapter 3). An antigen specific enzyme-linked immunosorbent assay (ELISA) is necessary to establish the antigen against which the antibodies are directed. The second main ANCA type, cytoplasmic ANCA (cANCA) (antiproteinase 3 or PR3) is present in a minority. Few patients are ANCA-negative (Gross, 1995; Lhote and Guillevin, 1995; Savage *et al.*, 1997). Patients suffering from PAN usually have no serum ANCAs.

Diagnosis

MPA differs clinically from PAN by early and progressive renal insufficiency. MPA resembles Wegener's granulomatosis (WG) by its predilection for kidneys and lungs, but is different in its histology and in being cANCA negative in the large majority of cases. MPA does not cause a granulomatous inflammation with vasculitis of the upper part of the respiratory tract as WG does.

Therapy

Therapy should aim primarily at the prevention of irreversible serious renal insufficiency. To this aim, the treatment scheme advocated by Savage *et al.* (1997) should be followed. They recommend prednisolone 1 mg/kg and oral cyclophosphamide 2 mg/kg daily until remission is obtained. Cyclophosphamide can then be replaced by a less toxic cytostatic agent, like azathioprine (see this Chapter, *Treatment and outcome of PAN*).

Neurology

No detailed descriptions or accurate figures on neurological aspects are available. The PNS is reported to be affected in approximately 30% of patients and the CNS in a minority. Headache and seizures are probably the most common CNS manifestations. (Serra *et al.*, 1984; Savage *et al.*, 1985; Adu *et al.*, 1987; Lhote and Guillevin, 1995).

CHURG-STRAUSS SYNDROME (CSS)

Definition and epidemiology

Churg-Strauss syndrome (CSS) or *allergic granulomatosis and angiitis* is a systemic vasculitis that was first decribed in 1951. It is now generally accepted as a distinct entity, different from PAN (Churg and Strauss, 1951). It is a disease predominantly, but not exclusively, of small vessels in patients with a history of allergic rhinitis and asthma (Masi *et al.*, 1990; Jennette *et al.*, 1994). Figures on incidence or prevalence are not available. In a large, tertiary referral centre, CSS was diagnosed from 1950–1974 in 30 patients and from 1974–1992 in 47 patients (Chumbley *et al.*, 1977; Sehgal *et al.*, 1995). In a series of 200 patients with necrotizing vasculitis, verified histologically by nerve or muscle biopsies, 11 (5%) had CSS (Said, 1998). Similar to MPA, CSS affects males more frequently than females (ratios of males to females vary in the literature from slightly more than 1 up to 3) (Lanham *et al.*, 1984; Lhote and Guillevin, 1995). A definite relation with age has not been established, though onset is mostly in the fourth or fifth decade and only rarely in the first decade.

Pathology and antibodies

The pathology of CSS encompasses two features. They are necrotizing vasculitis with or without fibrinoid necrosis or, in some biopsies, granulomatous vasculitis of small arteries and extravascular eosinophilic granulomas. Vasculitis is the consistent finding, the extravascular granulomas are present in 50% of the biopsies (Lie, 1995). A significant contribution of eosinophils is in favour of the diagnosis. Eosinophilia (more than 10% of circulating leukocytes) is another consistent laboratory finding. Serum ANCA, mostly pANCA, is positive in approximately 70% of patients (see Lhote and Guillevin, 1995).

Clinical features
Three phases are distinguished in the natural history of the disease.

1. The first stage is chronic and can exist for years. Patients have allergic rhinitis and asthma.
2. In the second stage patients have eosinophilic infiltrates in the lungs and other organs and blood eosinophilia.
3. Vasculitis develops in the third and last phase.

The organs that become affected are essentially similar to those in the other generalized necrotizing vascilitides, though there are a few characteristic features in the spectrum of severity and frequency of the affected organs (see Table 5.2). Pulmonary infiltrates are frequent, more so than in PAN, and involvement of the kidneys is less frequent and less severe than in MPA or WG. Coronary arteritis and myocarditis are notorious in this disease and are the main causes of death. The skin is frequently involved, as in MPA and PAN, but it has a special – though not disease specific – feature, which is the presence of subcutaneous nodules containing granulomas in 30% of patients.

Diagnosis
The American College of Rheumatology 1990 criteria (Table 5.8) are meant to distinguish CSS from other related diseases in patients in whom the presence of vas-

Table 5.8 American College of Rheumatology 1990 criteria for the classification of Churg-Strauss syndrome (traditional format)

Criterion	Definition
Asthma	History of wheezing or diffuse high-pitched rales on expiration
Eosinophilia	Eosinophilia > 10% on white blood cell differential count
Mononeuropathy or polyneuropathy	Development of mononeuropathy, multiple mononeuropathies, or polyneuropathy (*i.e.* glove/stocking distribution) attributable to a systemic vasculitis
Pulmonary infiltrates, non-fixed	Migratory or transitory pulmonary infiltrates on radiographs (not including fixed infiltrates), attributable to a systemic vasculitis
Paranasal sinus abnormality	History of acute or chronic paranasal sinus pain or tenderness or radiographic opacification of the paranasal sinuses
Extravascular eosinophils	Biopsy including artery, arteriole, or venule, showing accumulations of eosinophils in extravascular areas

For classification purposes, a patient shall be said to have Churg-Strauss syndrome (CSS) if at least 4 of these 6 criteria are positive. The presence of any 4 or more of the 6 criteria yields a sensitivity of 85% and a specificity of 99.7%.
From Masi *et al.* (1990), with permission.

culitis has been established already. Using these criteria, it is not possible to classify a patient in the second stage of CSS as such because by definition vasculitis has not developed yet. In practice, however, the disease may already be in the differential diagnosis when asthma with or without rhinitis or allergic rhinitis, eosinophilia, and multiple organ involvement (*e.g.*, the lungs with infiltrates, the heart with evidence of myocarditis, or the skin with eosinophilic infiltrations) are present (Rabusin *et al.*, 1998).

Therapy and outcome

Therapy is essentially similar as in MPA (see this Chapter, *Therapy* for MPA). The response to treatment, even of corticosteroids alone, may be dramatic, but in some cases cyclophosphamide is indispensable from the start to prevent serious organ (cardiac) damage. The five-year survival is approximately 75% according to Guillevin *et al.* (1987). Myocardial infarction and cardiac failure are the main causes of death. Other causes are renal failure, cerebral haemorrhage, gastrointestinal perforation and others (Lanham *et al.*, 1984). Abu-Shakra *et al.* (1994) studied the records in a vasculitis clinic of patients diagnosed with CSS during a 14-year period. All 12 patients went in remission and during the follow-up period there were only seven relapses in 1.154 patient-months. These results were markedly better than in 12 patients with PAN (see this Chapter, *Treatment and outcome of PAN*).

Neurology

Peripheral neuropathy. In different series, mononeuritis multiplex or polyneuropathy occur in approximately 50–70% of patients and are due to vasculitis–induced ischaemia. (Chumbley *et al.*, 1977; Lanham *et al.*, 1984; Lhote and Guillevin, 1995; Sehgal *et al.*, 1995). Although some inflammatory cells are present in some biopsies around small endoneurial vessels or in the subperineurial space, the vasculitis affects the epineurial vessels predominantly. The nerve fibres show axonal degeneration, differing in degree in different nerve fascicles, compatible with an ischaemic type of peripheral neuropathy. Recovery takes time (months), but is often better than expected even in patients who have been quadriplegic (Oh *et al.*, 1986; Heeg *et al.*, 1988; Marazzi *et al.*, 1992). Interestingly, there is a case report on a woman with asthma, eosinophilia, lung infiltrate, mild renal insufficiency, and paraesthesia at the feet who complained about proximal limb pain and stiffness and in whom a muscle biopsy revealed interstitial eosinophilic infiltrates and necrotizing vasculitis (De Vlam *et al.*, 1995).

CNS involvement. In the original, mainly autopsy-based study by Churg and Strauss (1951) of patients not treated with corticosteroids, evidence of a cerebral disorder was present in eight of 13 cases. Lanham *et al.* (1984) retrospectively analysed data from the English literature on 138 cases, mainly from the period when corticosteroids were not prescribed yet. Twenty of 82 cases had CNS manifestations. The cerebral features were described as ranging from disorientation to convulsions and coma. Cerebral haemorrhage and infarctions were a major cause of death. Only five of the 47 cases reviewed by Sehgal *et al.* (1995) had intracranial disorders. Three had cerebral infarctions: two women of 68 and 62 years had infarcts in the cerebral media territory and thalamus respectively, and a male patient had an infarct in the right parietal lobe, probably due to an embolus from a left ventricular thrombus. There was one case of bilateral trigeminal neuropathy and a further patient presumably with ischaemic, optic neuropathy. Case reports on patients with CSS in combination with intracerebral haemorrhage or multiple cerebral infarcts have been published (Liou *et al.*, 1994; Liou *et al.*, 1997). Of interest is the description of a 13-year-old girl with chronic sinusitis, asthma, eosinophilia, purpura, and livedo reticularis due to necrotizing vasculitis who developed bilateral chorea. MRI revealed lesions in the globus pallidus, compatible with bilateral, small infarcts or inflammatory processes. She reacted favourably to treatment with 0.6 mg/m²/d cyclophosphamide, prednisone 1 mg /kg/d, and triazipide 300 mg (Kok *et al.*, 1993).

Neuro-ophthalmology and otology. There are a number of rare neuro-ophthalmological manifestations of CSS, including eosinophilic granulomas in the eyelids, conjunctivitis, scleritis, episcleritis and uveitis, retinal ischaemia, IVth cranial nerve palsy, ischaemic optic neuropathy, and orbital pseudotumour (Weinstein *et al.*, 1983; Acheson *et al.*, 1993; Kattah *et al.*, 1994; Liou *et al.*, 1994; Bosch-Gil *et al.*, 1995). There is also a report on a patient with sudden right inner ear deafness, presumably due to VIIIth nerve palsy that developed during a relapse of CSS (Heeg *et al.*, 1988).

Mechanisms responsible for CNS manifestations. The mechanisms underlying the intracranial manifestations are heterogeneous. Some of the infarcts are probably due to vasculitis, and some others may be the result of emboli originating from the frequently affected heart. The cerebral haemorrhages may be explainable by weakening and aneurysmal dilatations due to vasculitis or in some cases to hypertension. Trigeminal neuropathy is in the ICTDs mostly due to inflammation of the ganglion Gasseri. The exact cause in CSS has not been established.

Prevention and management of neurological manifestations
Early diagnosis and treatment may prevent peripheral neuropathy from becoming severe. Comparison of the figures of Lanham *et al.* (1984) and Sehgal *et al.* (1995) indicates that similar to PAN, early and vigorous treatment may prevent development of CNS manifestations, thus reducing morbidity and mortality figures to a considerable degree.

WEGENER'S GRANULOMATOSIS (WG)

Definition and pathology
According to the Chapel Hill conference, WG is 'a granulomatous inflammation involving the respiratory tract and necrotizing vasculitis affecting small to medium-sized vessels (capillaries, venules, arterioles and arteries). Necrotizing glomerulonephritis is common' (Jennette *et al.*, 1994). The vasculitis is occasionally granulomatous and there is fibrinoid necrosis in up to 10%. The inflammatory infiltrate consists of polymorph nuclear cells including eosinophils, mononuclear cells with plasma cells, monocytes and CD4+ T-cells (Lie, 1995).

Epidemiology and aetiopathogenesis
According to the Norwich Health Authority in the UK, in a small area with a stable, mainly rural population of little more than 400,000, the annual incidence of WG in adults was calculated to be 8/10⁶ (Carruthers *et al.*, 1996). The prevalence of WG in the US was estimated to be at least 30/10⁶ (Cotch *et al.*, 1996). Males are affected somewhat more frequently than females, and children are spared. Though an auto-

immune origin of the disease is assumed, the aetiology and pathogenesis are unknown. Recently, progress concerning the underlying mechanisms of the disease has focused on a likely relation between relapses and nasal carriage of *Staphylococcus aureus* (Stegeman *et al.*, 1994; Stegeman *et al.*, 1996). Hereditary predisposition has not been shown so far. Antineutrophil cytoplasmic antibodies (cANCA, see Chapter 3) are present in more than 90% of patients with active disease and as of now are presumed to play an undefined role in the pathogenesis of WG (Duna *et al.*, 1995).

Clinical features

Onset of the disease is often insidious and its initial features are: nasal inflammation (Fig. 5.3), oral ulcers or gingivitis, sinusitis, otitis media with earpain and loss of hearing, fatigue, loss of appetite and weight, and unexplained fever (Cohen Tervaert *et al.*, 1987; Duna *et al.*, 1995; Savage *et al.*, 1997). Involvement of the larynx and trachea may lead to hoarseness, constrictures, stridor and obstruction of the air-

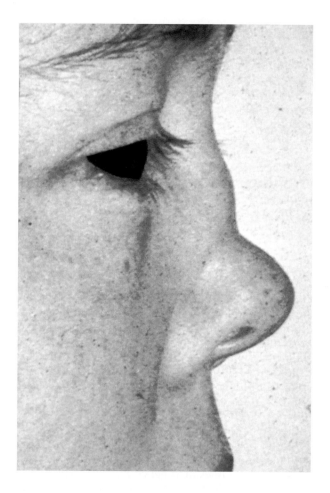

Figure 5.3 Wegener's granulomatosis. Saddle nose of a patient.

way. One of these constrictures, subglottis stenosis, is a notorious complication in youngsters predominantly. Lung abnormalities develop before long in nearly all patients and give rise to symptoms as cough, pleuritic pain and haemoptysis. X-rays and CT scans reveal infiltrates, nodules and, less frequently, pleuritic effusions and enlarged hilar or mediastinal lymph nodes. Secondary infections in the upper or lower respiratory tract may complicate the picture. When symptoms and signs are restricted to the upper and lower airways, WG is called limited.

Glomerulonephritis develops in the large majority of patients. When diagnosed and treated early, severe renal insufficiency, maintenance dialysis and kidney transplantation may be prevented. Every other segment of the urogenital tract in addition to the kidneys may become affected as well.

WG is a truly generalized disease and may involve almost all organs. Arthralgia, myalgia and synovitis occur commonly at some stage. Changes of the skin are common and comprise purpura, nodules, papules and ulcera. Involvement of the heart occurs only in a minority and presents mostly as pericarditis. Myocardial infarction, coronary vasculitis and valvulitis have been reported. The main gastrointestinal manifestations are pain, diarrhoea and bleeding. Fatal perforations have been described in case reports.

Diagnosis

Diagnosis is based on the involvement of the upper or lower airways, with vasculitis of preferentially small vessels and granulomatous tissue infiltration in biopsy material. There is often glomerulonephritis present, as well as evidence of a generalized disorder. Diagnosing WG may be difficult as histological confirmation is not always easily obtainable. Serum cANCA is positive in more than 90% of patients, particularly at active stages of the disease. The predictive value of testing for cANCA for diagnostic purposes and for relapses is disputed however (Duna *et al.*, 1995; Rao *et al.*, 1995; Franssen *et al.*, 1996; Rao *et al.*, 1996). The American College of Rheumatology criteria for WG (Table 5.9) are meant for the classification of patients with established vasculitis who are participating in clinical research projects (Leavitt *et al.*, 1990).

Treatment and outcome

Before the introduction of corticosteroids and cytotoxic agents, the average survival time of patients with WG was 5 months! Corticosteroids improved their fate, but cyclophosphamide changed their outlook drastically (Fauci *et al.*, 1983). Since then, as a rule treatment consists of cyclophosphamide 2–3 mg/kg/d orally in combination with prednisone 1 mg/kg/d orally (Fauci *et al.*, 1979; Fauci *et al.*, 1983). However, there is still considerable mortality (13%; Hoffman *et al.*, 1992) and morbidity (*e.g.*, side effects of medication) associated with the disease, as may be exemplified by the following. The figures on the incidence of bladder malignancy in patients treated with cyclophosphamide tend to become worse over time: incidence was stated to be 3% in 1988 (Stillwell *et al.*, 1988) but is now 16% (Talar-Williams *et al.*, 1996). According to Travis *et al.* (1995), patients treated with cyclophosphamide have, in general, a 4.5-fold increased risk of bladder malignancy. The risk is 2.4 times normal in patients who have had a cumulative dose of 20 g and 14.5 times normal after a cumulative dose of 50 g (Travis *et al.*, 1995) (see Chapter 4 for bladder toxicity and other side effects of cyclophosphamide). The main principles of treatment of WG are now as follows (Kallenberg, 1996):

Table 5.9 1990 criteria for the classification of Wegener's granulomatosis (traditional format)

Criterion	*Definition*
Nasal or oral inflammation	Development of painful or painless oral ulcers or purulent or bloody discharge
Abnormal chest radiograph	Chest radiograph showing the presence of nodules, fixed infiltrates or cavities
Urinary sediment	Microhaematuria (> red blood cells per high power field) or red cell casts in urine sediment
Granulomatous inflammation on biopsy	Histological changes showing granulomatous inflammation within the wall of an artery or in the perivascular or extravascular area (artery or arteriole)

For purposes of classification, a patient shall be said to have Wegener's granulomatosis if at least 2 of these 4 criteria are present. The presence of any 2 or more criteria yields a sensitivity of 88.25% and a specificity of 92%.
From Leavitt *et al.* (1990), with permission.

1. If the patient is not in a life or organ threatening situation, induce remission with prednisone (1 mg/kg/day) and methotrexate (20–25 mg weekly). This is successful in 70–75% of patients.
2. If there is a life or organ threatening situation, induce remission with prednisone (1 mg/kg/day) and cyclophosphamide (2–3 mg/kg/day). This also will succeed in approximately 75% of patients.
3. If not successful, try intravenous infuses of methylprednisolone (1 gram at three consecutive days), or in the case of organ threatening kidney disease, add plasma exchange (Pusey *et al.*, 1991).
4. When remission is induced, taper cyclophosphamide by steps of 25 mg once every three months, or replace cyclophosphamide within two months with azathioprine (see Chapter 4, *Azathioprine*). Prednisone can be tapered by 5 mg every two weeks.
5. Reduce the chance of relapses by treating patients for 24 months with trimethoprim/sulfamethoxazole (Stegeman *et al.*, 1994; Stegeman *et al.*, 1995).

Neurology

Neurological disorders are rarely presenting manifestations (see Dickey and Andrews, 1990; Nishino *et al.*, 1993a). They develop mostly during the course of the disease, in up to 25–35% of the patients (Fauci *et al.*, 1983; Hoffman *et al.*, 1992; Nishino *et al.*, 1993a). The incidence of peripheral nerve disorders is as high or higher than of CNS disease (varying from 10–28% of patients in different series; see Nishino *et al.*, 1993a). Previously, when patients were not treated yet with corticosteroids and cyclophosphamide, the percentage of patients with neurological disorders may have been higher (Drachman, 1963).

Peripheral neuropathy. Mononeuritis multiplex is by far the most frequent peripheral nerve syndrome in WG. Exactly as in PAN (Lhote and Guillevin, 1995), the peroneal nerve is most frequently affected, followed by the ulnar and tibial nerves and then the median nerve in that order (Lhote and Guillevin, 1995; Nishino *et al.*, 1993a; Said *et al.*, 1988). In other patients, peripheral nerve syndrome presents as distal symmetrical or asymmetrical polyneuropathy. Vasculitis in sural nerve biopsies has been demonstrated (Hawke *et al.*, 1991). As a rule, peripheral neuropathy responds favourably to treatment with corticosteroids, cyclophosphamide, or both (Nishino *et al.*, 1993a).

Headache. Headache is probably the least dramatic of the CNS symptoms in WG, though it is not the least frequent. In the series by Nishino *et al.* (1993a), 16% of patients had severe headache at one time, which was mostly attributed to sinusitis, orbital processes, or less often to intracranial changes.

Cranial neuropathy. Cranial neuropathy is reported in 10% or less of patients and in principle may involve all cranial nerves. The IInd and VIIth cranial nerve are affected the most often and the IXth–XIIth the least often (Nishino *et al.*, 1993a; Fauci *et al.*, 1983; Hadden *et al.*, 1998). Horner's syndrome is observed occasionally (Nishino *et al.*, 1993a).

Brain disorders. These are infrequent. They occurred in 13/324 patients reviewed by Nishino *et al.* (1993a) and in none of the 85 patients followed for years by Fauci *et al.* (1983). Five of 324 patients reviewed by Nishino *et al.* (1993a) were confused, had evidence of 'encephalopathy', and had seizures. All together, generalized seizures occurred in 10/324 patients, infarcts in 12 patients, and one patient had a subdural haematoma. Diabetes insipidus, with or without hyperprolactinaemia, was observed in several cases (Nishino *et al.*, 1993a; Fauci *et al.*, 1983; Czarnecki and Spickler, 1995; Rosete *et al.*, 1991; Hurst *et al.*, 1983; Haynes and Fauci, 1978).

The spinal cord. Spastic paraparesis, indicative of spinal cord involvement, was observed in 3/324 patients (Nishino *et al.*, 1993a). Another patient, a woman of 67, presented with lower limb weakness that appeared to be due to non-specific dural inflammation and cord compression. After seven months, she was diagnosed with WG (Nishino *et al.* 1993b).

Neuro-ophthalmology
WG differs from PAN and CSS by a more frequent involvement of the oculi and orbita (in up to 50%) (Duna *et al.*, 1995). Patients may present with, or develop, conjunctivitis, (epi)scleritis, keratitis, and uveitis, due to small vessel disease. Moreover, the granulomatous process in the nasal and paranasal spaces tends to break through the bordering walls into the orbita and to cause a series of abnormalities, including proptosis, optic neuropathy, oculomotor nerve lesions, muscular infiltration and retinal ischaemia (Fig. 5.4). Primary extraconal disease, without parasinusitis or nasal inflammation, may occur as well and may cause considerable diagnostic difficulties when it is the presenting manifestation of WG. Provenzale *et al.* (1996) reviewed orbital changes in 14 patients with 16 affected orbits. Paranasal sinusitis and evidence of nasal inflammation with bony erosion (saddlenose; see Fig. 5.2) were seen near 11 orbits. Nasal inflammation and paranasal sinusitis were not present near five other orbits, all with orbital masses. The orbital masses were frequently hypo-intense on T2-weighted MRI images, and appeared to consist at histological examination of inflamed vessels, granulomatous tissue, and necrotic material.

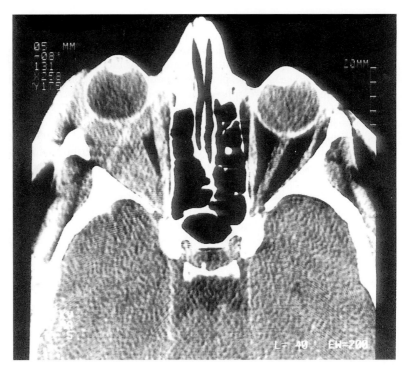

Figure 5.4 CT scan of a 29-year-old patient showing slight proptosis of the right eye and infiltration of the right orbita around the optical nerve and within the lateral rectus muscle. cANCA test was positive (see Chapter 3). A biopsy of the infiltrating mass revealed granulomatous inflammation without necrosis or vasculitis. Wegener's granulomatosus was diagnosed. The patient was treated with corticosteroids and a cytostatic agent and recovered well. (Courtesy of Dr. JW Cohen Tervaert.)

Neuro-otology

Hearing loss is frequent in WG and was initially described in approximately 40% of patients (Luqmani *et al.*, 1991). More recently, it has been described by Nishino *et al.* (1993a) in 16.7%. In most cases, it is due to middle ear abnormalities, *e.g.* mucosal oedema and serous exudate in the middle ear (Clements *et al.*, 1989; Luqmani *et al.*, 1991). In exceptional cases, granulomatous tissue in the middle ear cavity breaks through into the inner ear. The possibility of auditory nerve lesioning by vasculitis–induced ischaemia has been suggested but not demonstrated.

Mechanisms of CNS disease in WG

Drachman (1963) put forward three mechanisms to explain CNS disease in WG. The first one is invasion of the intracranial cavity by granulomatous tissue through continuity. Indeed, this has been documented, for instance by Satoh *et al.* (1988), but as shown by Provenzale and Allen (1996b), it is rare. These latter authors reviewed neuroradiological findings in a series of 100 patients with WG. Invasion through continuity was not seen in any case: not in 12 patients with nasal, paranasal, or orbital abnormalities nor in seven patients with intracranial neuroradiological changes.

Drachman's second mechanism is remote granulomatous infiltration of the meninges and the brain, independent of any changes in the nasal or auditory-vestibular spaces. CT scanning or MRI show diffuse, focal, plaque-like or nodular thickening of the meninges, as well as abnormal MR signals from nearby parts of the brain (Tishler *et al.*, 1993; Weinberger *et al.*, 1993; Nishino *et al.*, 1993b; Provenzale and Allen, 1996b; Hadden *et al.*, 1998; Katrib *et al.*, 1998). Biopsies from the meninges in such cases reveal granulomata, multinucleated giant cells and lymphocytic infiltration (Nishino *et al.*, 1993b; Tishler *et al.*, 1993; Weinberger *et al.*, 1993; Katrib *et al.*, 1998). Granulomata in brain tissue are commonly in a superficial position and in direct continuity to granulomatous inflammatory changes in the meninges covering the abnormal part of the brain (Oimomi *et al.*, 1980; Tishler *et al.*, 1993; Weinberger *et al.*, 1993; Provenzale and Allen, 1996b). Isolated granulomatous masses that are located deeply in the brain tissue are very rare (Scott Miller and Miller, 1993). In a case of diabetes insipidus, a sellar mass that extended into the suprasellar region with thickening of the infundibulum was seen, but apparently it was not associated with any changes in the sagittal sinus (Czarnecki and Spickler, 1995).

Drachman's third mechanism, which concerns intracerebral vasculitis unrelated to extravascular granulomatous tissue, has been observed only rarely (Fred *et al.*, 1964; Yamashita *et al.* 1986). Cerebral small vessel vasculitis is not easily established, however, because it escapes visualization by angiography and because brain biopsies are performed only rarely. The only possibility for a definite diagnosis that is left is post-mortem investigation. It is also very possible that the chance of cerebral small vessels becoming afflicted by WG is small. Nishino *et al.* (1993b) described a patient with subacute progressive memory loss, confusion, right sided hemiplegia, and at MRI, increased T2 signals in the pulvinar and thalamus at the left side, in the pons, and throughout the cerebral white matter. Such cases are not easily explainable by anything else than small vessel vasculitis. Intracerebral haemorrhage, as reported by Drachman, also may be due to vasculitis of brain vessels.

In the series of Nishino *et al.* (1993a), 12/324 patients had cerebral infarcts of undefined origin. In principle, the infarcts might have been due to intracranial vasculitis, compression by granulomatous masses, emboli from the heart afflicted with myocardial infarction due to coronary vasculitis or valvulitis, hypertension, or other causes unrelated to WG. Post-mortem studies of the brain in eight cases revealed no changes in two brains and one or multiple infarcts in six, apparently without any evidence of vasculitis or vascular lesions due to granulomata. Basilar artery occlusion in a 26-year-old man with WG was considered to be attributable to the presence of lupus anticoagulant (Savitz *et al.*, 1994).

Management of neurological manifestations

Peripheral neuropathy, neuro-ophthalmological, neuro-otologic, and meningeal processes are treated with corticosteroids and immunosuppressants and may require local symptomatic treatment, for example decompression. Secondary prevention is required for patients with cerebral infarcts and is dependent on the established or presumed cause (see Chapter 2, *Secondary prevention in patients with ischaemic stroke*). Specific studies on the effects of the different treatments for CNS manifestations in patients with WG have not been performed.

HENOCH-SCHÖNLEIN PURPURA (HSP)

HSP is a leukocytoclastic vasculitis of small vessels. Its special feature is the deposition of IgA-dominant immune complexes in the vessel walls (Jennette and Falk, 1997). A leukocytoclastic vasculitis is characterized by fibrinoid necrosis of the inner side of the vessel wall, infiltration of the vessel wall by polymorphonuclear neutrophils, and the presence of nuclear debris of these cells in the tissue (Fig. 5.5). HSP is a disease predominantly of children but may affect adults also. Following an upper airway infection, purpura appear on the skin of the lower legs and buttocks. Less often they appear elsewhere (Fig. 5.6) (see Callen and Kallenberg, 1995; Gibson and Su, 1995; Jennette and Falk, 1997). Other frequently affected systems or organs are the joints, the gastrointestinal tract and the kidneys. Patients may complain about pain in affected joints, colicky abdominal pain, vomiting and bloody diarrhoea. Examination may reveal periarticular oedema, melaena, proteinuria, microscopic or macroscopic haematuria, hypertension, nephrotic syndrome and nephritis. Less commonly, there is evidence of involvement of the lungs, the heart, the liver, the pancreas, the adrenals, and the PNS and CNS. HSP is diagnosed on the basis of the clinical presentation and is confirmed by demonstration of small vessel vasculitis and IgA deposition in cutaneous vessel walls in a skin biopsy.

Neurology

Belman *et al.* (1985) described three children, two of whom had partial seizures and two of whom also had transient pyramidal weakness. In addition, one of the children had a left brachial plexopathy that took four months to recover. The authors reviewed the neurological changes in 79 cases, all published in the literature. Headache occurred in 25–43% of the patients in different series and slight mental signs, as for instance increased irritability, were also frequent. Seizures were reported in 42/79 patients and focal deficits (chorea, cortical blindness, aphasia,

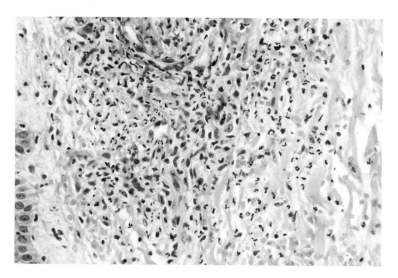

Figure 5.5 Leukocytoclastic vasculitis in skin showing nuclear debris (arrows).

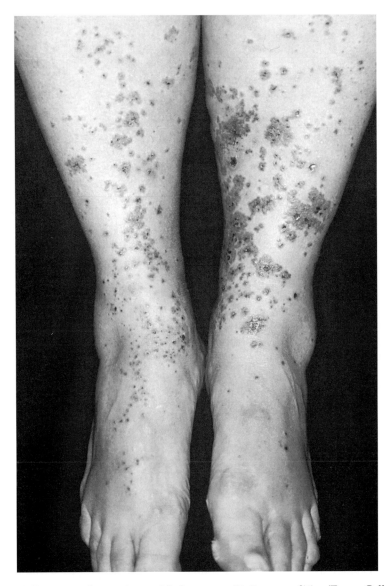

Figure 5.6 Purpura of a patient with hypersensitivity vasculitis. (From Callen and Kallenberg, 1995, with permission.)

hemiplegia, paraplegia, monoparesis, cerebellar dysfunction) in 26. Subarachnoid haemorrhage, intracerebral haemorrhage (Ng *et al.*, 1996), and subdural haematoma were also observed. Disorders of the PNS occurred less often in this group and comprised mononeuropathies and poly(radiculo)neuropathies. From this overview, one might obtain the impression that CNS manifestations in HSP are in fact frequent and occur much more often than generally realized. In this respect, Ostergard and Storm's study (1991) is of interest. These authors performed a prospective investigation for neurological and electroencephalographic abnormalities in 26 consecutive children with HSP. A hampering headache accompanied by behavioural changes was registered in eight patients. Neurological investigation disclosed no abnormalities. The electroencephalogram (EEG) showed several changes, including sharp wave paroxysms in 12 patients; these were mostly transient but persisted for at least one year in four children.

Therapy and outcome

HSP is a self-limited disease, and spontaneous recovery and resolution of pathological changes are the rule. Therefore, specific therapy is usually not required. However, progressive renal failure due to glomerulonephritis occurs occasionally and demands aggressive immunosuppressive therapy to prevent maintenance dialysis and renal transplantation (Goldstein *et al.*, 1992). Neurological disorders of the CNS and PNS justify, in our view, prescription of corticosteroids to prevent progress of nervous system vasculitis, antiepileptic medication to prevent recurrence of seizures, and other symptomatic treatment as required.

ESSENTIAL MIXED CRYOGLOBULINAEMIA (EC)

Cryoglobulins differ from other immunoglobulins by precipitation at cooling. Brouet *et al.* (1974) classified cryoglobulins into three groups on the basis of immunochemical heterogeneity (Box 5.1).

   The mixed cryoglobulins are designated as secondary when an associated disorder that can be held responsible for their presence is demonstrable. Examples of such associated diseases are lymphoproliferative disorders, infections and autoimmune diseases. When no such diseases are found, mixed cryoglobulin inaemio is designated as essential or primary. Now, it appears that there is a strong association between essential mixed cryoglobulins and hepatitis C virus (HCV) infections (Agnello and Romain, 1996; Agnello, 1995). HCV is transmitted sexually, by intravenous drug-use and transfusions.

Clinical features

EC occurs particularly in individuals of middle age and gives rise to vasculitis of the skin (purpura, ulcera, livedo reticularis in 60–80% of patients) (Fig. 5.6), liver dis-

Box 5.1 Classification of cryoglobulins

> Type I: Isolated monoclonal cryoglobulins without specificity, predominantly of IgM class (but also IgG and occasionally IgA and Bence Jones). These occur in 25%.
>
> Type II: Mixed cryoglobulins containing IgG and anti-IgG antibody of monoclonal type, predominantly IgM, but also IgG class and occasionally IgA. These also occur in 25%.
>
> Type III: Mixed cryoglobulins containing IgG and anti-IgG antibody of polyclonal type, predominantly IgM. These occur in 50%.
>
> The anti-IgG antibody in type II and type III is a rheumatoid factor.

ease, Raynaud's phenomenon, arthralgia, glomerulonephritis (proteinuria, microscopic haematuria and renal insufficiency), peripheral neuropathy and CNS manifestations (Gorevic *et al.*, 1980; Monti *et al.*, 1995).

Neurology
Peripheral neuropathy has been detected in approximately 20–70% of patients with EC, mostly as a chronic, chronic-relapsing, sensory, sensomotor polyneuropathy and less often as mononeuritis multiplex (Ferri *et al.*, 1991; Gemignani *et al.*, 1992; Cacoub *et al.*, 1994; Monti *et al.*, 1995). Biopsies of sural nerves in these patients reveal inflammatory infiltrates, consisting predominantly of mononuclear cells, around epineurial vessels, but rarely in vessel walls as in genuine vasculitis. Degeneration of nerve fibres is mainly axonal, though demyelination has been reported by some authors as well (Lippa *et al.*, 1986; Valli *et al.*, 1989; Khella *et al.*, 1995). Cell infiltrates in the endoneurial compartment are sparse. The mechanism responsible for neuropathy in EC is not clear at present, but in many cases it is not likely to be vasculitis-induced ischaemia (Monti *et al.*, 1995). Peripheral neuropathy is not present only in cases of EC in conjunction with HCV infection, but also in the HCV-negative cases (Cacoub *et al.*, 1994). CNS manifestations have been documented (seizures, intracranial haemorrhage), but are rare (Gorevic *et al.*, 1980).

Therapy and outcome
The usual therapy for peripheral neuropathy in patients with EC is a combination of corticosteroids and plasmapheresis or a cytostatic agent. Therapy has not always proven to be successful. In our experience, corticosteroids and cyclophosphamide (150 mg daily) are more effective than steroids alone or in combination with plasma exchange (Kater and Schuurman, 1981). Agnello (1995) suggests that, in patients with EC, one should test for HCV and, if present, treat with an antiviral agent. Interferon-alpha has been reported to be successful in HBV and HCV infections (Guillevin *et al.*, 1994; Di Bisceglie *et al.*, 1989) and has been used to treat peripheral neuropathy in patients with EC and HCV infection (Khella *et al.*, 1995; La Civita *et al.*, 1996; Ghini *et al.*, 1996; Zuber and Gause, 1997). At present, the experience during interferon-alpha administration is that cryoglobulin levels decrease. The effect on peripheral neuropathy is less obvious. In some cases, there is indeed improvement, which is apparently due to the effect on the cryoglobulins. Also, in few patients, the neurotoxicity of interferon-alpha induces or increases peripheral neuropathy (Zuber and Gause, 1997; Gastineau *et al.*, 1996). Other neurotoxic effects attributed to interferon-alpha are somnolence, headache, anterior ischaemic optic neuropathy and trigeminal neuropathy (Purvin, 1995; Read *et al.*, 1995).

IDIOPATHIC CUTANEOUS LEUKOCYTOCLASTIC VASCULITIS (IDIOPATHIC CLV)

Cutaneous leukocytoclastic vasculitis (CLV) (also known as hypersensitivity vasculitis, allergic vasculitis, small vessel vasculitis, and necrotizing vasculitis) of the skin, as defined in the section on Henoch-Schönlein disease, has many causes (Table 5.10), but in some cases is not related to another underlying disease or substance at all. So-called idiopathic, essential or primary CLV may be confined to the skin entirely or form part of a more generalized disorder that as a rule does not include

Table 5.10 Causes of cutaneous leukocytoclastic vasculitis (CLV)

Idiopathic
Henoch-Schönlein disease
No-IgA CLV vasculitis
Others
Inflammatory connective tissue disease
Infections
Streptococcus
Meningococcaemia
Hepatitis C
Others
Malignancies
Leukaemia
Lymphoma, Hodgkin's disease, multiple myeloma
Others
Drugs
Penicillin, sulfonamides
Quinidine, propylthiouracil, allopurinol

Data from Gibson and Su (1995), Callen and Kallenberg (1995), Calabrese and Duna (1996), and Roujeau and Stern (1994).

any neurological changes. Callen and Kallenberg (1995) refer to a study done by Liss and Wolverton (1991, not published) of 58 patients of whom 43% had renal disease, 32% had arthralgias, and 14% had liver, lung or gastrointestinal disorders. One patient had a CNS manifestation that was not specified.

MISCELLANEOUS

BEHÇET'S DISEASE

Introduction and epidemiology
This widespread, multisystem disorder was discovered in 1937 by the Turkish dermatologist Behçet, and was originally believed to occur predominantly in the Middle East and in Japan. Despite a considerable influx of individuals from Turkey, other Mediterranean countries and South East Asia, the prevalence in Northern Europe still seems to be very low, as suggested by the results of a Scottish study. The prevalence in Olmsted County in the USA is, however, not that much lower than in Japan (1:15000 versus 1:10000) (O'Duffy, 1994; Jankowski *et al.*, 1992). At present, reports on large series of patients are all form the Middle East, India and Japan. Behçet's disease affects predominantly young adults, and males more than females.

Aetiopathogenesis
The aetiology of Behçet's disease is not known. In Japan and the Middle East, a link has been established with HLA-B51, but this has not been confirmed in the USA (see O'Duffy, 1994). Data on twin studies are not available yet, and there are few studies

on the association of Behçet's disease with other disorders. A recent hypothesis expresses the view that the disease is based on immunological cross-reactivity to epitopes of certain heat-shock proteins of micro-organisms and humans (Hasan *et al.*, 1996).

Vessel pathology

Though vascular abnormalities initially did not receive too much attention, now vasculitis is recognized as one of the most important aspects of the pathology (O'Duffy and Hammill, 1996; Matsumoto *et al.*, 1991; Zelenski *et al.*, 1989; Lakhanpal *et al.*, 1985). Inflamed walls of arteriae show intense infiltration of adventitia and media especially, by polymorph nuclear cells, lymphocytes, plasma cells, eosinophils and a small number of giant cells (Matsumoto *et al.*, 1991). Fibrinoid necrosis is unusual. One of the peculiarities of this disease is that large veins are affected more frequently than large arteriae (Koc *et al.*, 1992), which gives Behçet's disease a special place in relation to the other vascular disorders discussed in this chapter. At the microscopical level, the affected veins show fibrous thickening of the intima, no more than slight infiltration by small round cells of the walls, and luminal obstruction by organized thrombi in the obstructed veins. Subcutaneous and submucosal biopsies from affected skin or mucosa reveal prominent swelling of the endothelial cells of capillaries, venules, and arterioles, as well as mixed cellular infiltrates consisting of lymphocytes and plasma cells in the walls of these vessels (O'Duffy *et al.*, 1971).

Clinical features

Members of the International Study Group for Behçet's disease (1990) agreed upon a set of five diagnostic criteria that are meant primarily for obtaining homogeneous populations in multicentre studies (Table 5.11). A peculiar criterion is the pathergy test: pricking the skin with a sterile needle results first in a papule and then in a

Table 5.11 International Study Group criteria for diagnosis of Behçet's disease

1. Recurrent oral ulceration	Minor aphthous, major aphthous or herpetiform ulceration observed by physician or patient, which has recurred at least 3 times in one 12-month period.
2. Recurrent genital ulceration	Aphthous ulceration or scarring observed by physician or patient.
Eye lesions	Anterior uveitis, posterior uveitis or cells in vitreous body on slit lamp examination; retinal vasculitis observed by ophthalmologist.
Skin lesions	Erythema nodosum, pseudofolliculitis, or papulopustular lesions, observed by physician or patient, acneiform nodules observed by physician in post-adolescent patients not on corticosteroid treatment
Positive pathergy test	Read by physician at 24–48 hours

Findings applicable only in absence of other clinical explanation. For diagnosis, number 1 is required and two of number 2.
From International Study Group for Behçet's Disease (1990), with permission.

small pustule. It is a useful criterion in Mediterranean countries where it is positive in 60–70% of patients. In Northern Europe and the USA it is mostly negative.

Many other organs not mentioned in the Table may become affected in the course of the disease. These include: the joints (predominantly the large joints); the intestines (ulcerative colitis); the heart (pericarditis, coronary arteriopathy and silent myocardial infarcts); the lungs (pulmonary vasculitis with infarcts, aneurysmal bleeding and haemoptysis); the kidneys (glomerulonephritis or interstitial nephritis); the epididymis; and the nervous system (Inaba, 1989). Large vessels are involved in up to 30% of patients (Koc *et al.*, 1992; Pande *et al.*, 1995). The most frequent type of large vessel disease is subcutaneous thrombophlebitis, but occlusion of large veins in the upper and lower limbs, of the superior and inferior vena cava, and of other veins is not rare; it is followed in frequency by occlusion and aneurysms of the arteries. Occlusion of the arteries may result in pulseless disease and subclavian stealing (Cooper *et al.*, 1994).

Diagnosis

At present, diagnosis is based solely on clinical criteria. The transient nature of the relevant symptoms and the fact that these symptoms are not necessarily present simultaneously increase the difficulty of an early correct diagnosis (Devlin *et al.*, 1995 and 1996). In addition, patients may present with neurological symptoms, for instance, before they have had any oral ulcers. A new laboratory test based on the proposed cross-reactivity to epitopes of the heat-shock proteins of micro-organisms and humans may prove to be a step forward (Hasan *et al.*, 1996). The ESR is raised in most cases and antiepithelial antibodies are present in a minority, particularly patients with retinal vasculitis. APL antibodies are absent, but there are reports on a pre-thrombotic state with increased levels of thrombin-antithrombin III complex, prothrombin fragments 1+2, and plasmin–α_2–antiplasmin complex (see Haznedaroglu *et al.*, 1997; Oner *et al.*, 1998).

Therapy

The prevailing notion is that Behçet's disease should be treated with corticosteroids or corticosteroids in combination with a cytostatic agent (Zelenski *et al.*, 1989; Bacon and Carruthers, 1995). Interferon-alpha is advocated for patients with mucocutaneous ulcers, skin ulcers, gastrointestinal ulcers and eye disease (see Grimbacher *et al.*, 1997). The reviving interest in thalidomide has led to studies on its effect in Behçet's disease (Hamuryudan *et al.*, 1998; Ehrlich, 1998).

Neurology

Disorders of the nervous system are present in < 5–10% of patients and nearly always concern the CNS (Pande *et al.*, 1995; Serdaroglu *et al.*, 1989). Mononeuritis multiplex and symmetrical distal polyneuropathies are exceptional, indicating that epineurial arteries and veins are affected little or not at all, in general (Chalk *et al.*, 1993; O'Duffy *et al.*, 1971). Myositis' has been reported (Worthmann *et al.*, 1996).

Symptoms and signs may originate from the whole CNS and comprise headache, seizures, organic brain syndrome, dementia, meningism, papilloedema, bulbar syndromes, cranial neuropathies, hemiplegia, aphasia, paraplegia and disturbance of micturition. Neurological symptoms develop insidiously (in 50%) or subacutely and may be transient or persistent (Inaba, 1989; Serdaroglu, 1998). Two points should be stressed. First, there is a predilection for brainstem syndromes, which is confirmed by radiological investigations. Secondly, cerebral venous sinus thrombosis (CVT) is surprisingly frequent. Wechsler *et al.* (1992) diagnosed CVT in 25/70 patients by means of angiography.

Forty-six out of 323 patients with Behçet's disease seen in one year in a Turkish university centre (63 new cases, 260 controls, 204 males) were referred for neurological evaluation (Serdaroglu *et al.*, 1989). Twenty-six patients had headache without any other neurological disorder and 17 had various neurological abnormalities, including aseptic meningitis (2), spinal cord syndrome (1), brainstem syndromes (3), and dementia with right-sided hemiplegia (1). Re-examination after approximately seven years showed that one patient in the headache group developed transient brainstem symptoms and one other patient had CVT (Akman-Demir *et al.*, 1996). Both recovered. Three patients from the group of 17 with neurological abnormalities died and five showed considerable progression of neurological abnormalities, with cognitive impairment in two. CVT occurred in two cases and transient partial (focal) neurological abnormalities in three.

CNS imaging
CT is considerably less informative than MRI and reveals in approximately 50% of neuro-Behçet's cases no abnormalities. The main abnormalities at MRI (leaving CVT out of consideration) are high-intensity lesions at T2 weighted images. The lesions vary in shape and are usually small, but occasionally they may be surprisingly large in comparison to the relative paucity of symptoms. They differ from similar lesions in MS because they are located in the white and grey matter and do not prefer periventricular regions. They tend to be most frequent in the brainstem (Banna and El-Ramahi, 1991; Al Kawi *et al.*, 1991; Kaneko *et al.*, 1995). Gadolinium enhancement may reveal lesions not seen on T1 and T2 weighted images. Enhancement disappears as symptoms resolve, indicating that the enhancement may have been due to oedema and a defective blood-brain barrier (Erden *et al.*, 1993). Neuro-Behçet's may also present as a space-occupying mass lesion both clinically and at imaging, but this is exceptional (Neudorfer *et al.*, 1993).

CNS pathology
There is a careful and very readable description in the literature of the CNS pathology of two cases of neuro-Behçet's from the pre-corticosteroid period (McMenemey and Lawrence, 1957). The main abnormality was the presence of a great number of small softenings and minute spongy areas in relation to blood vessels, showing perivascular cuffings and infiltrations by lymphocytes and microglial cells. Vessels in the 'active stage' of thrombosis were not seen. The softenings and spongy areas showed moderate microglia reaction, accumulation in histiocytes of breakdown products, loss of nerve cells and feeble astroglia proliferation. Though the nervous tissue at the site of the softenings was damaged, the lesions did not have the character of demyelinating plaques as in MS. Thickening of basal meninges with some round cell infiltration was described also.

The CSF
The CSF may be under increased pressure due to aseptic meningitis in some cases and to obstruction of venous blood flow in others. Cell content and protein content are raised in the case of aseptic meningitis and may be raised when brain tissue is

involved. There is evidence of intrathecal synthesis of immunoglobulins (Jongen *et al.*, 1992).

Management and outcome of patients with neurological manifestations

CVT should be searched for and excluded in all cases of neuro-Behçet's disease. If present, it should be treated for three weeks with low-weight molecular heparin, followed by warfarin (see Chapter 2, *Cerebral Venous Thrombosis*). Intervention studies in non-CVT cases of neuro-Behçet's have not been performed. A similar therapeutic regimen as for other patients with severe symptoms of Behçet's disease should be followed (see above, *Therapy*). The longitudinal study by Akman-Demir *et al.* (1996) strongly suggests that the prognosis of neuro-Behçet's is still serious from both the viewpoints of morbidity and mortality.

DEGOS' DISEASE OR MALIGNANT ATROPHIC PAPULOSIS

The lesion underlying the clinical manifestations of Degos' disease is a widespread vasculopathy of predominantly small vessels, characterized by intimal proliferation, narrowing of lumina, and thrombi and vessel obstruction. These result in haemorrhages and infarcts. Inflammatory changes are mild and infrequent. The mechanism responsible for this process is supposed to be immunological, though at present there is not much in support of this theory. The disease affects both sexes without obvious age preference and presents, in most cases, with a typical abnormality of the skin or infrequently with gastrointestinal symptoms or signs.

Malignant atrophic papulosis is recognized clinically by the development at the trunk and limbs of painless 'umbilicated papules' with porcelain-white centres at the top. The vasculopathy is not very selective and affects many organs or tissues. Five of 15 patients reported by Subbiah *et al.* (1996) had fatal strokes due to haemorrhagic or ischaemic infarcts and one had a disabling polyneuropathy. There is no therapeutic strategy to improve the disease or to slow down a progressive course. Antiplatelet agents, anticoagulation, fibrinolytic therapy, corticosteroids, cytostatic agents, and plasma exchange have all been tried and shown not to be consistently effective (Subbiah *et al.*, 1996; McFarland and Village, 1997). The course of the disease is not invariably down-hill, but outcome is often poor when the CNS (infarcts) or the gastrointestinal system (melaena, perforation) are involved.

COGAN'S SYNDROME

Cogan's syndrome is a rare disorder with acute or subacute (days to weeks) onset that affects predominantly young adults of either sex. Bilateral interstitial keratitis and vestibuloauditory dysfunction are its main clinical manifestations. Interstitial keratitis is often associated with other symptoms of eye disease, *e.g.* conjunctivitis, uveitis, scleritis and chorioiditis, while auditory dysfunction involves sensorineural hearing loss, vertigo and tinnitus. Systemic symptoms such as fever, fatigue and weight loss are present in some patients, and there is vasculitis of large and medium-sized vessels in probably a small minority of patients (<15%) (Raza *et al.*, 1998; Vollertsen *et al.*, 1986; Haynes *et al.*, 1980). The aorta, branches of the aorta and large limb vessels may be affected. Histological investigation of diseased vessels shows infiltration, mainly in the media and intima, by polymorphonuclear cells, mononuclear cells and occasionally giant cells. Cogan's disease is considered to be an auto-immune disorder and is treated with steroids and cytotoxic agents. Outcome is favourable as far as eye symptoms are concerned but hearing loss is usually irreversible. Vasculitis shows some overlap with Takayasu's disease both in distribution and histopathology. The disease.

VASCULITIS CONFINED TO THE NERVOUS SYSTEM

THE CENTRAL NERVOUS SYSTEM

Introduction
Vasculitis solely of the CNS without any generalized features was until the 1980s considered a rarity. At that time, methods to visualize the intracranial structures improved and CNS angiitis was diagnosed more often. Knowledge on the clinical features of the condition accumulated, and it gradually became clear that 'isolated CNS angiitis' might be more heterogeneous than initially conceived. Calabrese and Duna (1995) and Calabrese *et al.* (1993 and 1997) proposed that two entities should be distinguished: one, a chronic, progressive and often fatal form called primary angiitis of the CNS (PACNS) and another, a benign, monophasic form called benign angiopathy of the CNS (BACNS). There are no incidence figures yet, but there are data in the literature on 168 cases of 'isolated CNS vasculitis' (Calabrese *et al.*, 1997). PACNS occurs slightly more often in males than females and has little age preference. BACNS is more likely to occur in females. While there is some evidence indicating that PACNS is associated with viral infections and immunosuppressive states, the actual situation is that aetiology and pathogenesis are fully unknown (Calabrese *et al.*, 1997).

Primary angiitis of the central nervous system (PACNS)
The criteria for isolated angiitis of the CNS are: (1) a CNS syndrome that cannot be attributed to another cause; (2) lack of evidence of a generalized disorder, though anorexia, weight loss, vomiting and even fever are present in some cases (Vollmer *et al.*, 1993); (3) classic angiographic or histopathological features of CNS vasculitis (Box 5.2). The progressive clinical course is decisive for the differential diagnosis with BACNS.

The onset of PACNS is mostly insidious though it may be subacute or acute. An immunosuppressed state offers a favourable condition for the development of PACNS. There are 11 cases in the literature of PACNS in patients with Hodgkin's disease, two cases in patients with lymphocytic lymphoma, and one case in a trans-

---

Box 5.2 Criteria for the diagnosis primary angiitis of the CNS

1. A CNS syndrome that cannot be attributed to another cause.
2. No evidence for a generalized disorder.
3. Mild pleocytosis, raised protein content and normal glucose content of the CSF (present in approximately 80–90%).
4. Arteriographic features pointing to or compatible with brain vasculitis.
5. Histological confirmation of vasculitis in a brain biopsy.
6. Fluctuating or progressive course.

plant recipient (Wooten and Jasmin, 1996). Herpes zoster had been present or was present in five of the 13 cases with lymphoproliferative disorders.

Symptoms and signs are either non-focal, focal or both. Non-focal (diffuse) manifestations are headache of variable onset and degree, cognitive deterioration, confusion, and decreased consciousness. Focal manifestations are less common than non-focal and comprise seizures, TIAs, infrequently stroke, cranial neuropathies, bulbar symptoms, spasticity, and signs of mass lesions and intracerebral or subarachnoid haemorrhage. Some patients (15%) develop evidence of a spinal cord lesion (see Goldberg, 1997).

Diagnosis. Laboratory investigations do not offer a clue to the diagnosis. The ESR and acute phase reactants are entirely normal in a large minority of the patients, and ANAs, ANCAs, endothelial antibodies and RF are commonly not present (Calabrese and Mallek, 1988; Calabrese *et al.*, 1997). In patients with histologically proven PACNS (see below), the CSF is nearly always abnormal (in 80–90% of patients). There is usually a mild pleocytosis (mean number 70 white cells/mm^3) with a raised protein content and normal glucose as in aseptic meningitis.

CT scanning offers little help for diagnosis as it is normal in 50% of patients and the abnormalities have low specificity. In histologically proven cases, MRI appears very sensitive but not specific (Figs. 5.7 and 5.8). Angiography is normal in 40% of histologically proven cases, and when vascular abnormalities are present, they do not allow vasculitis to be distinguished from vasculopathy always (Duna and Calabrese, 1995) (Fig. 5.9). Even classical angiographic evidence of vasculitis (alternating segmental stenosis and ectasia in a diffuse fashion or in one area) is not fully reliable as it may occur in several non-vasculitic conditions, *e.g.* vasospasm by other causes and atherosclerosis (Duna and Calabrese, 1995). The typical micro-aneurysms of visceral vessels in PAN (Fig. 5.2) are seen seldom in cerebral vessels of patients with PACNS (Griffin *et al.*, 1973; Dunna and Calabrese, 1995).

Microscopy of affected parts of the brain shows a segmental vasculitis of medium- or small-sized arteries with granulomatous features in 80% of patients and PAN-like characteristics in the remaining 20%. Both types of changes often are present simultaneously in nearby vessels. In 50% of patients, venules are also involved (Lie, 1992; Calabrese *et al.*, 1997). Vasculitis occurs predominantly in the leptomeninx and cortex but may be confined largely to the white matter (Finelli *et al.*, 1997) (Figs. 5.10 to 5.13). It is widespread or local and may present as a mass lesion in one area. Due to the uneven distribution of the pathological changes, biopsies from definite cases of vasculitis are often not informative.

In some brain biopsies, taken from patients with possible PACNS, granulomatous angiitis and amyloid vasculopathy are both present, raising the question how to interpret this combination. Fountain and Eberhard (1996) compared clinical and laboratory findings in 13 cases with histopathological features of both PACNS and cerebral amyloid angiopathy (CAA), and those of PACNS only. They concluded that in patients with clinical and laboratory findings consistent with PACNS, the presence of CAA should not alter the intended treatment strategy (see under *Therapy and outcome*).

Benign angiopathy of the central nervous system (BACNS)

Decisive for the distinction from PACNS is the clinical course, which is often subacute or acute in onset and monophasic (Calabrese *et al.*, 1997). The neurological

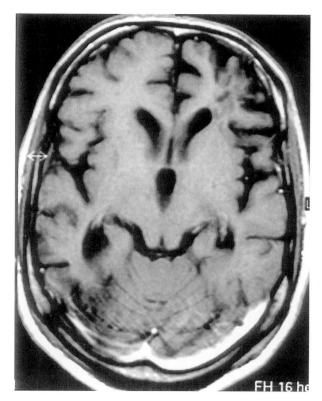

Figure 5.7 Cerebral vasculitis. Atrophy in the left frontal lobe secondary to an old (several weeks or more) ischaemic lesion in a 33-year-old male. Note marked hyperintensity of transverse sinus due to enhancement after intravenous contrast. Axial MRI, T1-Wi image. Same case as in Figures 5.8 to 5.13. (Courtesy of Dr. Lino Ramos.)

manifestations differ from those of PACNS in that non-focal clinical changes such as cognitive deterioration, confusion and decreased consciousness are in the background or absent. Patients complain about headache and develop signs compatible with focal lesions. In contrast to PACNS, the CSF is usually normal. Changes at angiography are compatible with segmental narrowing, or vasoconstriction. There is no doubt that such changes can occur in patients with cerebral vasculitis (Beresford *et al.*, 1979; Berger *et al.*, 1995), but they can also be induced by sympathicomimetic drugs, phaeochromocytoma, or may be seen in patients with migraine (Seradaru *et al.*, 1984; Tabbaa and Snyder, 1987; Lake *et al.*, 1990; Kapoor *et al.*, 1990; Solomon *et al.*, 1990; Kaufman *et al.*, 1998).

Diagnosis. At present, brain/spinal cord vasculitis is diagnosed mostly by the exclusion of other causes, notably infections, and by the demonstration of characteristic angiographic abnormalities. An immunosuppressed condition should be considered and ruled out. The chance of vasculitis in patients with normal CSF and MRI is remote (Calabrese, 1995).

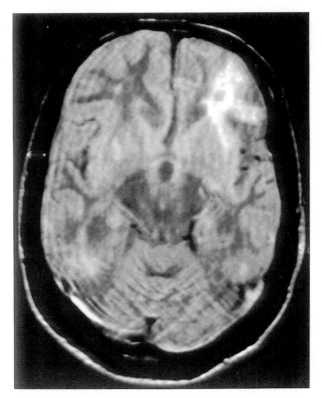

Figure 5.8 Cerebral vasculitis. High signal due to gliosis in an old (several weeks) ischaemic lesion in the left frontal lobe of a 33-year-old male. Lacunar infarct in right insular region. Axial MRI, T2- Wi. (Courtesy of Dr. Lino Ramos.)

As already discussed in the section on PACNS, a normal arteriogram does not exclude the possibility of vasculitis, as small vessels are not sufficiently visualized and as the characteristic angiographic abnormalities may not have developed by the time of investigation. MRI angiography has the advantage of being non-invasive but is less sensitive than conventional arteriography. Serial angiography is advocated by some to increase diagnostic sensitivity and to monitor the development and improvement of the vascular changes (Ozawa *et al.*, 1995).

The diagnostic yield of brain biopsies is often (in 20–50% of patients) disappointing (Javedan and Tamargo, 1997; Duna and Calabrese, 1995). The best results can be expected, according to most authors, with stereotactic biopsies from focal lesions demonstrated by MRI with contrast enhancement. When there is no focal target, an open biopsy is preferable and can best be taken from the anterior temporal pole or the mid-frontal lobe of the non-dominant hemisphere. Separate specimens should be removed from the grey and white matter and the dura and pia. Biopsy investigation offers a chance of a definite diagnosis and the ability to exclude conditions that mimic vasculitis, *e.g.* sarcoidosis and lymphoproliferative disorders. Biopsy investigation to confirm BACNS usually is not performed as long as the course of the disease is compatible with the diagnosis.

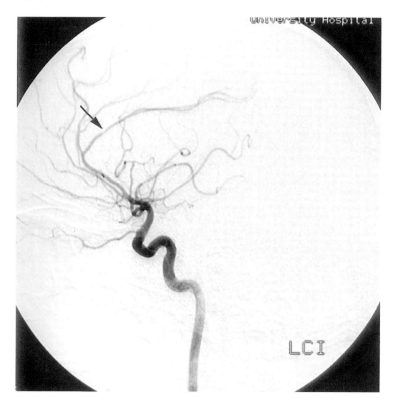

Figure 5.9 Cerebral vasculitis. Occasional, slight, segmental arterial narrowing (arrow), but no other obvious features of vasculitis. Carotis angiography of a 33-year-old male. (Courtesy of Dr. Lino Ramos.)

Therapy and outcome
PACNS is no longer considered as invariably fatal. Clinical experience suggests that it should be treated with high doses of corticosteroids or cyclophosphamide in combination with high-dose corticosteroids (see Chapter 4, *Side Effects of Cyclophosphamide*). Other authors prefer intravenous pulse doses (750–1000 mg) of methylprednisolone for 1–5 days. The duration of treatment of patients in remission is unknown but should be many months at least (Calabrese *et al.*, 1997). It is advised to treat BACNS less aggressively than PACNS (Crane *et al.*, 1991; Calabrese *et al.*, 1997), for instance, 3–6 weeks with high-dose corticosteroids and a calcium blocker. Drugs tending to induce vasoconstriction should be avoided.

VASCULITIS CONFINED TO PERIPHERAL NERVES (VPN)

Introduction and clinical features
The only two large studies of VPN were done by Dyck *et al.* in 1987, who named the disease as a separate entity, and by Davies *et al.* in 1996. The name of this presumed entity is not entirely correct, as only the symptoms are restricted to the PNS, not

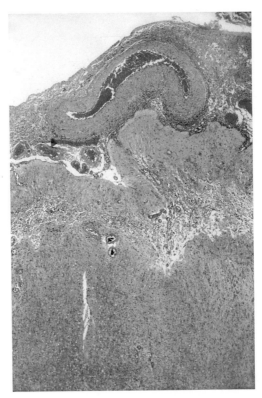

Figure 5.10 Cerebral vasculitis. Paraffin section of brain and meningeal biopsy of a 33-year-old male at low magnification showing thick-walled meningeal vessel and necrosis of superficial layer of underlying brain cortex. H&E. (Courtesy of Dr. Gerard H Jansen.)

vasculitis. Vasculitis in 'nonsystemic vasculitis neuropathy' (Dyck *et al.*, 1987) has been demonstrated also in skeletal muscle, but this remains subclinical by definition (Said *et al.*, 1988). The disease has no obvious sex preference and affects subjects of middle age or older. The clinical picture has the characteristics of mononeuritis multiplex or asymmetrical neuropathy. Less often and mostly at a more severe state of the disease, it has characteristics of predominantly distal, symmetrical senso-motor polyneuropathy. The ESR is, according to Davies *et al.* (1996), raised in 50–70% of the patients but can be entirely normal. ANA and RF are mostly negative.

Diagnosis
The decisive diagnostic investigation is, in nearly all cases, sural nerve biopsy and the observation, at microscopy, of a necrotic type of vasculitis, which often has fibrinoid necrosis of the intima and media of epineurial vessels (Fig. 5.14). VPN affects mainly arterioles, capillaries, and venulae, mostly in the epineurium or perineurium and sometimes in the endoneurium. Depositions of immunoglobulins, complement factors and fibrinogen as a rule are demonstrable in the vessel walls, even in those not or not yet inflamed.

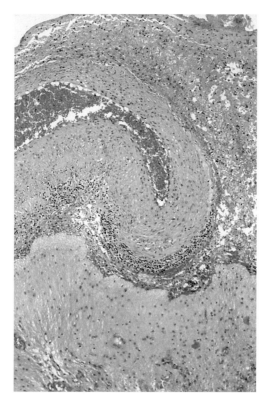

Figure 5.11 Cerebral vasculitis. Paraffin section of brain and meningeal biopsy of 33-year-old male at intermediate magnification showing thick-walled vessel lumen filled with blood cells. Note outward rim of small cells and underlying necrotic brain tissue.

Course and outcome

The course of the disease is monophasic, but a considerable minority of patients have a relapse. At nadir, the disability in the group assessed by Davies *et al.* (1996) varied from 2–5 on a five-point disability scale, and disability was, in 20% of the patients, at a maximum of 5. Although nerve fibres in sural nerve biopsies often show a severe degree of axonal degeneration, clinical recovery is much better than expected in such a condition. In the group of Davies *et al.* all 25 patients were alive at follow-up (mean follow-up time 176 weeks; range 12–435). This contrasts favourably to the survival rates of vasculitic neuropathy of all causes (Dyck *et al.*, 1987; Hawke *et al.*, 1991). Twenty of 23 patients seen at follow-up for disability grading were ambulant and self-caring. As well, as a group, the 23 patients had improved on the disability scale from an average of 3.25 to 1.9. Davies *et al.* suggest that the distinction of VPN from the systemic forms of vasculitis is justifiable in view of the relatively benign nature of the disease.

Treatment

Early diagnosis and treatment is required to prevent as much axonal degeneration and disability as possible. Treatment with high-dose prednisone (1–1.5 mg/

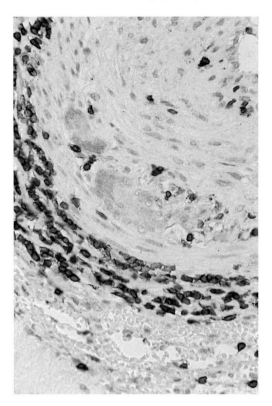

Figure 5.12 Cerebral vasculitis. Paraffin section of brain and meningeal biopsy of 33-year-old male at high magnification, showing part of thick wall of meningeal vessel. Immunohistochemistry reveals that outward rim of small vessels consists predominantly of CD3 positive T-lymphocytes. Note multinucleated giant cells in vessel wall, compatible with granulomatous vasculitis. (Courtesy of Dr. Gerard H Jansen.)

kg/day) is usually sufficient. Combination with another cytotoxic agent (methotrexate, see Chapter 4 for doses; cyclophosphamide at 2 mg/kg/day; see also Chapter 4) is justified when weakness is severe and the response to corticosteroid medication insufficient. The patients of Davies *et al.* (1996) were all treated with corticosteroids, and in 12 of 25 patients on oral medication, a 'cytotoxic agent' was added.

SECONDARY VASCULITIDES

Many of the primary vasculitides probably result from an immunological reaction to an external influence, most probably an infection, in an individual with a distinct hereditary predisposition. The difference from the secondary vasculitides, for which definite underlying causes are demonstrable, is therefore less marked than one would suppose in the first instance. The forms of secondary vasculitis, which

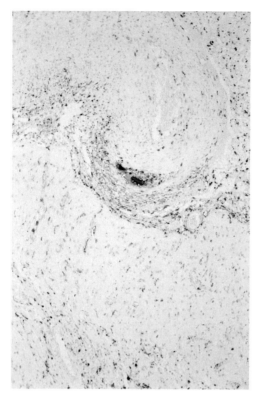

Figure 5.13 Cerebral vasculitis. Paraffin section of brain and meningeal biopsy of 33-year-old male at intermediate magnification showing that giant cells are CD 68 positive. (Courtesy of Dr. Gerard H Jansen.)

are at present distinguished, are summarized in Table 5.12. In the following, we indicate which of these disorders may be complicated by prominent neurological features and we provide references to relevant literature reviews. The vasculitides of the 'connective tissue diseases' are discussed in other chapters of this book.

VASCULITIDES SECONDARY TO INFECTIONS

For an extensive discussion of the complex and heterogeneous relations between infections and vasculitides, the reader is referred to Somer and Finegold (1995) and Lie (1996). The review by Gelber *et al.* (1997) concerns only neurological aspects and may be the most relevant for readers of this book. The following distinctions should be kept in mind:

1. The vessel walls may become infected from the outside, from an external adjacent site. The vasculitis of meningeal arteries and other vessels, complicating bacterial or fungal meningitis, may serve as an example (Roos, 1997; Gelber *et al.*, 1997).

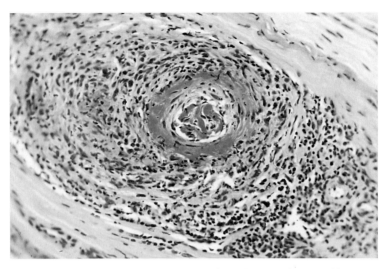

Figure 5.14 Necrotic arteritis. Cryostat section of sural nerve showing fibrinoid necrosis of inner part of the wall of a small artery with inflammatory infiltrate in the remaining part of the wall and around the vessel. There is also necrotic material with fibrinoid aspect in the vessel lumen. H & E.

2. The vessel walls may become infected by agents circulating in the blood stream, *e.g.* septic emboli in infectious endocarditis, tuberculosis, syphilitic vasculitis (Solenski and Haley, 1997).
3. Viral replication in and damage to endothelial cells is at the basis of some of the small vessel vasculitides (Grefte *et al.*, 1993).
4. Vasculitis may be the result of an immunological reaction to an infection. The best known example in this category is vasculitis due to an immune complex mediated process. Antigens derived from virus or bacteria have been demonstrated in such complexes. The immune complexes are deposited at the vessel walls and elicit an inflammatory reaction.

Some of the infection-related vasculitides are confined to the nervous system or cause prominent neurological manifestations. To this category, two already long-known disorders belong, syphilitic vasculitis and vasculitis in mycobacterium tuberculosis. As well, in this category are two more recently discovered disorders, vasculopathy of varicella zoster encephalitis and the vasculitis of Lyme neuro-borreliose.

Table 5.12 Secondary vasculitides

Secondary to connective tissue diseases
Secondary to infections
Secondary to malignancies
Secondary to drugs
Hypocomplementaemic urticarial vasculitis
Post-organ transplant vasculitis

Vasculopathy in varicella zoster encephalitis (VZV)

VZV is a disease of predominantly immunocompromised individuals (Amlie-Lefond *et al.*, 1995). It develops simultaneously with skin abnormalities or with a delay of months or weeks thereafter. Occasionally, a history of a zoster rash is not obtainable. The clinical manifestations comprise fever, seizures, partial (focal) deficit and mental changes. Imaging of the CNS reveals ischaemic or haemorrhagic infarctions and small lesions, predominantly demyelinative. Pathological studies have shown two types of vessel abnormalities:

1. large vessel vasculitis with mononuclear cells, fibrinoid necrosis and other changes, resulting in infarctions;
2. small, predominantly demyelinated lesions, in some cases with necrotic features, resulting from small-vessel vasculopathy characterized by endothelial swelling, scant cellular infiltration and viral inclusions in glia cells (Amlie-Lefond *et al.*, 1995).

VZV is treated with the antiviral agent acyclovir.

Vasculopathy in Lyme neuro-borreliose

Garcia-Monco and Benach (1995) published an extensive review of neuro-borreliose, and Oksi *et al.* (1996) a thorough analysis including pathology of three patients with CNS disorders. Halperin *et al.* (1996) have defined four neurological syndromes, causally related to Lyme borreliosis:

1. lymphocytic meningitis, often associated with cranial neuritis or painful radiculoneuritis in an early stage after infection;
2. encephalomyelitis due to unifocal or multifocal CNS disease;
3. peripheral neuropathy, usually not accompanied by meningitis;
4. an encephalopathic syndrome.

CNS manifestations occur only in a small minority of the patients.

Peripheral neuropathy may present in very different fashions, *e.g.* mono- or multiradiculitis, plexitis, mononeuritis multiplex, Bell's palsy, and infrequently other cranial neuropathies. As well, carpal tunnel syndrome, distal patchy paraesthesia, and distal symmetrical mainly sensory polyneuropathy may be present. The pathology is, however, always similar and therefore it is suggested that all these peripheral nerve diseases are expressions of one and the same underlying mechanism (Halperin *et al.*, 1990; Garcia-Monco and Benach, 1995). Microscopy of sural nerve biopsies have revealed axonal damage of the peripheral nerve fibres and perivascular infiltrates in endoneurium, perineurium and epineurium. There is no necrosis of vessel walls, and though thrombosis and recanalization are present, these are not frequent (Vallat *et al.*, 1987; Meier *et al.*, 1989).

Manifestations of brain and spinal cord involvement take longer to become manifest then lymphocytic meningitis and may occur or recur between months and several years after infection. Patients present with seizures, hemiplegia, paraplegia, ataxia, cranial neuropathy, disorders of micturition, other evidence of partial deficit, mood disorders and cognitive impairment. The CSF usually reveals a variable degree of pleocytosis of mononuclear cells, increased protein content, evidence for increased intrathecal synthesis of immunoglobulins and oligoclonal bands. It has been demonstrated that *Borrelia burgdorferi*, the spirochaete responsible for this disease, is able to penetrate at a very early stage into the CNS and to adhere to glial cells. MRI shows one or several, sometimes enhancing, focal lesions that may resolve with adequate antibiotic therapy and that may recur within months after a seemingly successful therapy. Extensive demyelination, in particular in periventricular areas, has also been observed. Microscopy of these brain lesions shows that endothelial cells of small intraparenchymal vessels are swollen and that the vessel walls and the perivascular space are infiltrated by lymphocytic cells (Oksi *et al.*, 1996). Similar changes may also be present in the meninges.

Diagnosis can be extremely difficult. Specific antibodies against Lyme borreliose may be present in the CSF or plasma, but the lack of such antibodies does not mean that Lyme borreliose can be ruled out. Cultures for *Borrelia burgdorferi* in CSF are only rarely positive. Polymerase chain reaction (PCR) for *Borrelia burgdorferi* DNA in CSF, plasma, or brain biopsy is the final diagnostic possibility, at present (Oksi *et al.*, 1996).

Patients are treated with intravenous penicillin (20 million units/d or ceftriaxone 2 g/day for 2–4 weeks, or longer if required.

VASCULITIS SECONDARY TO MALIGNANCIES

Paraneoplastic vasculitis is a rarity and restricted almost to the lymphoproliferative diseases. The reader is referred to Fortin (1996) for a short overview; to Wooten and Jasmin (1996) for an extensive review of vasculitis in patients with lymphoproliferative disease; and to Oh (1997) for paraneoplastic vasculitis of the PNS. The only combination that is not highly exceptional is vasculitic neuropathy in patients with cryoglobulinaemia and one of the following five lymphoproliferative disorders: lymphocyte lymphoma, Hodgkin's disease, Waldenström, angioimmunoblastic lymphadenopathy, and chronic lymphocytic leukaemia. Up to 1995, PAN has been described in 20 patients with hairy cell leukaemia. According to Wooten and Jasmin (1996), there are 11 cases with granulomatous angiitis and Hodgkin's disease in the literature; four of them had also herpes zoster! The association between giant cell arteritis and lymphocytic lymphoma has been described in three patients.

VASCULITIS SECONDARY TO DRUGS

A critical and very informative review on various aspects of drug-induced vasculitis is from Calabrese and Duna (1996). In the majority of patients with well-established, drug-induced vasculitis, symptoms are confined to the skin. In a minority, other organs are involved also and the CNS is not always spared.

More important, however, is a variety of drugs with sympathicomimetic properties that induce CNS events in particular. Drugs belonging to this category are: cocaine, heroine, oral or intravenous amphetamine, and phenylpropanolamine. These drugs have been demonstrated to cause, in a minority of users, infarcts or haemorrhages, either subarachnoidal or intraparenchymal. In a limited number of patients, the presence of vasculitis has been definitely established (see Krendel *et al.*, 1990), but the conclusion that vasculitis underlies all these cases is incorrect (Kaufman *et al.*, 1998). One of the difficulties is that the drugs used by addicts are often impure. In data on 3700 deceased cocaine users 13 cases of cocaine–related neurovascular complications were discovered. Seven had ischaemic brain injury, three subarachnoid haemorrhage, and three intraparenchymal haemorrhage. Aggarwal *et al.* (1996) examined sections of 14 brains from patients with cocaine-related cerebrovascular disease and in 12 cases, established intracerebral haemorrhage without finding any changes pointing to vasculitis.

HYPOCOMPLEMENTAEMIC URTICARIAL VASCULITIS

This uncommon illness is clinically considered to be related to systemic lupus erythematosus (SLE). Recently, it has been reviewed by Wisnieski *et al.* (1995). There are reports on at least 118 patients in the literature. The criteria for the diagnosis of the disease are urticarial lesions due to a leukocytoclastic vasculitis, a markedly decreased C1q, and antibody to C1q in serum. Other clinical features of the disease are arthralgia or arthritis; angioedema of periorbital tissues, lips, tongue, and hands; ocular inflammation; dyspnoea due to obstructive lung disease; and glomerulonephritis. Orbital pseudotumour with diplopia and other symptoms has been observed in one patient and pseudotumour cerebri in two.

POST-ORGANTRANSPLANT VASCULITIS

Vasculitis in transplant recipients can take the following forms:

- Necrotizing vasculitis in the graft presumably based on a mechanism that is characterized as the clinical equivalent of an organ-specific Shwartzman reaction (Burke *et al.*, 1995). This type of vasculitis does not involve the nervous system.
- Cytomegalus virus infection vasculitis. Cytomegalus virus infection occurs frequently in immunocompromised patients. The virus may replicate in endothelial cells of the vessels and thus cause a vasculitis. Meningo-encephalitis due to cytomegalus virus vasculitis has been described (Golden *et al.*, 1994).
- Recurrence of an auto-immune vasculitis, for instance in patients who developed renal insufficiency due to Wegener's granulomatosis. The chance of recurrence is small if patients are transplanted at a time that vasculitis is inactive (Nyberg *et al.*, 1997).
- De novo vasculitis not related to infections or previous auto-immune disease. Examples are PACNS and PAN (Schriner *et al.*, 1991).

REFERENCES

Abu-Shakra M, Smythe H, Lewtes J *et al* (1994) Outcome of polyarteritis nodosa and Churg-Strauss syndrome. An analysis of 25 patients. *Arthritis Rheum* **37**, 1798–1803.

Achar KN and Al-Nakib B (1986) Takayasu's arteritis and ulcerative colitis. *Am J Gastroenterol* **81**, 1215–1217.

Acheson JF, Cockerell OC, Bebtley CR *et al* (1993) Churg-Strauss syndrome presenting with severe visual loss due to bilateral sequential optic neuropathy. *Br J Ophthalmol* **77**, 118–119.

Adu D, Howe AJ, Scott DGI *et al* (1987) Polyarteritis and the kidney. *Quart J Med* **62**, 221–237.

Aggarwal SK, Williams V, Levine SR *et al* (1996) Cocaine-associated intracranial haemorrhage: Absence of vasculitis in 14 cases. *Neurology* **46**, 1741–1743.

Agnello V (1995) The aetiology of mixed cryoglobulinaemia associated with hepatitis C virus infection. *Scand J Immunol* **42**, 179–184.

Agnello V and Romain PL (1996) Mixed cryoglobulinemia secondary to hepatitis C virus infection. *Rheum Dis Clin North Am* **22**, 1–21.

Aiello PD, Trautman JC, McPhee TJ *et al.* (1993) Visual prognosis in giant cell arteritis. *Ophthalmology* **100**, 550–555.

Akman-Demir G, Baykan-Kurt B, Serdaglu P *et al* (1996) Seven-year follow-up of neurologic involvement in Behçet's syndrome. *Arch Neurol* **53**, 691–694.

Al Kawi MZ, Bohlega S and Banna M (1991) MRI findings in neuro-Behçet's disease. *Neurology* **41**, 405–408.

Amlie-Lefond C, Kleinschmidt-DeMasters BK, Mahalingam R *et al* (1995) The vasculopathy of varicella-zoster virus encephalitis. *Ann Neurol* **37**, 784–790.

Arend WP, Michel BA, Block DA *et al* (1990) The American College of Rheumatology Criteria for the determination of Takayasu's arteritis. *Arthritis Rheum* **33**, 1129–1134.

Bacon PA and Carruthers DM (1995) Vasculitis associated with connective tissue disorders. *Rheum Clin N Amer* **21**, 1077–1096.

Banna M and El-Ramahi K (1991) Neurologic involvement in Behçet disease; Imaging findings in 16 patients. *Amer J Neuroradiol* **12**, 791–796.

Barricks ME, Traviesa DB, Glaser JS *et al* (1977) Ophthalmoplegia in cranial arteritis. *Brain* **100**, 209–221.

Belman AL, Leicher CR, Moshe SL *et al* (1985) Neurologic manifestations of Schoenlein-Henoch purpura: Report of three cases and review of the literature. *Pediatrics* **75**, 687–692.

Bengtsson BA and Malmvall BE (1982) Giant cell arteritis. *Acta Med Scand Suppl*, 658.

Beresford HR, Hyman RA and Sharer L (1979) Self-limited granulomatous angiitis of the cerebellum. *Ann Neurol* **5**, 490–492.

Berger JR, Romano J, Menkin M *et al* (1995) Benign focal cerebral vasculitis: Case report. *Neurology* **45**, 1731–1734.

Bodker FS, Tessler HH, Shapiro MJ *et al* (1993) Ocular complications of Takayasu's arteritis in a hispanic woman. *Am J Ophthalmol* **115**, 676–678.

Boki KA, Dafni U, Karpouzas GA *et al* (1997) Necrotising vasculitis in Greece: Clinical, immunological and immunogenetic aspects. A study of 66 patients. *Brit J Rheumatol* **36**, 1059–1066.

Bondeson J and Asman P (1997) Giant cell arteritis presenting with oculomotor nerve palsy. *Scand J Rheumatol* **26**, 327–328.

Bosch-Gil JA, Falga-Tirado C, Simeon-Aznar CP *et al* (1995) Churg-Strauss syndrome with inflammatory orbital pseudotumour. *Brit J Rheumatol* **34**, 485–486.

Bowyer S, Mason WH, McCurdy DK *et al* (1994) Polyarteritis nodosa (PAN) with coronary aneurysms: The Kawasaki-PAN controversy revisited. *J Rheumatol* **21**, 1585.

Brouet JC, Clauvel JP, Danon F *et al* (1974) Biologic and clinical significance of cryoglobulins. A report on 86 cases. *Am J Med* **57**, 775–788.

Burke GW, Cirocco R, Markou M *et al* (1995) Acute graft loss secondary to necrotising vasculitis. *Transplantation* **59**, 1100–1104.

Cacoub P, Fabiani FL, Musset L *et al* (1994) Mixed cryoglobulinemia and hepatitis C virus. *Am J Med* **96**, 124–132.

Calabrese LH (1995) Vasculitis of the central nervous system. *Rheum Dis Clin N Amer* **21**, 1059–1076.

Calabrese LH, Gragg LA, Furlan AJ *et al* (1993) Benign angiopathy: A distinct subset of angiographically defined primary angiitis of the central nervous systems. *J Rheumatol* **20**, 2046–2050.

Calabrese LH and Duna GF (1995) Evaluation and treatment of central nervous system vasculitis. *Curr Opin Rheumatol* **7**, 37–44.

Calabrese LH and Duna GF (1996) Drug-induced vasculitis. *Curr Opin Rheumatol* **8**, 34–40.

Calabrese LH, Duna GF and Lie JT (1997) Vasculitis in the central nervous system. *Arthritis Rheum* **40**, 1189–1201.

Calabrese LH and Mallek JA (1988) Primary angiitis of the central nervous system. *Medicine* **67**, 20–39.

Callen JP and Kallenberg CGM (1995) The vasculitides: Relationship of cutaneous vasculitis to systemic disease. In: Kater L and Baart de la Faille H (eds) *Multi-Systemic Auto-Immune Diseases: An Integrated Approach*, pp 267–297. Amsterdam: Elsevier.

Carruthers DM, Watts RA, Symmons DPM *et al* (1996) Wegener's granulomatosis–increased incidence or increased recognition. *Brit J Rheumatol* **35**, 142–145.

Caselli RJ (1990) Giant cell (temporal) arteritis: A treatable cause of multi-infarct dementia. *Neurology* **40**, 753–755.

Caselli RJ, Hunder GG and Whisnant JP (1988a) Neurologic disease in biopsy-proven giant cell arteritis. *Neurology* **38**, 352–359.

Caselli RJ, Daube JR, Hunder GG *et al* (1988b) Peripheral neuropathic syndromes in giant cell (temporal) arteritis. *Neurology* **38**, 658–659.

Chalk CH, Dyck PJ and Conn DL (1993) Vasculitic neuropathy. In: Dyck PJ, Thomas PK, Griffin JW *et al* (eds) *Peripheral Neuropathy*, 3 ed, pp 1424–1436. Philadelphia: WB Saunders.

Cherin P, De Gennes C, Bletry O *et al* (1992) Ischaemic Vernet's syndrome in giant cell arteritis: First of two cases. *Am J Med* **93**, 349–352.

Chia L, Fernandeze A, Lacroix C *et al* (1996) Contribution of nerve biopsy findings to the diagnosis of disabling neuropathy in the elderly. A retrospective review of 100 consecutive patients. *Brain* **119**, 1091–1098.

Christian CL (1991) Hepatitis B virus (HBV) and systemic vasculitis (editorial). *Clin Exp Rheumatol* **9**, 1–2.

Chumbley L, Harrison EG Jr and DeRemee RA (1977) Allergic granulomatosis and angiitis (Churg-Strauss syndrome); Report and analysis of 30 cases. *Mayo Clin Proc* **52**, 477–484.

Churg J and Strauss L (1951) Allergic granulomatosis, allergic angiitis, and periarteritis nodosa. *Am J Pathol* **27**, 277–301.

Clements MR, Mistry CD, Keith AO *et al* (1989) Recovery from sensorineural deafness in Wegener's granulomatosis. *J Laryng Otol* **103**, 515–518.

Cohen RD, Conn DL and Ilstrup DM (1980) Clinical features, prognosis and response to treatment in polyarteritis. *Mayo Clin Proc* **55**, 146–155.

Cohen Tervaert JW, van der Wouden FJ and Kallenberg CGM (1987) Analyse van de symptomen voorafgaand aan de diagnose ziekte van Wegener. *Ned Tijdschr Geneesk* **131**, 1391–1394.

Cohen Tervaert JW and Kallenberg CGM (1993) Neurologic manifestations of systemic vasculitides. *Rheum Dis Clin N Amer* **19**, 913–940.

Cooper AM, Naughton MN and Williams BD (1994) Chronic arterial occlusions associated with Behçet's disease. *Brit J Rheumatol* **33**, 170–172.

Cotch MF and Rao JK (1996) New insights into the epidemiology of systemic vasculitis. *Curr Opin Rheumatol* **8**, 19–25.

Cotch MF, Hoffman GS, Yerg DE *et al* (1996) The epidemiology of Wegener's granulomatosis. *Arthritis Rheum* **39**, 87–92.

Crane R, Kerr LD and Spiera H (1991) Clinical analysis of isolated angiitis of the central nervous systems: A report of 11 cases. *Arch Intern Med* **151**, 2290–2294.

Czarnecki EJ and Spickler EM (1995) MR demonstration of Wegener granulomatosis of the infundibulum, a cause of diabetes insipidus. *Amer J Neuroradiol* **16**, 968–970.

Davies L, Spies JM, Pollard JD *et al* (1996) Vasculitis confined to peripheral nerves. *Brain* **119**, 1441–1448.

de Krom MCTF, Knipschild PG, Kester ADM *et al* (1992) Carpal tunnel syndrome. Prevalence in the general population. *J Clin Epidemiol* **45**, 373–375.

De Vlam K, De Keyser F, Goemaere S *et al* (1995) Churg-Strauss syndrome presenting as polymyositis. *Clin Exp Rheumatol* **13**, 505–507.

Devlin T, Gray L and Allen NB (1995) Neuro-Behçet's disease: Factors hampering proper diagnosis. *Neurology* **45**, 1754–1757.

Devlin T, Gray L, Allen NB (1996) Neuro-Behçet's disease in Japan. Reply from the authors. *Neurology* **47**, 614.

DiBisceglie AM, Martin P, Kassianides CK *et al* (1989) Recombinant interferon alfa therapy for chronic hepatitis C. A randomized, controlled trial. *N Engl J Med* **321**, 1501–1506.

Dickey W and Andrews WJ (1990) Wegener's granulomatosis presenting as peripheral neuropathy: Diagnosis confirmed by serum anti-neutrophil antibodies. *J Neurol Neurosurg Psychiat* **53**, 269–270.

Dillon MJ and Ansell BM (1995) Vasculitis in children and adolescents. *Rheum Dis Clin N Amer* **21**, 1115–1136.

Drachman DA (1963) Neurological complications of Wegener's granulomatosis. *Arch Neurol* **8**, 145–155.

Duna GF and Calabrese LH (1995) Limitations of invasive modalities in the diagnosis of primary angiitis of the central nervous system. *J Rheumatol* **22**, 662–667.

Duna GF, Galperin C and Hoffman GS (1995) Wegener's granulomatosis. *Rheum Clin N Amer* **21**, 949–986.

Dyck PJ, Benstead TJ, Conn DL *et al* (1987) Nonsystemic vasculitic neuropathy. *Brain* **110**, 843–853.

Edwards KK, Lindsley HB, Lai CW *et al* (1989) Takayasu's arteritis presenting as retinal and vertebrobasilar ischaemia. *J Rheumatol* **16**, 1000–1002.

Ehrlich GE (1998) Behçet's disease and the emergence of thalidomide. *Ann Intern Med* **128**, 494–495.

Engel DG, Gospe Jr SM, Tracy KA *et al* (1995) Fatal infantile polyarteritis nodosa with predominant central nervous system involvement. *Stroke* **26**, 699–701.

Erden E, Carlier R, Idiz ABC *et al* (1993) Gadolinium-enhanced MRI in central nervous system Behçet's disease. *Neuroradiol* **35**, 142–144.

Evans J and Hunder G (1997) The implications of recognizing large-vessel involvement in elderly patients with giant cell arteritis. *Curr Opin Rheumatol* **9**, 37–40.

Evans JM, O'Fallon WM and Hunder GG (1995) Increased incidence of aortic aneurysm and dissection in giant (temporal) arteritis. *Ann Intern Med* **122**, 502–507.

Fauci AS, Katz P, Haynes BF *et al* (1979) Cyclophosphamide therapy of severe systemic necrotising vasculitis. *N Engl J Med* **301**, 235–238.

Fauci AS, Haynes BF, Katz P *et al* (1983) Wegener's granulomatosis: Prospective clinical and therapeutic experience with 85 patients for 21 years. *Ann Intern Med* **98**, 76–85.

Feigal DW, Robbins DL and Leek JC (1985) Giant cell arteritis associated with mononeuritis multiplex and complement-activating 19S IgM rheumatoid factor. *Am J Med* **79**, 495–500.

Ferri C, Greco F, Longombardo G *et al* (1991) Antibodies to hepatitis C virus in patients with mixed cryoglobulinemia. *Arthritis Rheum* **34**, 1606–1610.

Finelli PF, Onyiuke HC and Uphoff DF (1997) Idiopathic granulomatous angiitis of the CNS manifesting as diffuse white matter disease. *Neurology* **49**, 1696–1699.

Fontana PE, Gabutti L, Piffaretti JC *et al* (1997) Antibiotic treatment for giant cell arteritis? *Lancet* **348**, 1630.

Fortin PR (1996) Vasculitides associated with malignancy. *Curr Opin Rheumatol* **8**, 30–33.

Fortin PR, Larson MG, Watters AK *et al* (1995) Prognostic factors in systemic necrotising vasculitis of the polyarthritis nodosa group – a review of 45 cases. *J Rheumatol* **22**, 78–84.

Fountain NB and Eberhard DA (1996) Primary angiitis of the central nervous system associated with cerebral amyloid angiopathy: Report of two cases and review of the literature. *Neurology* **46**, 190–197.

Franssen CFM, Cohen Tervaert JW, Stegeman CA *et al* (1996) c-ANCA as marker of Wegener's disease. *Lancet* **347**, 115–116.

Fred HL, Lynch EC, Greenberg SD *et al* (1964) A patient with Wegener's granulomatosis exhibiting unusual clinical and morphological features. *Am J Med* **37**, 311–319.

Frohnert PP and Sheps SG (1967) Longterm follow-up study of periarteritis nodosa. *Am J Med* **43**, 8–14.

Furlan AJ, Whisnant JP and Kearns TP (1979) Unilateral visual loss in bright light: An unusual symptom of carotid artery occlusive disease. *Arch Neurol* **36**, 675–676.

Galetta SL, Balcer LJ and Liu GT *et al* (1997a) Giant cell arteritis with unusual flow-related neuroophthalmologic manifestations. *Neurology* **49**, 1463–1465.

Galetta SL, Balcer LJ, Lieberman AP *et al* (1997b) Refractory giant cell arteritis with spinal cord infarction. *Neurology* **49**, 1720–1723.

Garcia-Monco JC and Benach JL (1995) Lyme neuroborreliose. *Ann Neurol* **37**, 691–702.

Gastineau DA, Habermann TM, Hermann RC (1989) Severe neuropathy associated with low-dose recombinant interferon-alpha (letter). *Am J Med* **89**, 116.

Gelber O, Roque C and Coyle PK (1997) Vasculitis owing to infection. *Neurol Clin* **15**, 903–925.

Gemignani F, Pavesi G, Focchi A *et al* (1992) Peripheral neuropathy in essential mixed cryoglobulinaemia. *J Neurol Neurosurg Psychiat* **55**, 116–120.

Gibson LE and Su WPD (1995) Cutaneous vasculitis. *Rheumatic Dis Clin N Amer* **21**, 1097–1113.

Ghini M, Mascia MT, Gentilini M *et al* (1996) Treatment of cryoglobulinemic neuropathy with alpha-interferon (letter). *Neurology* **46**, 588–589.

Golden MP, Hammer SM, Wanke CA *et al* (1994) Cytomegalovirus vasculitis. Case reports and review of the literature. *Medicine* **73**, 246–254.

Goldstein AR, White RHR, Akuse R *et al* (1992) Longterm follow-up of childhood Henoch-Schönlein nephritis. *Lancet* **339**, 280–282.

Goldberg JW (1997) Primary angiitis of the central nervous system. In: Rolak LA and Harati Y (eds) *Neuroimmunology for The Clinician*, pp 177–186. Boston: Butterworth-Heineman.

Gonzalez-Gay MA and Garcia-Porrua C (1998) Carotid tenderness: An ominous sign of giant cell arteritis? *Scand J Rheumatol* **27**, 154–156.

Gorevic PD, Kassab HJ, Levo Y *et al* (1980) Mixed cryoglobulinemia: Clinical aspects and long-term follow-up of 40 patients. *Am J Med* **69**, 287–308.

Gout O, Viala K and Lyon-Caen O (1998) Giant cell arteritis and Vernet's syndrome. *Neurology* **50**, 1862–1864.

Gran JT and Myklebust G (1997) The incidence of polymyalgia rheumatica and temporal arteritis in the county of Aust Agder, South Norway: A prospective study 1987–94. *J Rheumatol* **24**, 1739–1743.

Grefte A, van der Giessen M, van Son W *et al* (1993) Circulating cytomegalovirus (CMV)-infected endothelial cells in patients with an active CMV infection. *J Infect Dis* **167**, 270–277.

Griffin J, Price DL, Davis L *et al* (1973) Granulomatous angiitis of the central nervous system with aneurysms on multiple cerebral arteries. *Trans Am Neurol Assoc* **98**, 145–148.

Grimbacher B, Wenger B, Deibert P *et al* (1997) Loss of vision and diarrhoea. *Lancet* **350**, 1818.

Gross WL (1995) Antineutrophil cytoplasmic autoantibody testing in vasculitides. *Rheum Dis Clin N Amer* **21**, 987–1011.

Guillevin L, Tanter Y, Bletry O *et al* (1987) Systemic necrotising angiitis with asthma: Causes and precipitating factors. *Lung* **165**, 165–172.

Guillevin L, Fain O, Lhote F *et al* (1992) Lack of superiority of steroids and plasma exchanges to steroids in the treatment of polyarteritis nodosa and Churg-Strauss angiitis. A prospective randomized trial in 78 patients. *Arthritis Rheum* **35**, 208–215.

Guillevin L, Lhote F, Leon A *et al* (1993a) Treatment of polyarteritis nodosa related to hepatitis B virus with short term steroid therapy associated with antiviral agents and plasma exchanges. *J Rheumatol* **20**, 289–298.

Guillevin L, Visser H, Noël LH *et al* (1993b) Antineutrophil cytoplasm antibodies in systemic polyarteritis nodosa with and without hepatitis B virus infection and Churg-Strauss syndrome: 62 patients. *J Rheumatol* **20**, 1345–1349.

Guillevin L, Lhote F, Sauvaget F *et al* (1994) Treatment of severe polyarteritis nodosa related to hepatitis B virus with interferon-alpha and plasma exchanges. *Ann Rheum Dis* **53**, 334–337.

Guillevin L, Lhote F and Cohen P *et al* (1995) Polyarteritis nodosa related to hepatitis B virus. A prospective study with long-term observation of 41 patients. *Medicine* **74**, 238–253.

Guillevin L, Lhote F, Amouroux J *et al* (1996) Antineutrophil cytoplasmic antibodies, abnormal angiograms and pathological findings in polyarteritis nodosa and Churg-Strauss syndrome: Indications for the classification of vasculitides of the polyarteritis nodosa group. *Br J Rheumatol* **35**, 958–964.

Hadden RDM, Meikle D, Coulthard A *et al* (1998) Wegener's granulomatosis presenting with bulbar palsy and bilateral jugular vein compression. *Neurology* **50**, 1923–1924.

Hall S, Barr W, Lie JT *et al* (1985) Takayasu's arteritis. A study of 32 North American patients. *Medicine* **64**, 89–99.

Halperin JJ, Logigian EL, Finkel MF *et al* (1996) Practice parameters for the diagnosis of patients with nervous system Lyme borreliosis (Lyme disease). *Neurology* **46**, 619–627.

Hasan A, Fortune F, Wilson A *et al* (1996) Role of γδ cells in the pathogenesis and diagnosis of Behçet's disease. *Lancet* **347**, 789–794.

Hawke SHB, Davies L, Pamphlett R *et al* (1991) Vasculitic neuropathy. *Brain* **114**, 2175–2190.

Haynes BF and Fauci AS (1978) Diabetes insipidus associated with Wegener's granulomatosis successfully treated with cyclophosphamide. *N Engl J Med* **299**, 764.

Haynes BF, Kaiser-Kupfer MI, Mason P *et al* (1980) Cogan syndrome: Studies in 13 patients, long-term follow up and a review of the literature. *Medicine* **59**, 426–441.

Hamuryudan V, Mat C, Saip S *et al* (1998) Thalidomide in the treatment of the mucocutaneous lesions of the Behçet's syndrome. A randomized double-blind placebo-controlled trial. *Ann Intern Med* **128**, 443–450.

Haznedaroglu I, Buyukasik Y, Ozdemir O *et al* (1997) The prethrombotic/hypercoagulable state of Behçet's disease: Comment on the article by Golden *et al*. *Arthritis Rheum* **40**, 1915–1916.

Heeg JE, van Rijswijk MH, Hazenberg BPC *et al* (1988) Churg-Strauss syndrome with severe polyradiculopathy and unilateral nerve deafness. *Neth J Med* **32**, 185–193.

Hoffman GS, Kerr GS, Leavitt RY *et al* (1992) Wegener's granulomatosis: An analysis of 158 patients. *Ann Intern Med* **116**, 488–498.

Hoffman RM, Wheeler KJ and Deyo RA (1993) Surgery for herniated discs: A literature synthesis. *J Int Med* **8**, 487–496.

Hunder GG (1997) Giant cell arteritis and polymyalgia rheumatica. In: Kelly WN, Ruddy S, Harris Jr *et al. Textbook of Rheumatology*, 5 ed, pp 1123–1132. Philadelphia: WB Saunders Co.

Hunder GG, Arend WP, Bloch DA *et al* (1990) The American College of Rheumatology Criteria for the classification of vasculitis: Introduction. *Arthritis Rheum* **33**, 1065–1067.

Hunder GG, Bloch DA, Michel BA *et al* (1990) The American College of Rheumatology 1990 criteria for the classification of giant cell arteritis. *Arthritis Rheum* **33**, 122–128.

Hurst NP, Dunn NA and Chalders Th (1983) Wegener's granulomatosis complicated by diabetes insipidus. *Ann Rheum Dis* **42**, 600–601.

Inaba G (1989) Behçet's disease. *Handbook of Clinical Neurology* **56**, 593–610. Amsterdam: Elsevier.

International Study Group for Behçet's disease (1990) Criteria for diagnosis of Behçet's disease. *Lancet* **335**, 1078–1080.

Jacobs JC (1996) Kawasaki disease. *Curr Opin Rheumatol* **8**, 41–43.

Jankowski J, Crombie J and Jankowski R (1992) Behçet's syndrome in Scotland. *Postgrad Med* **68**, 566–570.

Javedan SP and Tamargo RJ (1997) Diagnostic yield of brain biopsy in neurodegenerative disorders. *Neurosurgery* **41**, 823–830.

Jongen PJH, Delmans HEM, Bruneel LB *et al* (1992) Humoral and cellular immunologic study of cerebrospinal fluid in a patient with Behçet's encephalitis. *Arch Neurol* **49**, 1075–1078.

Jennette JC and Falk RJ (1997) Small-vessel vasculitis. *N Engl J Med* **337**, 1512–1523.

Jennette JC, Falk RJ, Andrassy K *et al* (1994) Nomenclature of systemic vasculitis: Proposal of an international consensus conference. *Arthritis Rheum* **37**, 187–192.

Kallenberg CGM (1996) Treatment of Wegener's granulomatosis: New horizons? *Clin Exp Rheumatol* **14**, 1–4.

Kaneko K, Takahashi C, Terae S *et al* (1995) MRI of the brain in neuro-Behçet's disease. *Neuroradiol* **37**, 684.

Kapoor R, Kendall BE and Harrison MJG (1990) Persistent segmental cerebral artery constriction in coital cephalgia. *J Neurol Neurosurg Psychiat* **53**, 266–267.

Kater L and Schuurman HJ (1981) Immunobiology and clinical aspects of cryoglobulinaemia. *Plasma Therapy* **2**, 83–99.

Katrib A, Portek I, Corbett AJ *et al* (1998) Meningeal involvement in Wegener's granulomatosis. *J Rheumatol* **25**, 1009–1011.

Kattah JC, Chrousos GA, Katz PA *et al* (1994) Anterior ischaemic optic neuropathy in Churg-Strauss syndrome. *Neurology* **44**, 2200–2202.

Kaufman MJ, Levin JM, Ross MH *et al* (1998) Cocaine-induced cerebral vasoconstriction detected in humans with magnetic resonance angiography. *JAMA* **279**, 376–380.

Kerr G (1994) Takayasu's arteritis. *Curr Opin Rheumatol* **6**, 32–38.

Kerr GS (1995) Takayasu's arteritis. *Rheum Clin N Amer* **21**, 1041–1058.

Kerr G, Hallahan CW, Giordano J *et al* (1994) Takayasu's arteritis. *Ann Int Med* **120**, 919–929.

Khella SL, Frost S, Hermann GA *et al* (1995) Hepatitis C infection, cryoglobulinemia, and vasculitic neuropathy. Treatment with interferon alfa: Case report and literature review. *Neurology* **45**, 407–411.

Koc Y, Gullu I, Akpek G *et al* (1992) Vascular involvement in Behçet's disease. *J Rheumatol* **19**, 402–410.

Kok J, Bosseray A, Brion JP *et al* (1993) Chorea in a child with Churg-Strauss syndrome. *Stroke* **24**, 1263–1264.

Krendel DA, Ditter SM, Frankel MR *et al* (1990) Biopsy-proven cerebral vasculitis associated with cocaine abuse. *Neurology* **40**, 1092–1094.

La Civita L, Zignego AL, Lombardini F *et al* (1996) Exacerbation of peripheral neuropathy during alpha-interferon therapy in a patient with mixed cryoglobulinemia and hepatitis B virus infection. *J Rheumatol* **23**, 1641–1643.

Lake CR, Gallant S and Masson E (1990) Adverse drug effects attributed to phenyl propanolamine: A review of 142 cases. *Am J Med* **89**, 195–208.

Lakhanpal S, Tani K, Lie JT *et al* (1985) Pathologic features of Behçet's syndrome: A review of Japanese autopsy registry data. *Human Pathol* **16**, 790–795.

Lanham JG, Elkon KB, Pusey CD *et al* (1984) Systemic vasculitis with asthma and eosinophilia: A clinical approach to Churg-Strauss syndrome. *Medicine* **63**, 65–79.

Leavitt RY, Fauci AS, Bloch DA *et al* (1990) The American College of Rheumatology 1990 criteria for the classification of Wegener's granulomatosis. *Arthritis Rheum* **33**, 1101–1107.

Leib ES, Restivo C and Paulus HE (1979) Immunosuppressive corticosteroid therapy of polyarteritis nodosa. *Am J Med* **67**, 941–947.

Lhote F and Guillevin L (1995) Polyarteritis nodosa, microscopic polyangiitis, and Churg-Strauss syndrome: Clinical aspects and treatment. *Rheum Dis Clin North America* **21**, 911–947.

Lie JT (1992) Primary (granulomatous) angiitis of the central nervous system: a clinicopathologic analysis of 15 new cases and a review of the literature. *Human Pathol* **23**, 164–171.

Lie JT (1994) Nomenclature and classification of vasculitis: Plus ca change, plus c'est la meme chose. *Arthritis Rheum* **37**, 181–186.

Lie JT (1995) Histopathologic specificity of systemic vasculitis. *Rheum Dis Clin N Amer* **21**, 883–909.

Lie JT (1996) Vasculitis associated with infectious agents. *Curr Opin Rheumatol* **8**, 26–29.

Lie JT and Tokagawa DA (1995) Bilateral lower limb gangrene and stroke as initial manifestations of systemic giant cell arteritis in an African-American. *J Rheumatol* **22**, 363–366.

Lightfoot RW, Michel BA, Bloch DA *et al* (1990) The American College of Rheumatology 1990 criteria for the classification of polyarteritis nodosa. *Arthritis Rheum* **33**, 1088–1093.

Liou HH, Yip PK, Chang YC *et al* (1994) Allergic granulomatosis and angiitis (Churg-Strauss syndrome) presenting as prominent neurologic lesions and optic neuritis. *J Rheumatol* **21**, 2380–2384.

Liou H-H, Liu H-M, Chiang IP *et al* (1997) Case report. Churg-Strauss syndrome presented as multiple intracerebral hemorrhage. *Lupus* **6**, 279–282.

Lippa CF, Chad DA, Smith TW *et al* (1986) Neuropathy associated with cryoglobulinemia. *Muscle Nerve* **9**, 626–631.

Liu G, Shupak R and Chiu BKY (1995) Aortic dissection in giant cell arteritis. *Sem Arthritis Rheum* **25**, 160–171.

Loh M and Janner D (1996) Fever, aseptic meningitis and rash in a twenty-one month old male. *Pediatrc Infect Dis J* **15**, 97, 100–101.

Lupi-Herrera E, Sanchez-Torres G, Marcushamer J *et al* (1977) Takayasu's arteritis. Clinical study of 107 cases. *Amer Heart J* **93**, 94–103.

Luqmani R, Jubb R, Emery P *et al* (1991) Inner ear deafness in Wegener's granulomatosis. *J Rheumatol* **18**, 766–768.

Marazzi R, Pareyson D, Boiardi A *et al* (1992) Peripheral nerve involvement in Churg-Strauss syndrome. *J Neurol* **239**, 317–321.

Mason JC, Cowie MR, Davies KA *et al* (1994) Familial polyarteritis nodosa. *Arthritis Rheum* **37**, 1249–1253.

Masi AT, Hunder GG, Lie JT *et al* (1990) The American College of Rheumatology 1990 criteria for the classification of Churg-Strauss syndrome (allergic granulomatosis and angiitis). *Arthritis Rheum* **33**, 1094–1100.

Massey EW and Weed T (1978) Sciatic neuropathy with giant-cell arteritis. Letter. *N Engl J Med* **298**, 917.

Matsumoto H, Uekusa T, Fukuda Y *et al* (1991) Vasculo-Behçet's disease: A pathologic study of eight cases. *Human Pathol* **22**, 45–51.

McFarland HR and Village P (1997) Degos' disease. *Neurology* **49**, 308–309.

McMenemey WH and Lawrence BJ (1957) Encephalomyelopathy in Behçet's disease. *Lancet* **2**, 353–358.

Mehler MF and Rabinowich L (1988) The clinical neuro-ophthalmologic spectrum of temporal arteritis. *Am J Med* **85**, 839–844.

Meier C, Grahmann F, Engelhardt A *et al* (1989) Peripheral nerve disorders in Lyme-borreliosis. Nerve biopsy studies from eight cases. *Acta Neuropathol* **79**, 271–278.

Mercado U (1997) Classification of periarteritis nodosa and microscopic periarteritis: Comment on the article by Watts *et al*. *Arthritis Rheum* **40**, 788–789.

Michell BA and Hunder GG (1996) Clinical differentiation between giant cell (temporal) arteritis and Takayasu's arteritis. *J Rheumatol* **23**, 106–111.

Middlekauff HR, Fang MA and Hahn BH (1987) Polyarteritis nodosa of the epididymis in a patient with Whipple's disease. *J Rheumatol* **14**, 1193–1195.

Monti G, Galli M, Invernizzi F *et al* (1995) Cryoglobulinemias: A multi-centre study of the early clinical and laboratory manifestations of primary and secondary disease. *Quart J Med* **88**, 115–126.

Moore PM and Cupps TR (1983) Neurological complications of vasculitis. *Ann Neurol* **14**, 155–167.

Moore PM and Fauci AS (1981) Neurologic manifestations of systemic vasculitis. *Amer J Med* **71**, 517–524.

Myklebust G and Gran JT (1996) A prospective study of 287 patients with polymyalgia rheumatica and temporal arteritis. Clinical and laboratory manifestations at onset of disease and at the time of diagnosis. *Brit J Rheumatol* **35**, 1161–1168.

Neudorfer M, Feiler-Ofri V, Geyer O *et al* (1993) Behçet's disease presenting as a cerebral tumour. *Neuroradiol* **35**, 145.

Ng CG, Huang SC, Huang LT *et al* (1996) Henoch Schönlein purpura with intracerebral hemorrhage: Case report. *Pediatr Radiol* **26**, 276–277.

Nishino H, Rubino FA, DeRemee RA *et al* (1993a) Neurological involvement in Wegener's granulomatosis. An analysis of 324 consecutive patients at the Mayo Clinic. *Ann Neurol* **33**, 4–9.

Nishino H, Rubino FA and Parisi JE (1993b) The spectrum of neurologic involvement in Wegener's granulomatosis. *Neurology* **43**, 1334–1337.

Nordborg E and Bengtsson BA (1990) Epidemiology of biopsy-proven giant cell arteritis (GCA). *J Intern Med* **227**, 233–236.

Nordborg E and Nordborg C (1998) The inflammatory reaction in giant cell arteritis: An immunohistochemical investigation. *Clin Exp Rheumatol* **16**, 165–168.

Nordborg E, Nordborg C, Malmvall BO *et al* (1995) Giant cell arteritis. *Rheum Clin N Amer* **21**, 1013–1026.

Numano F (1997) Differences in clinical presentation and outcome in different countries for Takayasu's disease. *Curr Opin Rheumatol* **9**, 12–15.

Nyberg G, Akesson P, Norden G *et al* (1997) Systemic vasculitis in a kidney transplant population. *Transplantation* **63**, 1273–1277.

O'Duffy DJ (1994) Behçet's disease. *Curr Opin Rheumatol* **6**, 39–43.

O'Duffy JD, Carney JA and Deodhar S (1971) Behçet's disease. Report of 10 cases, 3 with new manifestations. *Ann Intern Med* **75**, 561–570.

O'Duffy JD and Hammill SC (1996) Silent myocardial ischaemia in Behçet's disease. *J Rheumatol* **23**, 211.

Oh SJ (1997) Paraneoplastic vasculitis of the peripheral nervous system. *Neurol Clin* **15**, 849–863.

Oh SJ, Herrara GA and Spalding DM (1986) Eosinophilic vasculitic neuropathy in the Churg-Strauss syndrome. *Arthritis Rheum* **29**, 1173–1175.

Oimomi M, Suehiro I, Mizuno N *et al* (1980) Wegener's granulomatosis with intracerebral granuloma and mammary manifestation. *Arch Int Med* **140**, 853–854.

Oksi J, Kalimo H, Marttila RJ *et al* (1996) Inflammatory brain changes in Lyme borreliosis. A report on three patients and review of the literature. *Brain* **119**, 2143–2154.

Oner AF, Gurgey A, Gurler A *et al* (1998) Factor V Leiden mutation in patients with Behçet's disease. *J Rheumatol* **25**, 496–498.

Ostergard JR and Storm K (1991) Neurologic manifestations of Schönlein-Henoch purpura. *Acta Paediatr Scand* **80**, 339–342.

Ozawa T, Sasaki O, Sorimachi T *et al* (1995) Primary angiitis of the central nervous system: Report of two cases and review of the literature. *Neurosurgery* **36**, 173–179.

Pande I, Uppal SS and Kailash S (1995) Behçet's disease in India: A clinical, immunogenetic and outcome study. *Brit J Rheumatol* **34**, 825–830.

Provenzale JM and Allen NB (1996a) Neuroradiologic findings in polyarteritis nodosa. *Am J Neuroradiol* **17**, 1119–1126.

Provenzale JM and Allen NB (1996b) Wegener granulomatosis: CT and MR findings. *Am J Neuroradiol* **17**, 785–792.

Provenzale JM, Mukherji S, Allen NB *et al* (1996) Orbital involvement by Wegener's granulomatosis: Imaging findings. *AJR* **166**, 929–934.

Pusey CD, Rees AJ, Evans DJ *et al* (1991) Plasma exchange in focal necrotizing glomerulonephritis without ant-GBM antibodies. *Kidney Int* **40**, 757–763.

Purvin VA (1995) Anterior ischaemic optic neuropathy secondary to interferon alpha. *Arch Ophthalmol* **113**, 1041–1044.

Rabusin M, Lepore L, Costantnides F *et al* (1998) A child with severe asthma. *Lancet* **351**, 32.

Rao JK, Allen NB, Feussner JR, *et al* (1995) A prospective study of antineutrophil cytoplasmic antibody (c-ANCA) and clinical criteria in diagnosing Wegener's granulomatosis. *Lancet* **346**, 926–931.

Rao JK, Weinberger M, Allen NB *et al* (1996) c-ANCA as marker of Wegener's disease. Author's reply. *Lancet* **347**, 118–119.

Raza K, Karokis D and Kitas GD (1998) Cogan's syndrome with Takayasu's arteritis. *Br J Rheumatol* **37**, 369–372.

Read SJ, Crawford DH and Pender MP (1995) Trigeminal sensory neuropathy induced by interferon-alpha therapy (letter). *Aust NZ J Med* **25**, 54.

Rodriguez-Pla A, de Miguel G, Lopez-Contreras J *et al* (1996) Bilateral blindness in Takayasu's disease. *Scand J Rheumatol* **25**, 394–395.

Roos KL (1997) Bacterial meningitis. In: Roos KL (ed) *Central Nervous System Infectious Diseases and Therapy*, pp 99–126. New York: Marcel Dekker Inc.

Rose CD, Eichenfield AH, Goldsmith DP *et al* (1990) Early onset sarcoidosis with aortitis – 'juvenile systemic granulomatosis.' *J Rheumatol* **17**, 102–106.

Rosete A, Cabral AR, Kraus A *et al* (1991) Diabetes insipidus secondary to Wegener's granulomatosis: Report and review of the literature. *J Rheumatol* **18**, 761–765.

Roujeau JC and Stern RS (1994) Severe adverse cutaneous reactions to drugs. *N Engl J Med* **331**, 1272–1285.

Russo MG, Waxman J, Abdoh A *et al* (1995) Correlation between infection and the onset of the giant cell (temporal) arteritis syndrome. *Arthritis Rheum* **38**, 374–380.

Sack M, Cassidy JT and Bole GG (1975) Prognostic factors in polyarteritis. *J Rheumatol* **2**, 411–420.

Said G (1998) Vasculitic neuropathies. In: Latov N, Wokke JHJ and Kelly JJ (eds) *Immunological and Infectious Diseases of The Peripheral Nerves*, pp 158–167. Cambridge: Cambridge University Press.

Said G, Lacroix-Ciaudo C, Fujimura H *et al* (1988) The peripheral neuropathy of necrotizing arteritis: A clinicopathological study. *Ann Neurol* **23**, 461–465.

Salvarini C, Gabriel SE, O'Fallon WM *et al* (1995) The incidence of giant cell arteritis in Olmsted County, Minnesota: Apparent fluctuations in cyclic pattern. *Ann Int Med* **123**, 192–194.

Satoh J, Miyasaka N, Yamada T *et al* (1988) Extensive cerebral infarction due to involvement of both anterior cerebral arteries by Wegener's granulomatosis. *Ann Rheum Dis* **47**, 606–611.

Savage COS, Winearls CG, Evans DJ *et al* (1985) Microscopic polyarteritis: Presentation, pathology and prognosis. *Quart J Med* **56**, 467–483.

Savage COS, Harper L and Adu D (1997) Primary systemic vasculitis. *Lancet* **349**, 553–558.

Savitz JM, Young MA, Ratan RR (1994) Basilar artery occlusion in a young patient with Wegener's granulomatosis. *Stroke* **25**, 214–216.

Schmidt WA, Kraft HE, Vorpahl K *et al* (1997) Color duplex ultrasonography in the diagnosis of temporal arteritis. *N Engl J Med* **337**, 1336–1342.

Schriner RW, Nada AK, Lie JT *et al* (1991) De novo systemic vasculitis in a renal transplant recipient. *Mayo Clin Proc* **66**, 183–186.

Scott DGI, Bacon PA and Elliott PJ (1982) Systemic vasculitis in a district general hospital 1972–1980: Clinical and laboratory features, classification and prognosis in 80 cases. *Q J Med* **203**, 292–311.

Scott Miller K and Miller JM (1993) Wegener's granulomatosis presenting as a primary seizure disorder with brain lesions demonstrated by magnetic resonance imaging. *Chest* **103**, 316–318.

Sehgal M, Swanson JW, DeRemee RA *et al* (1995) Neurologic manifestations of Churg-Strauss syndrome. *Mayo Clin Proc* **70**, 337–341.

Serdaroglu P (1998) Behçet's disease and the nervous system. *J Neurol* **245**, 197–205.

Serdaroglu P, Yazici H, Ozdemir C *et al* (1989) Neurologic involvement in Behçet's syndrome: A prospective study. *Arch Neurol* **46**, 265–269.

Seradaru M, Chiras J, Cujas M *et al* (1984) Isolated benign cerebral vasculitis or migrainous vasospasm? *J Neurol Neurosurg Psychiat* **47**, 73–76.

Serra A, Cameron JS, Turner DR *et al* (1984) Vasculitis affecting the kidney: Presentation, histopathology and longterm outcome. *Quart J Med* **53**, 181–207.

Silva JE, Brown JD, Watson BV *et al* (1998) Temporal arteritis (TA) presenting as bilateral brachial plexopathy (Parsonage-Turner syndrome) and ophthalmoparesis. *Neurology* **50**, A122–A123.

Sima D, Thiele B, Turowski A *et al* (1994) Anti-endothelial antibodies in Takayasu arteritis. *Arthritis Rheum* **37**, 441–443.

Solenski NJ and Haley Jr EC (1997) Neurological complications of infectious endocarditis. In: Roos KL (ed) *Central Nervous System Infectious Diseases and Therapy*, pp 331–363. New York: Marcel Dekker Inc.

Solomon S, Lipton RB and Harris PH (1990) Arterial stenosis in migraine: spasm or arteriopathy? *Headache* **30**, 52–61.

Somer T and Finegold SM (1995) Vasculitides associated with infections, immunization and antimicrobial drugs. *Clin Infect Dis* **20**, 1010–1036.

Stegeman CA, Cohen Tervaert JW, Sluiter WJ *et al* (1994) Association of chronic nasal carriage of

Staphylococcus aureus and higher relapse rates in Wegener granulomatosis. *Ann Intern Med* **120**, 12–17.

Stegeman CA, Cohen Tervaert JW, de Jong PE *et al* (1995) Prevention of relapses of Wegener's granulomatosis by treatment with trimethoprim-sulfamethoxazole. A placebo-controlled trial. *J Am Soc Nephrol* **6**, 930.

Stegeman CA, Cohen Tervaert JW, de Jong PE *et al* (1996) Trimethoprim-sulfamethoxazole (co-trimoxazole) for the prevention of relapses of Wegener's granulomatosis. *N Engl J Med* **335**, 16–20.

Stillwell THJ, Benson RC, DeRemee RA *et al* (1988) Cyclophosphamide-induced bladder toxicity in Wegener's granulomatosis. *Arthritis Rheum* **31**, 465–470.

Subbiah P, Wijdicks E, Muenter M *et al* (1996) Skin lesion with a fatal neurologic outcome (Degos' disease). *Neurology* **46**, 636–640.

Subramanyan R, Joy J and Balakrishnan KG (1989) Natural history of aorta arteritis (Takayasu's disease). *Circulation* **80**, 429–437.

Tabbaa MA and Snyder BD (1987) Vasospasm versus vasculitis in cases of benign cerebral vasculitis (letter). *Ann Neurol* **21**, 109.

Talar-Williams C, Hijazi TM, Schnaubec A *et al* (1996) Cyclophosphamide-induced cystitis and bladder cancer in patients with Wegener's granulomatosis. *Ann Intern Med* **124**, 477–484.

The Italian General Practioner Study Group (1995) Chronic symmetric symptomatic polyneuropathy in the elderly: A field screening investigation in two Italian regions. I. Prevalence and general characteristics of the sample. *Neurology* **45**, 1832–1836.

Thomson GT, Johston JL, Sharpe JA *et al* (1989) Internuclear ophthalmoplegia in giant cell arteritis. *J Rheumatol* **16**, 693–695.

Tishler S, Williamson T, Mira SS *et al* (1993) Wegener granulomatosis with meningeal involvement. *Amer J Neuroradiol* **14**, 1248–1252.

Travis LB, Curtis RE, Glimclius B *et al* (1995) Bladder and kidney cancer following cyclophosphamide therapy for non-Hodgkin's lymphoma. *J Natl Cancer Inst* **87**, 524–530.

Vallat JM, Hugon J, Lubeau M *et al* (1987) Tick-bite meningoradiculoneuritis: Clinical, electrophysiologic and histologic findings in 10 cases. *Neurology* **37**, 749–753.

Valli G, De Vecchi A, Gaddi L *et al* (1989) Peripheral nervous system involvement in essential cryoglobulinemia and nephropathy. *Clin Exp Rheumatol* **7**, 479–483.

Vollertsen RS, McDonald TJ, Younge BR *et al* (1986) Cogan's syndrome: 18 cases and a review of the literature. *Mayo Clin Proc* **61**, 344–361.

Vollmer TL, Guarnaccia J, Harrington W *et al* (1993) Idiopathic granulomatous angiitis of the central nervous system: diagnostic challenges. *Arch Neurol* **50**, 925–930.

Watts RA, Joliffe VA and Scott DGI (1995) Has PAN been classified out of existence? *Brit J Rheumatol* **34**, (supplement) 25 (abstract).

Watts RA, Jolliffe VA, Carruthers DM *et al* (1996) Effect of classification on the incidence of polyarteritis nodosa and microscopic polyangiitis. *Arthritis Rheum* **39**, 1208–1212.

Wechsler B, Vidailhet M, Piette JC *et al* (1992) Cerebral venous thrombosis in Behçet's disease: Clinical study and long-term follow-up of 25 cases. *Neurology* **42**, 614–618.

Weinberger LM, Cohen ML, Remler BF *et al* (1993) Intracranial Wegener's granulomatosis. *Neurology* **43**, 1831–1834.

Weinstein JM, Chui H, Lane S *et al* (1983) Churg-Strauss syndrome (allergic granulomatous angiitis). Neuro-ophthalmologic manifestations. *Arch Ophthalmol* **101**, 1217–1220.

Wells KK, Folberg R, Goeken JA *et al* (1989) Temporal artery biopsy: correlation of light microscopy and immunofluorescence microscopy. *Ophthalmology* 96: 1058–1064.

Weyand CM and Goronzy JJ (1995) Giant cell arteritis as an antigen driven disease. *Rheum Dis Clin N Am* **21**, 1027–1040.

Weyand CM, Hunder NN, Hicok KC *et al* (1994) HLA-DRB1 alleles in polymyalgia rheumatica, giant cell arteritis and rheumatoid arthritis. *Arthritis Rheum* **37**, 514–520.

Wisnieski JJ, Baer AN, Christensen J *et al* (1995) Hypocomplementemic urticarial vasculitis syndrome. Clinical and serologic findings in 18 patients. *Medicine* **74**, 24–41.

Wooten MD and Jasmin HE (1996) Vasculitis and lymphoproliferative diseases. *Sem Arthritis Rheum* **26**, 564–574.

Worthmann F, Bruns J, Turker T *et al* (1996) Muscular involvement in Behçet's disease: case report and review of the literature. *Neuromuscular Dis* **6**, 247–253.

Yamashita Y, Takahashi M, Bussaka H *et al* (1986) Cerebral vasculitis secondary to Wegener's granulomatosis: computed tomography and angiographic findings. *J Comp Assist Tomogr* **10**, 115–120.

Zelenski JD, Capraro JA, Holden D *et al* (1989) Cerebral nervous system vasculitis in Behçet's syndrome. Angiographic improvement after therapy with cytotoxic agents. *Arthritis Rheum* **32**, 217–220.

Zuber M and Gause A (1997) Peripheral neuropathy during interferon-alpha therapy in patients with cryogobulinemia and hepatitis virus infection. *J Rheumatol* **24**, 2488.

6

Inflammatory Myopathies

INTRODUCTION

The classification of the inflammatory myopathies has caused major problems in the past and is still not entirely satisfactory. Similar to the vasculitides (Chapter 5), a distinction can be made between the primary, idiopathic, and secondary forms. Dermatomyositis (DM), polymyositis (PM), and inclusion body myositis (IBM) all belong to the first category. Other entities within this group are the eosinophilic and granulomatous myositides, orbital myositis, and focal myositis (Table 6.1). The infectious and iatrogenic/toxic forms constitute the second category. In recent years, excellent reviews on the inflammatory myopathies have been published (Engel *et al*, 1994; Dalakas, 1991; Mastaglia and Ojeda, 1985a,b). In this chapter, we summarize what is known about the aetiology and pathogenesis of these diseases and concentrate on recent developments in clinical, diagnostic, and therapeutic aspects.

THE IDIOPATHIC INFLAMMATORY MYOPATHIES

EPIDEMIOLOGY OF DERMATOMYOSITIS, POLYMYOSITIS AND INCLUSION BODY MYOSITIS

Figures on the incidence of the main inflammatory myopathies in adults vary from approximately $10/10^6$ in the USA to $7.6/10^6$ and $7.7/10^6$ in Sweden and Singapore (Medsger *et al.*, 1970; Plotz, 1989; Koh *et al.*, 1993; Weitoft *et al.*, 1997). Dermatomyositis (DM) occurs at all ages with peaks in frequency in youngsters between 5–15 and in individuals around 50 years. In a large, population-based cohort of 392 DM patients, approximately 20% were below the age of 16 years (childhood or juvenile dermatomyositis, cDM) (Sigurgeirsson *et al.*, 1992).

Estimates on the incidence of cDM in the USA and the UK are slightly below or above $2/10^6$ (Symmons *et al.*, 1995). Girls are more affected than boys. However, a

Table 6.1 The inflammatory myopathies

Primary or idiopathic	Dermatomyositis in adults
	Dermatomyositis in childhood
	Polymyositis
	Inclusion body myositis
	Eosinophilic myositis
	Granulomatous myositis
	Orbital myositis
	Focal myositis
Secondary	Drug-induced myositis
	Infectious myositis

recent study in Finland mentions an incidence in that country of $5/10^6$ (Kaipainen-Seppanen and Savolaimen, 1996). Polymyositis (PM) is predominantly a disease of adults and is very rare in children. Inclusion body myositis (IBM), on the other hand, is typically a disease of the middle aged, older individuals, and males especially. DM and PM affect females more often than males and are more frequent in blacks than in whites (Medsger *et al.*, 1970). The other idiopathic myositides are rare; no figures on the incidence of these diseases are available. Myositis is estimated to be associated with one of the main inflammatory connective tissue diseases (ICTDs) in approximately 20% of patients (Targoff, 1998). In mixed connective tissue disease (MCTD), this percentage is much higher, however, up to approximately 65% (see Chapter 12). There are case reports on the combination of IBM and ICTDs.

DERMATOMYOSITIS

Aetiology
The origin of DM is probably multifactorial, as are most of the other ICTDs. The association of the disease with the human leukocyte antigens (HLA) B38 and DR3 points to a genetic factor (see Garlepp, 1996). These antigens are markers for a limited number of ancestral haplotypes that have been associated with auto-immune diseases. Familial cases are, however, very rare (Hennekam *et al.*, 1990) and results of twin studies are not available. For a long time, viral infections have been thought to be the cause of the inflammatory myositides, but polymerase chain reaction and *in situ* hybridization have not provided any support for this theory, as no viral genomic material has been detected in muscle fibres (Leff *et al.*, 1992; Leon-Monzon and Dalakas, 1992; see Dalakas and Sivakumar, 1996). This does not exclude, however, that inflammatory myopathies may be an abnormal reaction towards a viral or bacterial infection. In some cases, DM is associated with a malignancy (Airio *et al.*, 1995; Sigurgeirsson *et al.*, 1992; see this Chapter *Paraneoplastic DM*). In these conditions, antibodies to epitopes of malignant cells may conceivably cross-react with epitopes in the capillaries of muscle and skin, which is comparable to the mechanism underlying Lambert-Eaton myasthenic syndrome (LEMS) in patients with small-cell bronchus carcinoma (Lennon *et al.*, 1995; see also Chapter 2). Though childhood and adult DM are not considered separate diseases, there are a number of differences in clinical and pathological aspects, indicating that there may be differences in the constellation of aetiological factors as well.

Pathogenesis

Banker and Victor (1966) already suggested in the sixties that DM might essentially be an angiopathy. Subsequent investigations showed that capillaries in muscle tissue were damaged and lost before any changes of muscle fibres could be observed. Damage to the capillaries was mediated by the complement C5b-C9 membrane attack complex (MAC), as was demonstrated by immuno-histochemical studies with antibodies against neoantigens of the C5b-C9 MAC (Kissel *et al.*, 1986, 1991; Emslie-Smith and Engel, 1990). Dermal capillaries in skin biopsies, especially those in the superficial vascular plexus, were also reduced in density (Crowson and Magro, 1996). The reason for the attack on the vascular endothelium has not been discovered yet. Intravenous immunoglobulins (IVIG) inhibit the assembly and deposition of MAC in endomysial capillaries (Basta and Dalakas, 1994).

Pathology

The histopathological changes in the skin comprise hypovascularity particularly in the superficial capillary plexus, deposition of lymphocytes along the dermal-epidermal junction (interface dermatitis), basilar vacuolopathy, dyskeratosis, deposition of mucin in the mesenchym, and slight thickening of the basement membrane in some cases. Perivascular mononuclear cell infiltration is slight or absent. Immuno-histochemistry reveals C5b-C9 MAC deposition in dermal, preferentially superficial, vessels and along the dermal-epidermal junction (Crowson and Magro, 1996).

The changes in muscular tissue are confined to the capillaries at onset and concern swelling and vacuolization of endothelial cells and microtubular inclusions within these cells (de Visser *et al.*, 1989). In some areas, C5b-C9 MAC is deposited in the capillaries in between muscle fibres and in perimysial arterioles (Fig. 6.1). Staining of capillaries and other vessels clearly shows hypovascularity, often in a strikingly uneven fashion (Fig. 6.2) (Emslie-Smith and Engel, 1990). When muscle pathology is somewhat more advanced, inflammatory cell infiltrates are present and consist of macrophages and lymphocytes (B-cells more than T-cells). The infiltrates are located predominantly in the widened perimysial spaces, often perivascular, and extend into the perifascicular zone of the fascicles at some places (Fig. 6.3). All the changes of the muscle fibres are attributed to ischaemia. A highly characteristic abnormality is the so-called *perifascicular atrophy* that is observed to a variable degree in some fascicles in approximately 75% of the biopsies (Fig. 6.4) (Griggs *et al.*, 1994; Mendell *et al.*, 1996). The fibres are atrophic because of the loss of myofibrils and are less stainable because of the decrease of oxidative enzymes. There is also necrosis of isolated fibres or groups of fibres. Some fascicles or parts of fascicles may be severely affected and consist only of atrophic and necrotic fibres, while other nearby fascicles are much better preserved.

Clinical features of DM in adults (aDM)

Onset of the disease is usually insidious over the course of weeks, though it may occasionally be subacute or even acute (days). The acute form can cause rhabdomyolysis and may be life threatening (Caccamo *et al.*, 1993). The first symptoms and signs concern the skin. The first symptoms appearing in the muscles before the skin is very unusual (Bohan *et al.*, 1973; Rockerbie *et al.*, 1989; Drake *et al.*, 1996).

Cutaneous abnormalities in DM. The cutaneous lesions are comprised of at least five distinct changes, and they may cause considerable discomfort from intractable

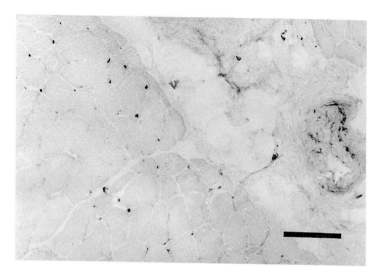

Figure 6.1 Dermatomyositis. C5b-C9 complement membrane attack complex (MAC)-positive capillaries. Black dots representing MAC-positive capillaries are seen in between some muscle fibres and in the wall of an arteriole in the perimysium. Transverse cryostat section. Bar: 100 μm. [From Jennekens, *et al.* (1995), with permission.]

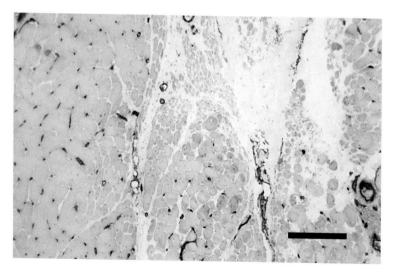

Figure 6.2 Dermatomyositis. Vessels in this transverse cryostat section are labelled with an immunoperoxidase method using *ulex europeus*. Capillaries are scarce or absent in perifascicular zones with atrophic muscle fibres. Bar: 100 μm.

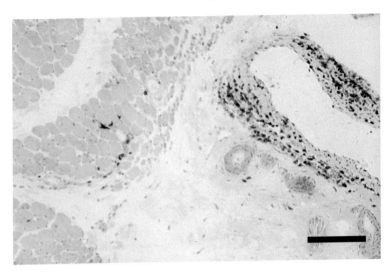

Figure 6.3 Dermatomyositis. CD3 positive lymphocytes are present in and around a venous vessel wall in the perimysium. Some lymphocytes are located in between muscle fibres. Note perifascicular atrophy. Transverse cryostat section. Bar: 100 μm.

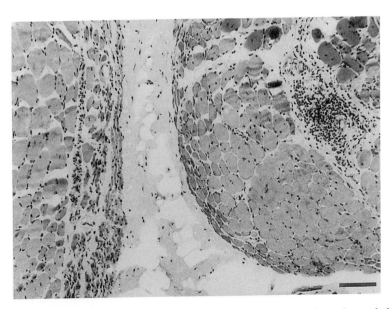

Figure 6.4 Dermatomyositis. H & E stained transverse cryostat section of muscle biopsy from a child. There is a marked degree of perifascicular atrophy of muscle fibres, particularly of the fascicle at the left side. Note inflammatory cell infiltrate at the right side. Bar: 100 μm. [From Jennekens *et al.* (1995), with permission.]

pruritus. One of these five changes (*Gottron's sign*) is considered sufficiently specific to justify the diagnosis according to the American Academy of Dermatology (Box 6.1).

Clinical signs of muscle involvement in DM. The symptoms of muscle inflammation are pain and weakness. They may cause a considerable discomfort in some cases (Box 6.2).

Other manifestations of DM in adults. Patients often feel unwell and lose body-weight. They may have fever, arthralgia and Raynaud's phenomenon. Cardiomyositis has been documented (Haupt and Hutchins, 1982), but is, in our experience and that of others, rarely symptomatic (Askari and Huettner, 1982) and attracts little attention in the literature.

Amyopathic DM
Some patients have typical skin lesions but remain free from muscular symptoms for some time (Euwer and Sontheimer, 1991). Mostly, muscles eventually become involved after months or even years, but there are patients who after periods of 4–11 years still have no signs of muscle disease (Stonecipher *et al.*, 1993). In such cases, the muscle capillaries may be affected but muscle fibre pathology is scarse or absent (Otero and Dalakas, 1992; Crowson and Magro, 1996). Amyopathic DM is considered a stage in a disease that is primarily directed against dermal and muscular endothelium; some patients remain at this stage. In the rheumatological literature, approximately 10% of DM is estimated to be amyopathic. In a dermatological

---

Box 6.1 Cutaneous lesions in dermatomyositis

1. Heliotrope erythema: symmetrical lilac discolouration of the eyelids, predominantly the upper eyelids, and the area around the eyelids (Callen, 1987; Jennekens *et al.*, 1995; Drake *et al.*, 1996). Oedema of the eyelids can cause swelling to such a degree that the patient is unable to open the eyes. More often, however, the discolouration is subtle and oedematous swelling is slight or not present.
2. Erythema: this can have a butterfly-shape on the face as in SLE. A diffuse, macular or streak-like erythema may appear in light exposed areas, on the neck, on the coeur, and on the back. There is often erythema at the extensor aspects of the upper limbs, hands, and less often the lower limbs.
3. Periungual erythema with capillary dilatation: this is a characteristic phenomenon but not very specific.
4. Gottron's sign: well-defined, livid red plaques that become pale and atrophic may appear on bony prominencies, *e.g.* the knuckles, elbows, ankles, and knees. Gottron's papules are more elevated than Gottron's signs (Fig. 6.5).
5. Photosensitive poikiloderma: characterized by a complicated pattern of atrophy, pigmentation and depigmentation, and teleangiectasias. Photosensitivity is not very prominent.
6. Diffuse erythematous scaly dermatosis of the scalp with or without alopecia.
7. Subcutaneous calcinosis: this is rare in adult DM.

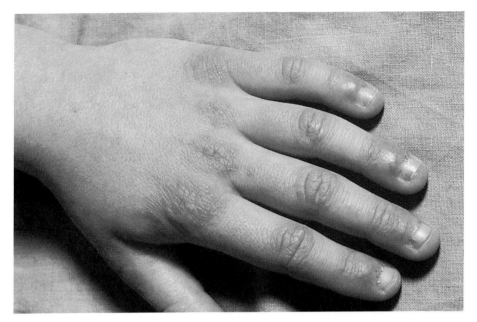

Figure 6.5 Dermatomyositis. Gottron's sign: livid red, well-circumscribed infiltrations on the knuckles of the proximal interphalangeal joints. Note periungual erythema: this is a characteristic but not a very specific phenomenon that may occur also in lupus erythematosus and scleroderma. [From Jennekens *et al.* (1995), with permission.]

Box 6.2 Symptoms of muscle involvement in dermatomyositis

1. Pain: this is experienced mainly or only during muscle activity, not when resting nor while in bed. The exception is the spontaneous pain of patients with the more severe subacute or acute form of DM. Pain is felt usually in the proximal muscles of the limbs, e.g. the thigh and upper arm muscles. Examination reveals that the musculature is painful to a variable degree at palpation.
2. Muscle weakness: this is experienced by patients during activities for which proximal limb muscles are used, *e.g.* going up staircases, standing up from a chair, or lifting ones arms. Up to 50 or 60% of patients complain that they have to swallow repeatedly before food passes slowly downwards. Examination reveals symmetrical weakness of predominantly the proximal limb muscles and the musculature of the neck, especially the neck flexors. Shoulder and upper arm muscles can be affected more than pelvic and thigh muscles or vice versa. Facial muscles are rarely involved and the extraocular muscles are spared. Dysphagia is attributed to cricopharyngeal muscle obstruction and oesophageal muscle obstruction (Sonies, 1997). More generalized weakness occurs in severe cases. Tendon reflexes usually remain elicitable and sensibility is unaffected.

referral centre with established interest in DM, 19 patients were diagnosed in a seven-year period; seven had classic DM and 12 had amyopathic DM (no muscle weakness and normal CK serum levels). Two of these latter cases developed myositis after 18 and 28 months, and three others had transient elevation of serum CK levels (Whitmore *et al.*, 1996). Exactly how frequent amyopathic DM is in comparison to classic DM remains to be established.

Interstitial lung fibrosis and aDM
The data on interstitial lung fibrosis in DM will be presented together with those in PM (see below).

Malignancy and aDM
Population-based studies into the relation of myositis and malignancy show an increased incidence of cancer and an increased cancer mortality rate in DM, particularly in patients older than 50 years (Sigurgeirsson *et al.*, 1992; Airio *et al.*, 1995). Cancer of the breast, reproductive organs, gastrointestinal tract, and lungs, as well as other cancers have been registered. Several studies point to a strong association with ovarian cancer (Sigurgeirsson *et al.*, 1992; Whitmore *et al.*, 1994; Airio *et al.*, 1995). Ovarian cancer has been reported also in amyopathic DM (Whitmore *et al.*, 1996).

CHILDHOOD DERMATOMYOSITIS

Aetiological and pathological differences from aDM
The aetiology of cDM is not better understood than of DM in general. There is a strong association with HLA-DQA1*0501 (Reed *et al.*, 1991) that points to a genetic predisposition, but in contrast to many other ICTDs, there is no increased frequency of auto-immune disease among relatives (Pachman *et al.*, 1997). Environmental conditions are not different from controls, and antibodies to potential infectious agents are not more frequent or increased in children with DM (Pachman *et al.*, 1997). Muscle pathology in cDM is not different in type but some changes are more frequent and severe. Perifascicular atrophy is generally more obvious in children than in adults, and deposition of C3 and IgG and IgM in small vessels, as observed by Whitaker and Engel (1972), occurs more frequently in children. The incidence of muscle specific antibodies (MSAs) in serum is lower than in DM of adults (see Rider, 1995; see also Chapter 3, *Antibodies*).

Clinical differences from aDM
cDM presents, in 20% of patients (Pachman, 1986; Pachman *et al.*, 1998) or less (Norris, 1989; Symmons *et al.*, 1995), with muscle symptoms, while in adults, onset is nearly always with cutaneous symptoms (see this Chapter *DM in Adults*). The study of Pachman *et al* (1998) shows that it may take 10 months (in Caucasians) to 20 months (in minority groups) before cutaneous symptoms appear in a child that first presents with weakness. It is not definitely known whether amyopathic DM occurs in childhood, though the Pachman *et al.* (1998) study revealed a long delay of up to one year until muscle weakness developed in some children with cutaneous symptoms. Onset with fever is common in cDM and unusual in aDM (Pachman *et al.*, 1998). In cDM, secondary changes due to hypovascularization are probably more prominent, and involvement of other organs is more frequent (Box 6.3)

Box 6.3 Clinical features of childhood dermatomyositis. Differences from the disease in adults

1. Digital ulceration (Pachman, 1986) and white patches of the skin due to compromised perfusion (Norris, 1989) are observed in cDM and are exceptional in aDM.
2. Calcinosis is one of the most dreaded complications in cDM, but is rarely observed and not prominent in aDM (Figs. 6.6 and 6.7). Calcinosis in cDM develops during the course of the disease and can present as nodules of variable size in the dermal tissue. A long delay until diagnosis is associated with a higher incidence of subcutaneous calcinosis (Pachman *et al.*, 1998). The white colour of the calcium in the nodule may show through the skin and when the nodule causes ulceration of the skin a white chalky material may be extruded gradually from it. Calcium deposits can also occur in deeper layers and are then often plaque-like and larger than the dermal nodules. Generalized calcinosis can lead to wheelchair dependency (Maugars *et al.*, 1996).
3. Contractures secondary to muscle weakness are well known in cDM and unusual in aDM. Once present, they are difficult or impossible to get rid of (Norris, 1989).
4. Involvement of other organs is probably more frequent in cDM than in aDM and includes: ulcers in the gastrointestinal tract causing maelena, haematemesis and perforation (Pachman, 1986 and Pachman *et al.*, 1998), arthritis (Pachman *et al.*, 1998), pancreatitis (See *et al.*, 1997), aspiration and pneumonia, interstitial lung fibrosis, electrocardiographic abnormalities, and small vessel occlusions in the retina causing cotton wool spots and visual loss (Yeo *et al.*, 1995; Pachman, 1986).

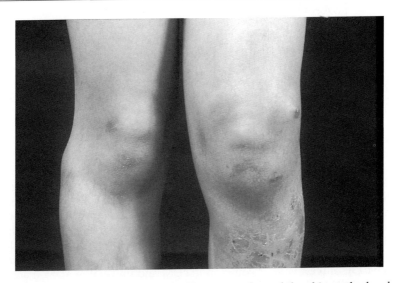

Figure 6.6 Childhood dermatomyositis. Uneven surface of the skin at the level of the knees due to subcutaneous calcinosis. (Courtesy of Professor Wietse Kuis.)

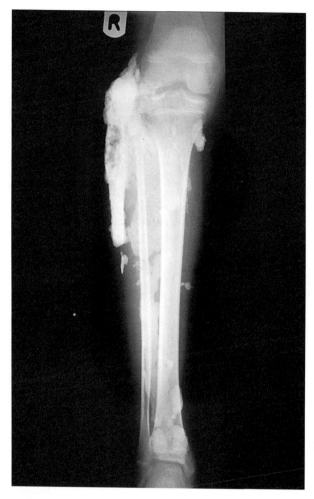

Figure 6.7 Childhood dermatomyositis. Massive subcutaneous calcinosis. Same case as in Figure 6.6. (Courtesy of Professor Wietse Kuis.)

Lipoatrophy and cDM
Total or partial lipoatrophy can precede cDM or develop when it is already present. Lipoatrophy has also been described in association with myasthenia gravis (MG) and other ICTDs and has been suggested to be immunologically mediated (Kavanagh *et al.*, 1993; Laxer and Feldman, 1997).

Malignancy and cDM
Though the association with malignancies could not be established in a large retrospective study (Hiketa *et al.*, 1992), at least 11 cases have been described, mostly with lymphoma or leukaemia and in single cases with neuroblastoma, nasopharyngeal carcinoma, or primary hepatocarcinoma. In some cases, DM behaved as

a paraneoplastic process in that clinical signs improved when the tumour was treated or eradicated and worsened when the tumour recurred (Plotz, 1995; Leaute-Labreze *et al.*, 1995).

POLYMYOSITIS (PM)

Introduction
The distinction of PM from IBM is a recent one, and it is still not always made in the literature. Some cases of IBM must have been diagnosed previously as PM. The consequence of the discovery of IBM can only be that PM (not associated with, or part of another ICTD) is diagnosed now much less often than previously. It is not yet known how rare isolated PM really is. PM has few characteristic clinical features that facilitate the diagnosis. Proximal limb muscle weakness and elevation of CK activity in serum occur in many myopathies, and even the inflammatory cell infiltrations in muscle biopsies are not decisive for diagnosis, as they occur as a secondary phenomenon in several of the muscular dystrophies. The whole constellation of symptoms, signs, and laboratory features decisive for the diagnosis.

Aetiology and pathogenesis
The present knowledge on the aetiology of PM is just as limited as that of DM. Evidence for a hereditary predisposition is weak and familial occurrence is rare. Association of PM with HLA-B38 and DR3 has been reported (see Garlepp, 1996). PM is not a viral infection (Leff *et al.*, 1992; Leon-Monzon and Dalakas, 1992), though it may be a reaction towards an infectious agent, as in Guillain-Barré syndrome (see Chapter 2). The association with malignancies is contested. The results of studies on the immunopathogenesis of PM can be summarized as follows (Plotz, 1995; Hohlfeld *et al.*, 1997): for reasons not yet clear, a number of muscle fibres express HLA class I antigen on their surface, which they normally do not. In the endomysial space in between the muscle fibres, an inflammatory cell infiltrate consisting of lymphocytes and macrophages is present. The lymphocytes are mostly CD8+ T-cells and include cytotoxic T-cells. There are also some natural killer cells and a few B-cells. The CD8+ T-cells and macrophages pervade the basal lamina of some HLA class I expressing muscle fibres and invade the muscle fibres. The cell adhesion molecule, ICAM-1, is expressed on the surface of invaded muscle fibres and is likely to serve as a ligand for the invading cells (de Bleecker and Engel, 1994).

Pathology
A prerequisite for the histological diagnosis of PM is the presence of inflammatory cell infiltrates that are located mostly in the endomysium, less often in the perimysium, and sometimes in the perivascular regions (Griggs *et al.*, 1994). The inflammatory cells often surround healthy-looking muscle fibres and may penetrate into otherwise healthy muscle fibres (Fig. 6.8). Necrotic fibres containing mononuclear cells, mostly macrophages and some T-cells, are also present and may be C5b-C9 MAC-positive. In affected parts of the muscle sections, many fibres generally have internal nuclei and some, usually small fibres, show regenerative activity. In some muscle fibres, the oxidative enzyme activity is irregularly distributed and an occasional ragged red fibre may be observed (Carpenter and Karpati, 1992). In more advanced stages, a number of muscle fibres has disappeared and others are

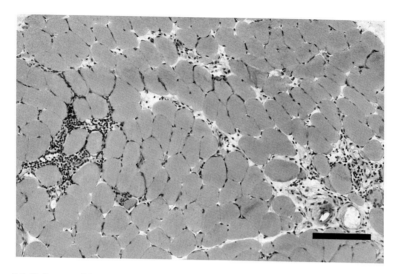

Figure 6.8 Polymyositis. Healthy-looking muscle fibres at the mid-left side of the figure are surrounded by an inflammatory infiltrate. Other fibres are infiltrated by inflammatory cells or have already disappeared. Transverse cryostat section. H & E. Bar: 100 μm.

atrophic, thus creating widened endomysial and perimysial spaces with proliferated connective tissue.

Clinical features
Onset is usually insidious, within months or less often weeks. Patients feel unwell and may have fever, myalgia at exertion, and arthralgia. Activities involving proximal limb muscles either require more time than usual or cannot be performed. As well, swallowing requires an effort. When in bed, lifting the head may not be possible (see Box 6.2). Though focal onset followed by 'generalization' has been described (Flaisler *et al.*, 1993), the clinical picture is usually approximately symmetrical from the start.

Examination reveals no skin lesions, some pain at palpation of muscles, and weakness of predominantly proximal limb muscles, neck flexors, and muscles involved in swallowing. The erector trunci muscles and the neck extensors may also be affected. The facial musculature is commonly not involved and extraocular muscles are spared, exactly as in dermatomyositis. PM may be associated with Raynaud's phenomenon and one of the other ICTDs (see this Chapter, *PM and other disorders*).

Interstitial lung fibrosis and PM
Interstitial lung fibrosis is recognized by different groups in 5–40% of patients with PM or DM during the course of the disease. Dyspnoea and unproductive cough are its main symptoms. Biopsies of lung tissue show interstitial pneumonia with inflammatory infiltrates and focal areas of fibrosis (Marie *et al.*, 1998). Patients are treated with corticosteroids and immunosuppressants with variable results (Marie *et al.*, 1998; Tazelaar *et al.*, 1990; Maddison and Jablonska, 1995). Interstitial lung

fibrosis is notorious for its unfavourable effect on morbidity and mortality of patients with myositis.

Anti-Jo-1 antibodies (anti-histidyl-tRNA synthetase) occur in 20% of patients with myositis, and occur more often in PM than in DM (Nishikai *et al.*, 1998; Vazquez-Abad and Rothfield, 1996). These antibodies are in 50–70% of patients associated with antisynthetase syndrome, which includes interstitial lung fibrosis (see Chapter 3, *Antibodies in Patients with Myositis*). The main elements of this syndrome are Raynaud's phenomenon, mechanic's hands, arthritis, interstitial lung fibrosis, myositis, and low-grade fever. Often, not all elements are present simultaneously. Mechanic's hands is a hyperkeratotic non-pruritic eruption and its appearance resembles the working hands of a labourer. Not all patients with interstitial lung fibrosis and myositis have anti-Jo-1 antibodies. Interstitial lung disease with fibrosis and inflammatory cell infiltrates causes dyspnoea and nonproductive cough, and it has an unfavourable prognosis.

Malignancy and PM
A relation with malignancies has been less firmly established than in DM (Manchul *et al.*, 1985; Sigurgeirsson *et al.*, 1992; Zantos *et al.*, 1994; Airio *et al.*, 1995). Airio *et al.* (1995) found an increased risk on haematological malignancies among patients with PM (four in a group of 175 patients; one could have been expected), but could not draw more firm conclusions in view of the limited number of affected cases. According to Sigurgeirsson *et al.* (1992) the relative risk on malignancy is 1.8 for men and 1.7 for women in PM compared to 2.4 for men and 3.4 for women in DM.

PM and other disorders
The main ICTDs (SLE, rheumatoid arthritis (RA), systemic sclerosis, Sjögren's syndrome and MCTD) are associated with myositis in variable frequency, usually without skin rash (see this Chapter, *Epidemiology*). One should not assume that this form of myositis is always identical to PM, as described in the foregoing. The histopathology of myositis in SLE is, according to Engel *et al.* (1994), similar to that of dermatomyositis (see also Chapter 7, *Myositis in SLE*).

The association of primary biliary sclerosis and myopathy has been documented in 15 cases (Varga *et al.*, 1993; Bondeson *et al.*, 1998). Inflammatory infiltrations are, with few exceptions, a dominating histological feature of this myopathy (Varga *et al.*, 1993). Mitochondrial abnormalities in muscle fibres were described in 4 cases.

There are case histories on the association of PM with a variety of other disorders, *e.g.* Hashimoto's disease (Dahan *et al.*, 1984), myasthenia gravis (MG) (Behan *et al.*, 1982), thymoma (Rowland *et al.*, 1973), thymomectomy (Hassel *et al.*, 1992), thymoma and T-cell lymphocytosis (Cranney *et al.*, 1997), benign monoclonal gammopathy (Telerman-Toppet *et al.*, 1982; Miller and Kiprov, 1984), and cryoglobulinaemia (Voll *et al.*, 1993).

PM in childhood
PM in children is heterogeneous and very rare. The following conditions have to be distinguished:

1. Juvenile dermatomyositis may present for some time (up to 10 to 20 months) as polymyositis (Pachman *et al.*, 1998).
2. PM in children may form part of an overlap syndrome (Singsen *et al.*, 1977).

3. PM can also occur in children with hereditary agammaglobulinaemia (Mease *et al.*, 1981). In one such case in our centre, proximal limb weakness was slight and muscle biopsy revealed inflammatory cell infiltration in the endomysial space.
4. There are case reports on the association of polymyositis and malignancy in children (Sherry *et al.*, 1993).
5. So-called 'benign acute childhood myositis' or 'myalgia cruris epidemica' may be less benign in our experience than the name of the disorder suggests. In the recovery period of an influenza-like infection, tenderness, and in some cases, swelling of lower limb muscles develop, especially of calf muscles. Serum CK activity is raised 10–20 times normal and even more, and there may be red-brown discolouration of the urine, indicative of myoglobinuria. Muscle biopsies show muscle fibre necrosis and regeneration with few if any inflammatory cell infiltrations. Recovery follows spontaneously, but there may be a relapse after the next bout of influenza (Dietzman *et al.*, 1976; Carpenter and Karpati, 1984).
6. Neonates or infants in the first year of life who present with muscle hypotonia may show in their muscle biopsies endomysial fibrosis, muscle fibre necrosis and regeneration, and mononuclear cell infiltrates in the endomysial and perimysial spaces (Roddy *et al.*, 1986). In retrospect, most of these cases may have had congenital muscular dystrophy (Pegoraro *et al.*, 1996). Therefore, it may be that neonatal or infantile PM does not exist.

Graft-versus-host polymyositis

A graft can launch an immunological reaction against unknown antigens in the host, provided it functions long enough and contains the immunocompetent cells required for the reaction. There are two phases in this immune reaction: the first is 'acute' and occurs within a time period of 100 days after transplantation, and the second is chronic and begins after 80 days. The main manifestations of the chronic phase are a cutaneous rash or scleroderma-like change, a sicca syndrome, obstructive and restrictive pulmonary disorders, liver dysfunction with cholangitis as in primary biliary cirrhosis, MG, probably an inflammatory neuropathy, and polymyositis. Polymyositis can also be the only manifestation of the syndrome (Parker *et al.*, 1996; Parker *et al.*, 1997). Graft-versus-host disease is a delayed type hypersensitivity reaction against cells of the host and is mediated by cytotoxic T-cells and T-helper cells of the donor. Muscle biopsies from patients with this form of polymyositis show inflammatory cell infiltrates, muscle fibres infiltrated by CD8+ T-cells of the cytotoxic subclass, and macrophages as in PM. The clinical symptoms are also similar as those in PM. Therapy with corticosteroids has a favourable effect and results in return of muscle function (see this Chapter, *Therapy*).

LABORATORY INVESTIGATIONS IN DM AND PM

Antibodies and other serum factors

Anti-Mi-2 and anti-Jo-1 belong to the *myositis specific autoantibodies* (MSAs), and are of great theoretical interest even though their significance for the pathogenesis of the myositides is not known (Miller, 1993; Targoff, 1995). Anti-Mi-2 (see Chapter 3) recognizes a 218-kDa nuclear protein involved in transcriptional activities, and is present in approximately 20% of patients with aDM as well as in a few cases of cDM.

The prevalence of this antibody in PM is low and varies from 0–3.5% (Seelig *et al.*, 1995; Drake *et al.*, 1996; Feldman *et al.*, 1996; Mierau *et al.*, 1996; Roux *et al.*, 1998).

Anti-Jo-1 antibody is the most common MSA in PM and DM and is present in approximately 20% of patients with myositis, including myositis in overlap syndromes. It is not present in systemic sclerosis and other rheumatic diseases (Vazquez-Abad and Rothfield, 1996; Nishikai *et al.*, 1998). It belongs, together with four other antibodies, to a small group of anti-aminoacyl-tRNA synthetases (Provost and Kater, 1995; see also Chapter 3). Anti-Jo-1 is by far the most common of these antibodies and 5–10 times more frequent than any of the others. Anti-Jo-1 antibodies are found in 50–70% of patients who have interstitial lung disease and other manifestations of the antisynthetase syndrome (see this Chapter, *DM and PM with interstitial lung fibrosis*).

Antinuclear antibodies (ANAs) are positive in 50–80% of patients (Drake *et al.*, 1996; Uthman *et al.*, 1996; Feldman *et al.*, 1996). Polymyositis scleroderma (PM Scl) antibodies occur occasionally in cDM and were initially suggested to be predictive for development of scleromyositis (see Chapter 12), but this was not confirmed (see Laxer and Feldman, 1997). Von Willebrand factor (VWF) is a glycoprotein that augments adherence of platelets to injured vascular endothelium. Serum levels of VWF are increased in DM but not in a consistent fashion, and therefore are not recommended for routine testing in DM (Bloom *et al.*, 1995). Serum levels of neopterin are reported to be related to DM disease activity, but they are also raised in other conditions, *e.g.* intercurrent infections (Pachman, 1995).

Muscle enzymes

Creatine kinase (CK) activity is, in general, elevated in patients with myositis, and may attain values of 200 times normal or more, especially in acute cases. However, myositis can not be ruled out when CK activity is normal or only slightly raised. This is true especially in DM, when ischaemia of the muscle fibres is slight and causes little if any elevation of CK activity. In the study of Pachman *et al.* (1998) on cDM, 27 of 76 (36%) patients had normal CK activity in serum at diagnosis. From the data gathered by Japanese physicians on a few hundred patients, it appears that in 10% CK activity was normal (Tanimoto *et al.*, 1995). Determination of other muscle enzymes or myoglobin to assess muscle fibre leakage provides no additional information and is therefore superfluous.

Systemic inflammatory signs

Systemic inflammatory signs, expressed by elevated serum CRP levels, accelerated ESR (> 20 mm/h Westergren method), or fever are, according to Japanese clinicians, present in a high percentage of patients (approximately 85%) (Tanimoto *et al.*, 1995).

Electromyography

Electromyography of affected muscles reveals two kinds of changes: (1) short-duration, low-amplitude, polyphasic motor unit potentials, indicating that motor units have lost a number of muscle fibres; and (2) spontaneous activity with fibrillation potentials, positive waves, and less often complex repetitive discharges probably due to changes in muscle fibre membranes. The combination of 'myopathic' motor unit potentials and abnormal spontaneous activity is not specific to inflammatory myopathies and may be observed in a variety of active myopathies (*e.g.*, Becker muscular dystrophy, Pompe's disease, amyloid myopathy). Electromyographic abnormalities in proven PM may, in exceptional cases, be restricted to paraspinal musculature (Barkhaus *et al.*, 1990; Robinson, 1991).

Muscle imaging

Most authors prefer magnetic resonance (MR) for imaging. Computer tomography's advantage is high sensitivity for depicting calcifications, and its drawback is the exposure of patients to ionizing radiation. MRI is more sensitive than myosonography for detecting changes in PM and DM, and allows differentiation between increase in muscle oedema and fat or connective tissue, which is not well differentiated by myosonography. MRI is also more expensive than myosonography (see Reimers *et al.*, 1994; Park *et al.*, 1995; Reimers and Finkenstaedt, 1997). On their own, MRI findings do not allow diagnosis of myositis, as muscle oedema and replacement of muscle tissue by fat or connective tissue are not specific for the inflammatory myopathies. The value of MRI for the assessment of the effect of therapy is still disputed at present.

THE DIAGNOSIS OF DM AND PM

Introduction

When Bohan and Peter published their landmark study on polymyositis and dermatomyositis in 1975, IBM had already been described but was considered very rare and was not generally accepted as a distinct entity (see Carpenter, 1996). Bohan and Peter proposed five diagnostic criteria. The first concerns skin lesions and is crucial for DM, but irrelevant for PM. The next three (proximal limb muscle weakness, elevated CK activity, and myopathic EMG) do not differentiate PM from a long list of other myopathies. The final criterion, muscle biopsy (inflammatory cell infiltrations and degeneration and regeneration of muscle fibres), cannot be considered as decisive any more, as inflammatory cell infiltrations are a feature of some of the hereditary muscular dystrophies (congenital muscular dystrophy, facioscapulohumeral muscular dystrophy, limb girdle muscular dystrophy, and Duchenne muscular dystrophy) and as they occur in a similar fashion in IBM (Engel, 1986; Munsat, 1986; Griggs *et al.*, 1994; Pegoraro *et al.*, 1996; van der Kooi *et al.*, 1998).

To compensate for the lack of sensitivity and specificity in the Bohan and Peter criteria, a group of Japanese authors searched for some additional criteria and analysed data from a large number of patients gathered retrospectively by Japanese specialists in 31 centres. They suggested four other criteria that might be useful: systemic inflammatory signs, muscle pain, non-destructive arthritis or arthralgia, and the presence of MSAs. As appears in the following, the Japanese criteria were accepted only in part.

Diagnosing DM

DM is diagnosed only when there are cutaneous lesions. In children with muscle symptoms, one may have to wait for the skin lesions, which occasionally may not appear (van Rossum *et al.*, 1994; see this Chapter, *Clinical Aspects of cDM*). In adults, myositis without skin lesions is not likely to evolve into DM. The American Academy of Dermatology advises one to distinguish between two kinds of cutaneous lesions: those that confirm the diagnosis (Gottron's sign or papules) and those that support the diagnosis (Box 6.4).

Box 6.4 The contribution of cutaneous lesions to the diagnosis of DM

---

1. Characteristic skin lesions that confirm the diagnosis: Gottron's sign and Gottron's papulae.
2. Diagnosis is confirmed by the combination of characteristic muscle findings and less specific cutaneous changes: periorbital heliotrope erythema often associated with oedema; photosensitive poikiloderma; violaceous erythema over the extensor aspects of the arms and hands; teleangiectasia and erythema of the proximal nailfolds; and diffuse pruritic erythematous scaly dermatosis of the scalp with or without alopecia.

From Drake *et al.* (1996), with permission.

In a group of 159 patients with DM, 82 had Gottron's sign and 50 did not (Tanimoto *et al.*, 1995). In a control group of 234 patients with SLE and scleroderma, Gottron's sign was registered in three patients (Tanimoto *et al.*, 1995). When there is doubt about the nature of the cutaneous lesions, it can be helpful to examine a skin biopsy of an affected part of the skin for reduced density (hypovascularity) of the superficial capillary plexus of the dermis and for deposition of the C5b-C9 MAC in vessel walls in the dermis. The presence of the muscle-specific antibody, anti-Mi-2, strongly supports the diagnosis DM, and the presence of anti-Jo-1 supports the diagnosis of myositis (Targoff *et al.*, 1997).

Characteristic muscle findings in DM are, according to Bohan and Peter (1975), proximal muscle weakness, elevated CK levels, myopathic EMG, and a pathological muscle biopsy with inflammatory mononuclear cell infiltrations as well as necrosis and regeneration of muscle fibres. Characteristic for the muscle pathology of DM are also perifascicular muscle fibre atrophy (present in approximately 75% of muscle biopsies) and lack of invasion of healthy-looking muscle fibres by lymphocytes (see this Chapter, *Pathology of DM*). MRI may reveal muscle involvement even when serum CK activity is normal and muscle biopsy is not informative (Stonecipher *et al.*, 1994). MRI may be helpful also for deciding from which muscle a biopsy can best be taken.

Diagnosing PM

At present, there is no unanimity on the criteria for PM. Targoff *et al.* (1997) do not follow the suggestion of Japanese authors (see *Introduction* above) (Tanimoto *et al.*, 1995), and propose that to the four widely accepted criteria for PM outlined by Bohan and Peter (1975) three others should be added:

- Presence of muscle-specific antibodies
- MR changes indicative of myositis
- Exclusion of other myopathies

Examination for MSAs implies, at present, looking for the presence of anti-Jo-1, as the incidence of the other MSAs is very low (see this Chapter, *Laboratory Investigations*). MRI may be valuable to demonstrate the presence of muscle involvement and to reveal which muscle is most suited for biopsy. Other myopathies that have to be excluded are primarily the hereditary muscular dystrophies with inflammatory features: Duchenne and Becker muscular dystrophy, facioscapulohumeral muscular dystrophy, congenital muscular dystrophy with merosin deficiency, and limb girdle muscular dystrophy. Inflammatory infiltrates can occur in sections of each of these dystrophies.

We suggest that the diagnostic value of MSAs and MRI requires confirmation, preferably in prospective studies. Until results from such studies are available, one of the requirements for a definite diagnosis of PM remains the presence of mononuclear inflammatory cell infiltrates in a muscle biopsy. Recent onset of muscle disease, systemic inflammatory signs, muscle pain, and non-destructive arthritis or arthralgia (Tanimoto *et al.*, 1995), all support the diagnosis (Table 6.2).

Diagnosing malignancies in patients with DM or PM
Screening for malignancy in adults includes, according to the guidelines of the American Academy of Dermatology, a thorough physical examination, chest X-ray and mammography, pelvic ultrasonography, measurement of serum C-125 (an ovarian cancer tumour marker), stool examination for occult blood, complete blood cell count, serum chemistry screen, and urine analysis. Re-evaluation for malignancy at time intervals of 6 or 12 months for a period of two years after diagnosis of DM is advised (Drake *et al.*, 1996). No special screening program is required in cDM.

The screening program in PM is similar to that in DM, with the exception of pelvic ultrasonography and serum C-125 measurement.

TREATMENT AND OUTCOME OF DM AND PM

Measurement of effects of treatment
The effect of therapy is best measured by visual evaluation of the dermatological abnormalities and by assessment of muscle function. Muscle function is assessed by functional and timed tests, examination of the forced vital capacity of respiration, manual muscle testing (MMT), or hand-held myometry. Functional and timed tests (standing up from a chair, climbing stairs, reaching for high-placed objects, lifting the head from a horizontal position, drinking a certain volume of fluid) reflect daily activities and therefore offer an essential type of information. MMT, graded accord-

Table 6.2 Criteria for the diagnosis of polymyositis

Required for diagnosis	Typical mononuclear cell infiltrates in muscle biopsy
	Other forms of myositis or myopathy are excluded:
	  sarcoid myositis, drug-induced myositis, and
	  hereditary dystrophies with cellular infiltrates

Supporting the diagnosis	Recent onset Weakness of proximal limb muscles, neck flexors and other muscles Muscle pain at exertion Elevated serum CK activity MSA is present MRI reveals muscle oedema
Compatible with the diagnosis	Systemic inflammatory signs Raynaud's phenomenon Non-destructive arthritis or arthralgia

ing to the Medical Research Council (MRC) scale from 0–5 and hand-held myometry are both reliable and reasonably sensitive tests for measuring muscle strength (Mendell and Florence, 1990; Louwerse *et al.*, 1995). MMT has the additional advantage of not being dependent on the availability of a device. MMT and hand-held myometry require training and experience, and can best be performed on a limited number of muscles or muscle groups in each patient, preferably by the same investigator at repeat examinations.

Serum CK activity offers valuable information on the changes and the effects of the inflammatory process to the muscle fibres. CK activity cannot replace assessment of muscle function, but it reveals the decrease or increase of leakage of enzymes from the muscle fibres reliably.

Treatment of dermatitis in DM
The skin should be protected from sunlight and some form of antipruritic therapy may be required. Aminoquinoline antimalarials are reputed to induce partial improvement in some patients [oral hydroxychloroquine (plaquenil[R]) 200–400 mg/day is preferred above chloroquine] (Drake *et al.*, 1996; Kasteler and Callen, 1997; Block, 1998; see also Chapter 4). When antimalarials are not of sufficient benefit or when cutaneous lesions are severe, treatment with corticosteroids, approximately 1 mg prednisone/kg/day, should be considered (Drake *et al.*, 1996). Weekly low-dose methotrexate (average maximal dose, 7.5 mg/week; range for maximal doses may vary from 2.5–25 mg) can be added in order to spare corticosteroids and is advised by experienced authors on the basis of observations in a small series of patients (Kasteler and Callen, 1997). Skin disease is in some cases much more resistant to therapy than myositis.

Treatment of myositis
Corticosteroids are still considered the best choice for initiation of treatment, in doses of approximately 1–1.5 mg prednisone/kg/day for 4 weeks (see Chapter 4, *Corticosteroids*). The benefit of treatment becomes apparent with the fall in serum CK levels and the improvement of muscle function after some delay. Tapering of corticosteroid doses is then allowed, according to the scheme discussed in Chapter 4. While tapering, muscle function should continue to improve gradually. Low-dose corticosteroid treatment should be continued for at least a year after complete remission is obtained. More often than not, there will be a renewed increase of weakness and elevation of serum CK activity; adjustment of corticosteroids to a higher dose will then be necessary.

If the scheme given here is not sufficiently effective, combination with azathioprine or methotrexate should be considered (azathioprine oral doses of 2–3 mg/kg/day; methotrexate oral doses of 7.5–25 mg/week. See this Chapter, *Treatment of Dermatitis*). Cyclosporin and cyclophosphamide have been used in some studies, but sufficient data on results are not available and intervention studies have not been performed. A favourable effect has been observed with pulsed high-dose dexamethasone therapy in an uncontrolled pilot study (van der Meulen *et al.*, 1998a).

Intravenous infusions of immunoglobulin (IVIG) are of interest for scientific and therapeutic reasons (see this Chapter, *Pathogenesis*) and initially seemed very promising, even in patients resistant to more conventional forms of treatment

(Cherin *et al.*, 1991; Dalakas *et al.*, 1993). However, subsequent investigations did not support the choice of IVIG as initial treatment (Cherin *et al.*, 1994; Mastaglia *et al.*, 1997). As it stands now, IVIG should be attempted when the previously discussed lines of treatment have failed (see Chapter 4 for dosages). Plasmapheresis and leukapheresis had no better effect than sham-apheresis as shown in a double-blind placebo controlled study of 39 patients (Miller *et al.*, 1992).

Treatment of childhood dermatomyositis

Treatment strategies are essentially similar as those in aDM. Corticosteroids are the drugs of choice for initiation of treatment because they are powerful and can induce remission. The choice of the daily dose is a matter of opinion: Sansome and Dubowitz (1995) prefer 1 mg prednisone/kg/day, with or without azathioprine or methotrexate, and others prefer 2 mg prednisone/kg/day. There are also advocates of pulse therapy with intravenous prednisolone, 30 mg/kg/day at three successive days. Retrospectively analysed results of treatment with intermittent high-dose intravenous methylprednisolone in 14 children indicate that it prevents calcinosis, shortens course of the disease, and is associated with less morbidity than oral medication (Callen *et al.*, 1994). IVIG can be administered in the corticosteroid resistant cases (Sansome and Dubowitz, 1995; see Chapter 4 for dosages).

Symptomatic treatment

Passive physiotherapy is required for bed-ridden patients to prevent contractures. In this respect, patients with cDM require much attention. Early diagnosis and medical treatment (not physiotherapy!) may possibly help to prevent the development of calcinosis in cDM (Pachman *et al.*, 1998). Once calcinosis is present, no effective medical treatment is available. Attention should be given to the nutritional status of patients with dysphagia. Cardiac rhythm disorders and involvement of other organs require the appropriate care.

Outcome of DM and PM in adults

Patients tend to improve when they are treated (Joffe *et al.*, 1993); therapy resistance should be reason to reconsider the diagnosis. So far, studies on 'outcome' have not distinguished between PM and IBM yet. Some or many of the therapy-resistant patients in these studies may therefore concern cases of IBM (Amato *et al.*, 1996).

In general, the prognosis of aDM is reputed to be better than of PM (Dalakas, 1991). In a study of inflammatory myopathies with a mean follow-up period of 62 months, therapy could be discontinued in five of 30 patients because of remission (Uthman *et al.*, 1996). Koh *et al.* (1993) reported that in a five-year period, 27 of 75 patients with PM (the authors did not distinguish from IBM) or DM achieved remission and had no relapse. These figures indicate that full remission is obtained in a more or less large minority and that there is a tendency to chronicity in the remaining cases. A relapse after complete remission remains possible, even after many years (Lee *et al.*, 1997).

In different studies, the survival rate of patients with 'inflammatory myopathy' varied after 8–11.6 years, from approximately 56–85% (Hochberg *et al.*, 1986; Maugars *et al.*, 1996; Uthman *et al.*, 1996). Only few patients died from the effects of muscle weakness. Causes of death that were mentioned were old age, infection, malignancies, and interstitial lung fibrosis.

Outcome of cDM

Childhood DM burns out or is under control in approximately two years (Banker and Victor, 1966; Mastaglia *et al.*, 1997). In a retrospective study in two centres of 33 patients (30 with cDM and three with childhood PM) who had been followed for a mean period of 4 years, complete recovery of functional capacity was obtained in 19 patients, 10 kept a mild functional handicap, two were wheelchair dependent, one died by respiratory insufficiency and viral pneumonia within months after onset of the disease, and one was not available for follow-up (van Rossum *et al.*, 1994). Twelve patients had some degree of calcinosis, two patients developed SLE, and one other child developed MCTD. These figures reveal that the prognosis *quoad vitam* is not unfavourable, but that there is a considerable risk of a permanent handicap or another ICTD.

PREGNANCY AND DM OR PM

The literature on this subject concerns only a few patients and does not distinguish between DM and PM (Gutierrez *et al.*, 1984; da Rocha *et al.*, 1992; Otero and Dalakas, 1992). Our own experience is also limited. Onset of DM or PM during pregnancy has been reported (Papapetropoulos *et al.*, 1998). A minority of patients (15% according to da Rocha *et al.*, 1992) with DM or PM experience progress of disease manifestations during pregnancy. Abortion and premature delivery are suggested to occur more frequently in patients with DM or PM. Neonates from diseased mothers do not show evidence of dermatomyositis. In our view, pregnancy in patients with DM or PM need not be discouraged.

INCLUSION BODY MYOSITIS (IBM)

Introduction

This disease was first described by the American author, S-M Chou, in 1967 and received its name, inclusion body myositis, from Yunis and Samaha in 1971. IBM has a number of distinctive clinical and pathological characteristics, and is now generally accepted as an inflammatory myopathy that is different from PM and DM. Though figures on incidence or prevalence are not available yet, IBM is assumed to be the most frequently acquired myopathy after the age of 50 and is diagnosed 2–4 times more often in males than females (Lotz *et al.*, 1989; Lindberg *et al.*, 1994). Sporadic IBM (sIBM) is distinguished from hereditary inclusion body myopathy (hIBM) (Griggs *et al.*, 1995; Sivakumar *et al.*, 1997). The latter comprises a number of hereditary myopathies with pathological changes in muscle fibres resembling those in sIBM, but without inflammation. The clinical phenotypes of the hIBMs also differ from sIBM (Askanas, 1997).

Aetiology and pathogenesis

The demonstration of packed filaments in muscle nuclei or near degenerating nuclei was the reason that sIBM was considered to be of viral origin. This theory became uninteresting when subsequent investigations failed to provide any support for it. The pathology of sIBM then gave rise to two other diverging theories. One proposed that sIBM might be an auto-immune disease and the other suggested that it could be a degenerative disorder, the Alzheimer's disease of the skeletal musculature (Barohn *et al.*, 1995; Sivakumar *et al.*, 1997).

The first and main reason for the auto-immune hypothesis was the presence of mononuclear inflammatory cell infiltrates in the endomysium in muscle biopsies and the attack by some of these cells on histologically normal fibres. The muscle fibres under attack and some other fibres, though not as widespread as in PM, expressed MHC class I antigen and adhesion molecule ICAM-1; the cells invading the muscle fibres were mostly of CD8+ cytotoxic T-cell phenotype (see Askanas and Engel, 1995; Carpenter, 1996). Of interest was that sIBM was occasionally observed in patients with auto-immune conditions such as Sjögren's syndrome, scleroderma, dermatomyositis, lupus erythematosus, and chronic immune thrombocytopenia (Rugiero *et al.*, 1995). The strong association of sIBM and the HLA-DR3 phenotype (incidence in sIBM 92% and in controls 25%) (Garlepp *et al.*, 1994; see also this Chapter, *Aetiology of DM*) also supports an auto-immune mechanism, especially in view of the association of the ancestral haplotypes of DR3 with other auto-immune diseases (Garlepp, 1996).

The theory of a degenerative Alzheimer's-like disorder stems from the fact that, structurally, abnormal muscle fibres in the muscle biopsies appeared to be stainable, by immuno-histochemical methods, for a number of 'dementia proteins'. Investigations in this direction were initiated by Mendell *et al.* (1991) who searched for an explanation of the bundles of unbranched intracellular filaments in the abnormal muscle fibres (see this Chapter, *Pathology of sIBM*) and decided to look for the presence of amyloid. Congo-red staining indeed revealed typical green birefringence at polarization microscopy in some fibres in all cases examined. The amyloid deposits were small (2–8 µm) and not always easily detectable, though it appeared that visualization of Congo-red staining could be facilitated by the use of fluoresence microscopy eventually (Askanas *et al.*, 1993). The deposits were potassium permanganate resistant and showed no immuno-staining for transthyretin, immunoglobulin light chains, or human P component, and differed from amyloid in systemic amyloidosis in this respect. The deposits did stain, however, with antibodies to β-amyloid, a protein known by its presence in amyloid in cerebral blood vessels of patients with Alzheimer's disease. Since then, Askanas and co-workers (1996) demonstrated the presence of – or at least, immuno-histochemical staining for – a series of unusual proteins in the sarcoplasm of structurally abnormal fibres, *e.g.* β-amyloid protein, β-amyloid precursor protein, hyperphosphorylated τ, α1-antichymotrypsin, apolipoprotein E, and ubiquitin. These proteins accumulate also in Alzheimer's disease. β-amyloid precursor protein and ubiquitin occur normally only in the neuromuscular junction, and β-amyloid precursor protein is expressed in the envelopes of some nuclei. Carpenter (1996) suggested that the breakdown of muscle nuclei is the essential step in sIBM.

The accumulation of 'Alzheimer's-associated' proteins in the muscle fibres and the lack of response of most patients to any form of immune suppression (see this Chapter, *Therapy of sIBM*) led to the concept that sIBM might be a degenerative disease in origin (Barohn *et al.*, 1995).

Pathology

For many authors, sIBM is still primarily a histopathological diagnosis (Griggs *et al.*, 1995; see, however, Verschuuren *et al.*, 1997). The following changes are observed in the muscle sections:

- Mononuclear inflammatory cell infiltrates, mainly in the endomysium. Occasionally in biopsies or sections, inflammatory infiltrates are scarce or absent (Lotz *et al.*, 1989).
- Invasion of non-necrotic muscle fibres by activated CD8+ cytotoxic T-cells and some macrophages. The muscle fibres under attack, and a few others, express MHC class I antigen on their surface (Carpenter, 1996).
- Rimmed vacuoles are present in muscle fibres, as shown in cryostat sections, in percentages of cross-sectioned muscle fibres varying from less than 1% up to 70% (Fig. 6.9). The vacuoles are round or slit-like, jagged spaces and contain or are surrounded by basophilic (in haematoxylin and eosin stained sections) or red (in Gomori trichrome) granules. In paraffin sections, the granules are not preserved and the vacuoles lack an important diagnostic feature. In semi-thin sections, the vacuoles are often not visible as such because they are filled with osmiophilic material, which is best seen in paraphenylene stainings (Carpenter, 1996). Rimmed vacuoles are not specific for sIBM and occur in a limited number of other diseases (Jongen *et al.*, 1995).
- Occasionally, fibres show a ragged red aspect with increased activity of succinic dehydrogenase and decreased activity of cytochrome oxidase. Large mitochondrial DNA deletions have been demonstrated in mitochondria from muscle fibres in sIBM (Oldfors *et al.*, 1993).
- Congo-red-positive material showing green birefringence on polarization microscopy and orange-like fluorescence under the fluorescent microscope (using the customary filters for fluorescein isothiocyanate staining) is present

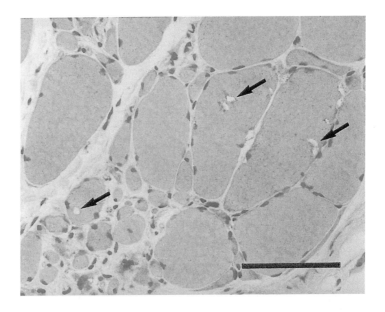

Figure 6.9 Inclusion body myositis. Rimmed vacuoles are present in several large transversely sectioned muscle fibres. There is a small group of atrophic fibres at the bottom left. Other atrophic fibres are located in between large fibres. Bar: 100 μm. Transverse cryostat section, H. & E. [From Jennekens *et al.* (1995), with permission.]

in few or many fibres dependent on the stage of the disease and is probably absent in some biopsies (Fig. 6.10) (Amato *et al.*, 1996; Carpenter, 1996).

- Electron microscopy reveals that the osmiophilic granules consist largely of membranous whorls (Fig. 6.11). Fibres with such membranous whorls often contain collections or bundles of filaments of 15–21 nm in the vicinity of debris of uncertain origin (Fig. 6.12). Somewhat thinner filaments are occasionally seen in the sarcoplasmic nuclei. An immuno-histochemical procedure allows identification of these filaments at the light microscopical level by a commercially available antibody, SM1-31 (Fig. 6.13) (Askanas *et al.*, 1996; Carpenter, 1996).
- In addition to these more or less characteristic changes, there are also a series of unspecific abnormalities.

Not all the abnormalities described here are always present, certainly not in the beginning when patients have to be diagnosed. Patients have been reported who were first considered to suffer from PM and from whom a second biopsy was taken after months or years because they were therapy resistant. This second biopsy revealed the typical features of sIBM, which had not been present in the first biopsy even in retrospect (van der Meulen *et al.*, 1998b; Amato *et al.*, 1996; Lotz *et al.*, 1989).

Clinical features and course of the disease
The presenting symptom is weakness, not pain, though some patients complain about pain at a later stage of the disease. Onset is commonly in the lower limbs, often asymmetrical, and develops slowly (Griggs *et al.*, 1995; Verschuuren *et al.*,

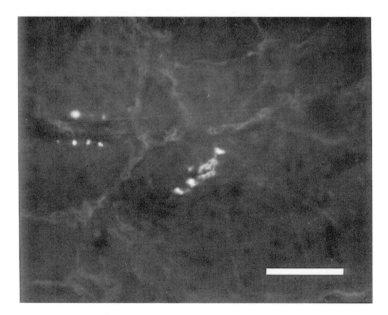

Figure 6.10 Inclusion body myositis. Fluorescence of Congo-red-stained amyloid in muscle fibres of formalin-fixed, transverse cryostat section, from a biopsy obtained at autopsy from a patient with inclusion body myositis. Bar: 50 μm. [From Jennekens *et al.* (1995), with permission.]

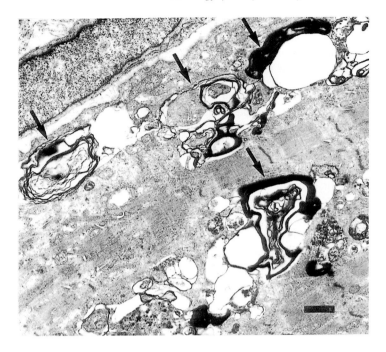

Figure 6.11 Inclusion body myositis. Electron micrograph of ultrathin muscle section showing several large membranous whorls (arrows) and other debris. Same biopsy as in Figure 6.9. Bar: 1 μm. [From Jennekens *et al.* (1995), with permission.]

1997). Knee extensors are preferentially involved, more than hip flexors, hamstrings, and foot extensors. In the upper limbs, finger flexors and wrist flexors are weaker in general than shoulder abductors (Amato *et al.*, 1996). Biceps and triceps muscles and other proximal muscles are also involved. It is not definitely established yet whether the forearm flexors are already affected at an earlier stage of the disease, though weakness of these muscles may be the presenting symptom (Lotz *et al.*, 1989). Dysphagia is common and can also be a presenting symptom (Wintzen *et al.*, 1988; Lotz *et al.*, 1989; Riminton *et al.*, 1993). Facial muscles may be involved, even markedly; external eye muscles are spared however, exactly as in DM and PM. Tendon reflexes of weak muscles can be decreased or may be abolished. The course of the disease is slowly progressive. Patients may become wheelchair dependent and expire from aspiration pneumonia or respiratory insufficiency. The differential diagnosis from motor neuron disease may create difficulties because IBM affects elderly subjects, is purely motor, CK activity is not always raised, and electromyography may simulate a neurogenic disorder (see below). IBM does not, however, give rise to fasciculations or muscle cramps. The muscle biopsy is decisive in case of doubt (see previous section).

Associated diseases
Distal, mainly sensory neuropathy has been reported in some patients (Lotz *et al.*, 1989; Amato *et al.*, 1996). Cardiovascular abnormalities are frequent and are at least

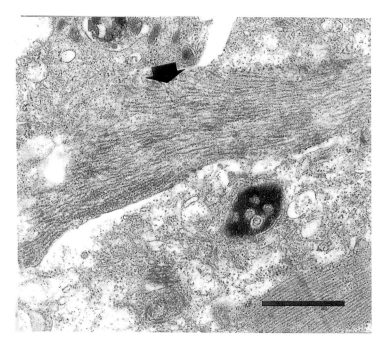

Figure 6.12 Inclusion body myositis. Electron micrograph of ultrathin section showing in the centre a bundle of rectilinear 18 nm filaments (arrow). At the bottom right of the figure, part of a myofibril is depicted. Same biopsy as in Figure 6.9. Bar: 1 µm. [From Jennekens *et al.* (1995), with permission.]

in part age related, though it cannot be excluded that sIBM affects the cardiac muscle to some degree. Malignancies in patients with sIBM have also been observed, but at present there is no evidence for a causal relation. There are reports on auto-immune diseases in patients with sIBM (see also this Chapter, *Aetiology and Pathogenesis of IBM*) (Rugiero *et al.*, 1995).

Laboratory findings in sIBM

Antibodies and other serum factors. Results of investigations for MSAs in sIBM are not yet available. ANAs and RFs are usually not detectable.

Serum CK activity. CK activity was normal in eight of 40 patients (20%) (Lotz *et al.*, 1989). Mean values for the whole group were two to three times normal, which is low in comparison to the mean values at diagnosis in DM and PM (Amato *et al.*, 1996).

Electromyography. Features often considered as 'neurogenic' (fibrillation potentials, positive waves, long-duration polyphasic potentials) are frequent in sIBM and may erroneously lead to the conclusion of a neurogenic muscular disorder. Similar changes are also observed in PM and DM but are less prominent. An investigation of whole motor units by macro EMG provided no evidence for a 'coexisting neurogenic component' (Luciano and Dalakas, 1997).

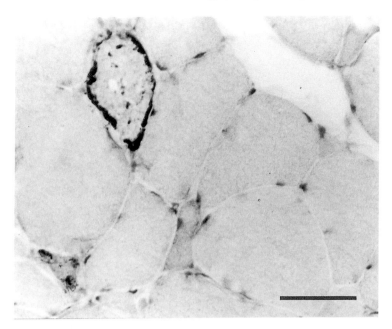

Figure 6.13 Staining of IBM muscle fibres with an immunoperoxidase method using SMI-31. Bar: 50 μm. (Courtesy of Drs. MG van der Meulen and Jessica E Hoogendijk.) (See Spuler and Engel, 1997).

Magnetic resonance imaging. Twenty of 21 randomly chosen patients with sIBM in a large referral centre showed evidence of muscle tissue replacement by fat or fibrosis in the flexor digitorum profundus (FDP) muscle. The flexor digitorum superficialis muscle and most other forearm muscles were also affected but less frequently and extensively than the FDP (Sekul *et al.*, 1997). MRI investigation of the forearm musculature may be helpful when there is doubt about the diagnosis.

Muscle biopsy. The histopathological findings have been described in the section on *Pathology.*

Therapy
The results of treatment with corticosteroids, cytostatic agents, and intravenous immunoglobulins are disappointing (Griggs *et al.*, 1995; Barohn, 1997). Most authors refrain therefore from any attempt at 'causative treatment' in order to avoid the harmful side effects of the drugs. Others have registered partial improvement or delay in progression in some cases (Leff *et al.*, 1993; Dalakas *et al.*, 1997; see also Lotz *et al.*, 1989). Mastaglia *et al.* (1997) recommend a 3–6 month trial of oral corticosteroids (see Chapter 4, *Corticosteroids*) alone or in combination with methotrexate or azathioprine, as well as an assessment of the effect of therapy by quantitative muscle testing and functional scales. The question for the near future is whether intervention studies can demonstrate delay in progress of the disease by treatment with immunosuppressive or myotrophic agents and whether this is sufficient to counterbalance the side effects of these agents. It is of interest that strength training against

resistance done by patients with sIBM during a 12 week period resulted in some improvement in strength compared to baseline and that adverse effects were not discovered (Spector *et al.*, 1997). This indicates that patients need not refrain from exercise.

NECROTIZING MYOPATHY WITH PIPESTEM CAPILLARIES

A myopathy was described by Emslie-Smith and Engel (1991) and Authier *et al.* (1996) in two males and two females that had scattered atrophic, necrotic, and regenerating muscle fibres and thickened hyalinized capillaries in muscle biopsies. Vessel walls in the muscle biopsies were thickened and resembled pipestems. The capillary density was decreased and MAC was detected in the walls of some capillaries and arterioles. Ultrastructural investigation showed the thickening to be due to amorphous material that partially or completely replaced the original structure. Inflammatory cells were few, if any, and were localized in the endomysium. Microtubular inclusions in endothelial cells, as observed in dermatomyositis, were not present.

The patients varied in age from 48 to 65 years, and had proximal limb muscle weakness in three cases and recurrent episodes of pain and weakness in one other case. Outcome was unfavourable in each case (Table 6.3). Authier *et al.* (1996) suggested that this myopathy might be an unusual form of dermatomyositis.

EOSINOPHILIC MYOSITIS

Inflammatory cell infiltrates in eosinophilic myositis differ from infiltrates in other forms of myositis by the presence of many eosinophils. The infiltrates are localized in the endomysium and associated with necrosis of muscle fibres. Eosinophilia in the circulation and bone marrow may also be present but are not required for the diagnosis. Eosinophilic myositis is, in some cases, well-localized and nodular. In others it is diffuse or widespread and is therefore a heterogeneous condition. It has to be distinguished from eosinophilic perimyositis, a disorder with eosinophilic infiltrates in epimysium and perimysium but without necrosis of muscle fibres (Kaufman *et al.*, 1993; Espino-Montoro *et al.*, 1997; see this Chapter, *Fasciitis and perimyositis with eosinophilia*). The eosinophilic granule major basophilic protein is cytotoxic and degranulation of the cells might induce tissue damage by this protein. Two idiopathic forms of eosinophilic myositis have to be distinguished from the secondary forms:

1. Hypereosinophilic syndrome (HES): this idiopathic condition is diagnosed when (1) an eosinophilic blood cell count of at least 1500/l is sustained (2) for at least 6 months, (3) and is complicated by dysfunction of several organs (Editorial, 1983). Eosinophilic myositis in this condition is infrequent (Fauci *et al.*, 1982).
2. Idiopathic eosinophilic myositis (IEM).
3. Infectious eosinophilic myositis: helminth infections, *e.g.* trichinosis, cysticercosis and echinoccus, and some cases of pyomyositis (Mastaglia and Walton, 1992).
4. A toxic variety: eosinophilia-myalgia syndrome due to contaminated L-tryptophan (Varga and Kähäri, 1997).

Table 6.3 Clinical features of necrotizing myopathy with pipestem capillaries in 4 patients

Gender/age	Onset	Presenting symptom	Muscle signs	Serum CK elevation	Other manifestations	Outcome
*female, 58 yrs	Subacute	Respiratory distress	Proximal myopathy and pain	15–50 fold	Fibrosing alveolitis, myocarditis	Death after 14 months, cardiovascular
*female, 65 yrs	Subacute	Weakness	Proximal myopathy	15–50 fold	Cerebral vasculitis, multiple infarcts	Death after 11 months, bronchopneumonia
*male, 67 yrs	Subacute	Carcinoma – gall bladder	Proximal myopathy	15–50 fold	Dissemination of carcinoma	Death after 6 months
**male, 48 yrs	Recurrent episodes for 7 yrs	Weakness, muscle pain	Transient myopathy	3–10 fold	Mild cutaneous changes as in DM	Multiple cerebral infarcts 4 yrs after diagnosis

*Described by Emslie-Smith and Engel (1991).
**Described by Authier *et al.* (1996).

There are now at least 20 cases of IEM in the literature (perimyositis not included) (Kaufman *et al.*, 1993; Nagar and Bar-Ziv, 1993; Espino-Montoro *et al.*, 1997). It appears that the disorder is more frequent in males than females and that age at onset varies from 14 to 79 years. Some patients develop proximal limb weakness with elevation of CK activity. In many others, symptoms are focal or multiple and concern unilateral or bilateral swelling and myalgia or cramps of the calves, thighs, arms, shoulder, neck, chest wall, or multiple sites. The course of the disorder may be chronic, relapsing, or cyclic. The disorder need not be confined to the skeletal musculature. In some cases, there is pericardial effusion, heart block, myocarditis, and arthralgia. Association of eosinophilic myositis with vasculitis and poly-neuropathy has been described and demands distinction from Churg-Strauss syndrome (Espino-Montoro *et al.*, 1997). Systemic symptoms such as fever and malaise are present in a few cases and the ESR may be raised.

Management and outcome. The short-term prognosis of the condition is very good. With few exceptions, patients react favourably to moderate doses of corticosteroids. Sufficient data on long-term outcome are not available however.

FASCIITIS AND PERIMYOSITIS WITH EOSINOPHILIA

This disorder was first described by Shulman in 1975. It is clinically characterized by painful swelling and induration of the skin and underlying tissue diffuse or locally, in particular of the forearms and below the knees (Serratrice *et al.*, 1990; Kaufman *et al.*, 1993). Serum CK activity need not be raised. Eosinophilia may be present, but is not a prerequisite for the diagnosis, and hypergammaglobulinaemia is frequent. Biopsies show collagenous hypertrophy of the fascia and the tissue above it, as well as infiltration by mononuclear cells and by eosinophils, the latter in percentages varying from 5–50%. The collagen hypertrophy and the inflammatory infiltrates may extend into the epimysial and perimysial spaces (perimyositis). Eosinophilic fasciitis is considered by rheumatologists as a disorder belonging to the 'scleroderma-spectrum', in view of the swelling of the skin and underlying tis-sue and the collagen hypertrophy. Most patients respond favourably to treatment with corticosteroids but the condition may relapse.

GRANULOMATOUS MYOSITIS

Granulomatous myositis has several causes including tuberculosis, leprosy, intra-muscular injections, and sarcoid myositis (Mrak, 1982; Brumback and Staton, 1983; Job, 1994). We discuss sarcoid myositis in view of its practical interest in this section.

Sarcoid myositis

Based on data from several decades ago, an asymptomatic form of sarcoidosis is stated to occur in up to 50% of patients in the acute diagnostic stage of the disease. Serum CK activity is usually not raised, and it is only when a random muscle biopsy is taken that involvement of the musculature can be demonstrated by the presence of non-caseating granulomas with epitheloid cells and giant cells (Mastaglia and Walton, 1992). Data on MRI of this form of muscle involvement are not available yet. Symptomatic sarcoid myositis is very unusual. A focal or multifocal presenta-tion with swelling of one or both calves (or of the calves and thighs) or with nodules is observed occasionally (Douglas *et al.*, 1973; Jennekens and Kater, not published). Sarcoid myositis may also present with predominant proximal limb muscle weakness and, in some cases, involvement of the respiratory muscles including the diaphragm (Pringle and Dewar, 1997; Mozaffar *et al.*, 1998).

Diagnosis and management. Serum CK activity can be raised markedly and in these cases, electromyography reveals typical low-amplitude, short-motor unit potentials and spontaneous activity with fibrillation potentials and positive waves (see also section on *Electromyography*). Muscle biopsy may not only reveal cellular infiltration with noncaseating granulomas but also some degree of atrophy and necrosis of muscle fibres (Dewberry *et al.*, 1993; Fonseca *et al.*, 1993; Pringle and Dewar, 1997). Symptomatic sarcoid myositis is treated with corticosteroids (see Chapter 4).

ORBITAL MYOSITIS

Idiopathic orbital myositis
This disease has no sex preference and affects individuals of all ages, although there is a preference for young and middle-aged adults (see Scott and Siatkowski, 1997). The aetiology is not known; however, there are reports on a preceding upper airway infection in some cases, indicating that an abnormal reaction to an infection in perhaps genetically predisposed individuals might be involved. The association of idiopathic orbital myositis with other auto-immune diseases, in some cases, is also in favour of an auto-immune mechanism.

Onset varies from acute to insidious. Patients develop pain, diplopia, slight proptosis, eyelid oedema and periorbital oedema, chemosis, conjunctival injection and blepharoptosis, at one or both sides. In the acute phase, the involved muscles are paretic; in the chronic stage, they are not only paretic but inhibit by fibrosis movements in the opposite direction. The condition may be unilateral or bilateral. MRI reveals that involved extraocular muscles are enlarged (Fig. 6.14). Histological studies have shown that this is due to inflammatory infiltration of the affected muscles by predominantly mononuclear white blood cells and by oedema (Figs 6.15 and 6.16). Muscle fibres are damaged and at a later stage fibrosis follows.

Diagnosis and management. Diagnosis is based on the clinical features and the results of imaging. Idiopathic orbital myositis responds favourably to treatment with corticosteroids but may relapse.

Graves' ophthalmopathy
Graves' disease consists of a complex of three disorders: hyperthyroidism with goitre, ophthalmopathy, and dermopathy. Ophthalmopathy is usually bilateral but may be entirely unilateral, and is due to the inflammation of the elements in the orbita, excluding the eyeball. Antibodies against retro-orbital fibroblasts and eye muscles have been discovered and may be involved in the pathogenesis (Bahn and Heufelder, 1993). The three main clinical differences with idiopathic orbital myositis are (1) the more severe proptosis, (2) the optic neuritis and atrophy due to compression of the optic nerve by the swollen and inflamed content of the orbita, and (3) the lid retraction and lid lag, which can be improved by adrenergic antagonists

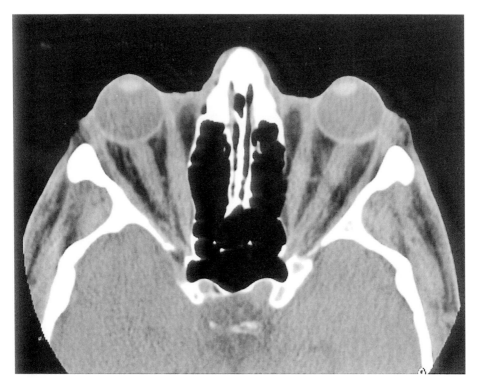

Figure 6.14 Enlargement of extraocular muscles by myositis. Compare with normal thickness of extraocular muscles in Fig. 5.3. Note also, proptosis. (Courtesy of Dr. Lino Ramos.)

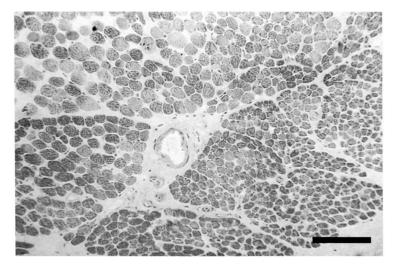

Figure 6.15 M. obliquus inferior. Transverse cryostat section of a control case, Gomori trichome. Bar: 100 μm. (Courtesy of Dr. Tjaard U Hoogenraad.)

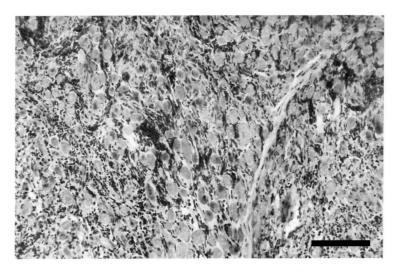

Figure 6.16 Orbital myositis. Transverse cryostat section of m obliquus inferior showing dense inflammatory infiltrate. H & E. Bar: 100 μm. (Courtesy of Dr. Tjaard U Hoogenraad.)

(Scott and Siatkowski, 1997). MRI and muscle biopsy confirm that eye muscles are enlarged and inflamed as in idiopathic orbital myositis (Figs 6.14–6.16).

Diagnosis and treatment. The differential diagnosis with idiopathic orbital myositis depends on the clinical features and the demonstration of thyroid diseases. Treatment is symptomatic, in mild cases; in severe cases, corticosteroids are given in doses of 1–2 mg prednisone/kg/day.

Acquired Brown syndrome
This is not a myositis but an inflammatory disorder of the posterior part of the superior oblique muscle tendon. The swelling impedes sliding of the tendon and as a consequence the affected eye cannot be raised sufficiently. Patients complain about vertical diplopia on upward and inward gaze. In some patients, gazing upward and inwardly gives rise to a palpable click, which is a sign that may be helpful for diagnosis. The swelling of the tendon has been visualized on CT scans. Acquired Brown syndrome has been described in patients with SLE (Chapter 7), RA, juvenile chronic arthritis, and adult Still's disease (Chapter 9). The syndrome may disappear spontaneously or can be treated with a non-steroidal anti-inflammatory drug (NSAIDs) or a low dose (20 mg/day) of prednisone.

FOCAL MYOSITIS

There are a number of local forms of myositis. All occur seldom but are worth knowing. Sarcoid and eosinophilic myositis may present with a local swelling or nodule(s) as described in the foregoing sections. Infectious disorders such as pyomyositis of bacterial origin and parasitic infections are, or can be, local (see this

Chapter, *Infectious Myositis*). Fasciitis, which is not a myositis but which may include a perimyositis and cause myopathic changes, is also a local disorder. The inflammatory changes in the underlying muscular tissue in local scleroderma are focal (see Chapter 10, *Localized Scleroderma*). Onset of polymyositis may be local (see below). There is, finally, an idiopathic genuine focal myositis that is different from all the foregoing conditions.

Focal myositis sensu stricti (ss)

Focal myositis, as described here, is a rare entity of unknown origin. It does not have a clear preference for a certain age or for one of the sexes. The most common presentation is a painful mass in one of the muscles of the lower limb that enlarges within a matter of months. There are several variations on this theme: enlargement can take place over a long time period – years instead of months; there can be several enlarging masses; or the enlarging masses can develop at other sites, *e.g.* in the abdomen, forearm, neck, tongue, or perioral muscle, and pain can be absent. Some patients have systemic symptoms (fever, raised ESR, and C-reactive protein) and slightly increased activity of serum CK, which may reflect the activity of the local process or predict progress to PM (Flaisler *et al.*, 1993; Marie *et al.*, 1998). MRI is more informative than CT and reveals muscle enlargement, fatty infiltration, and changes compatible with oedema. Histology shows a variable, often mild, degree of mononuclear, mainly lymphocytic infiltration; no invasion of healthy muscle fibres by inflammatory cells; no vasculitis; increased variation in fibre sizes with fibre hypertrophy and atrophy; fibre splitting; internal nuclei; fibre necrosis, which is usually not prominent; fibre regeneration; and some degree of vacuolation. Spontaneous remission is the rule, but chronic progression and relapses have been reported. In some patients, the mass has been removed surgically because of doubt on its benign nature (Caldwell *et al.*, 1995; Garcia-Consuegra *et al.*, 1995; Macchioni *et al.*, 1995; Mastaglia and Walton, 1992; Smith *et al.*, 1997). Treatment with a moderate dose of corticosteroids has a rapid beneficial effect on the pain and local swelling (Marie *et al.*, 1998).

SECONDARY FORMS OF MYOSITIS

DRUG-INDUCED MYOSITIS

D-penicillamine. In therapy with D-penicillamine, PM is a rare complication in genetically predisposed individuals (Swartz and Silver, 1984; Carrol *et al.*, 1987). Patients recover when the drug is withdrawn.

Simvastatine. Cholesterol-lowering hydroxymethylglutaryl co-enzyme A-reductase inhibitors, such as simvastatine and others, may induce an inflammatory myopathy, which may necessitate withdrawal of the drug (Giordano *et al.*, 1997).

Streptokinase. This is a thrombolytic agent with antigenic properties. Intravenous administration may lead to the formation of antibodies and to circulating immune complexes. Few patients develop 5–10 days or more after injection of streptokinase, fever, rash, arthralgia, arthritis, cutaneous vasculitis, glomerulonephritis, and myalgia or myositis. Myositis may cause proximal limb weakness and dysphagia predominantly. Serum CK activity is markedly raised and muscle biopsy shows necrotic muscle fibres, thickened arterioles with prominent endothelial cells, and mononuclear inflammatory cell infiltrates, often in a perivascular position. There is a favourable response to treatment with corticosteroids (Muzio *et al.*, 1997).

Other medical drugs. There are occasional reports on various forms of myositis in patients treated with penicillin, sulphonamides, propylthiouracil, cimetidine, procainamide hydralazine, phenytoin, mesantoin, and levodopa (see Argov and Mastaglia, 1994).

Ciguatera toxin. This toxin derives from the dinoflagellate *Gambierdiscus toxicus* and accumulates upwards in the marine food chain. Ciguatera poisoning in humans may occur by eating fish in tropical areas of the Pacific and Atlantic oceans. In the acute phase of intoxication, patients complain about myalgia and have a raised serum CK activity. A PM has been described in several individuals months to years after severe poisoning (Stommel and Parsonnet, 1993).

Contaminated L-tryptophan. The eosinophilia-myalgia syndrome is attributed to the tryptophan-dimer amino acid analogue, 1,1'ethylidene–bis–(L-tryptophan) (EBT). This product has been found in lots of L-tryptophan, destined for consumption by 1-tryptophan users. EBT stimulates fibroblast proliferation *in vitro* and increases collagen synthesis and α1-pro-collagen mRNA levels. It has also a strong effect on eosinophil-vascular cell interactions (see Varga and Kähäri, 1997).

Patients who have used EBT-containing L-tryptophan develop symptoms of myalgia, muscle weakness, cutaneous oedema and induration, paraesthesia, and other symptoms. They also show signs at examination of fasciitis, myopathy, neuropathy, and less often of disorders of other organs. Laboratory examination reveals a marked peripheral eosinophilia. Symptoms vanish at least in part when L-tryptophan is not used any more. Eosinophilia-myalgia closely resembles the toxic-oil syndrome.

INFECTIOUS MYOSITIS

Virus and myositis
Virus infections of muscle fibres have not been demonstrated despite systematic attempts by several groups. However, the association of viral infection with myositis is undeniable and is likely to be based on immunological mechanisms. The PM of human immunodeficiency virus (HIV) and human T-cell leukaemia-lymphoma virus type 1 (HTLV-1) infection is also virus-associated and not due to infection of muscle fibres (see for review Ytterberg, 1996). Viruses may elicit a sudden and unexpected rhabdomyolysis; the mechanism underlying this calamity is not clear (Singh and Scheid, 1996).

Bacterial infections

Borrelia burgdorferi. Myositis in Lyme disease is either localized near involved joints or skin or generalized as in DM. Muscle biopsies reveal inflammatory mononuclear cell infiltrations, and may demonstrate spirochaetes with immuno-gold staining. A case of rhabdomyolysis during *Borrelia burgdorferi* infection has been reported (Reimers *et al.*, 1993; Jeandel *et al.*, 1994).

Legionellosis. Myalgia and increased serum CK activity due to muscle fibre necrosis and inflammatory cell infiltrations in muscle are not uncommon in legionellosis (Warner *et al.*, 1991). Legionellosis is one of the most frequently reported causes of rhabdomyolysis (Singh and Scheid, 1996).

Bacterial rhabdomyolysis. Many bacteria can elicit a rhabdomyolysis. The pathogenesis is a mystery. See Singh and Scheid (1996) for a list of 20 different bacteria that have been associated with rhabdomyolysis.

Pyomyositis. This is a bacterial infection of skeletal muscle with abscess formation. Clinical manifestations of an abscess in a muscle are tenderness, swelling, induration, and overlying erythema as local symptoms. Fever and raised ESR are systemic phenomena. Imaging by CT or MRI can reveal fluid collection(s) and may thus facilitate the diagnosis. Pyomyositis is mostly caused by *Staphylococcus aureus* infection, and according to the literature, is not uncommon in tropical regions (Gordon *et al.*, 1995; Ytterberg, 1996). In Western countries, it occurs mostly in immunocompromised individuals (Carpenter and Karpati, 1984; Schwartzman *et al.*, 1991; Deodhar *et al.*, 1997). However, there are exceptions. Reports demonstrate pyomyositis in six children and two men caused by polymicrobial, anaerobic, *Streptococcus pneumoniae*, and other bacteria (Gamboa *et al.*, 1993; Gonzalez-Gay *et al.*, 1993; Brook, 1996). Treatment consists of drainage of the abscess and antibiotic medication.

Toxoplasmosis gondii infection
This is a complication in immunocompromised patients (Grove, 1988). Toxoplasma antibodies were previously stated to be more frequent in patients with PM and DM than in controls. However, more recent investigations lend no support to this claim (Pachman *et al.*, 1997).

Infections by fungi and helminths
For an extensive description of these disorders, the reader is referred to Banker (1994).

CONCLUSION

The inflammatory myopathies are far more heterogeneous than realized a decade ago. The primary, idiopathic disorders have to be distinguished from secondary diseases due to bacterial, fungal, or other infections and to toxic or drug-reaction. DM is likely to be primarily a vasculopathy and should probably be distinguished in intervention studies from inflammatory polymyositis, which is a true muscle disease. IBM is another true muscle disease and differs from PM in clinical and pathological features and in outcome. The incidence of IBM is higher than initially expected: it is probably the main form of myositis in middle-aged and old people. Patients with 'therapy resistant myositis' may be suffering from IBM.

REFERENCES

Airio A, Pukkala E and Isomaki H (1995) Elevated cancer incidence in patients with dermatomyositis – a population-based study. *J Rheumatol* **22**, 1300–1303.

Amato AA, Gronseth GS, Jackson CE *et al* (1996) Inclusion body myositis: Clinical and pathological boundaries. *Ann Neurol* **40**, 581–586.

Argov Z and Mastaglia FL (1994) Drug-induced neuromuscular disorder in man. In: Walton JN, Karpati G and Hilton-Jones D (eds) *Disorders of Voluntary Muscle*, 6ed, pp 989–1029. Edinburgh: Churchill Livingstone.

Askanas V (1997) New developments in hereditary inclusion body myopathies. *Ann Neurol* **41**, 421–422.

Askanas V, Alvarez RB, Mirabella M *et al* (1996) Use of anti-neurofilament antibody to identify paired-helical filaments in inclusion-body myositis. *Ann Neurol* **39**, 389–391.

Askanas V and Engel WK (1995) New advances in the understanding of sporadic inclusion-body myositis and hereditary inclusion body myopathies (Review). *Curr Opin Rheumatol* **7**, 486–496.

Askanas V, Engel WK and Alvarez RB (1993) Enhanced detection of congo red – positive amyloid deposits in muscle fibres of inclusion body myositis and brain of Alzheimer's disease using fluorescence technique. *Neurology* **43**, 1265–1267.

Askari AD and Huettner TL (1982) Cardiac abnormalities in polymyositis/dermatomyositis. *Semin Arthritis Rheum* **12**, 208–219.

Authier FJ, Kondo H, Ghnassia MD *et al* (1996) Necrotising myopathy with pipestem capillaries and minimal cellular infiltration: A case associated with cutaneous signs of dermatomyositis. *Neurology* **46**, 1448–1451.

Bahn RS and Heufelder AE (1993) Pathogenesis of Graves' ophthalmopathy. *N Engl J Med* **329**, 1468–1475.

Banker BQ (1994) Parasitic infections. In: Engel AG and Franzini-Armstrong C (eds) *Myology*, 2ed, pp 1438–1460. New York: McGraw-Hill.

Banker BQ and Victor M (1966) Dermatomyositis (systemic angiopathy) of childhood. *Medicine* **45**, 261–289.

Barkhaus PE, Nandekar SD and Sanders DB (1990) Qualitative EMG in inflammatory myopathy. *Muscle Nerve* **13**, 247–253.

Barohn RJ (1997) The therapeutic dilemma of inclusion body myositis. *Neurology* **48**, 567–568.

Barohn RJ, Amato AA, Sahenk Z *et al* (1995) Inclusion body myositis: Explanation for poor response to immunosuppressive therapy. *Neurology* **45**, 1302–1304.

Basta M and Dalakas MC (1994) High dose intravenous immunoglobulin exerts its beneficial effect in patients with dermatomyositis by blocking endomysial deposition of activated complement fragments. *J Clin Invest* **94**, 1729–1735.

Behan WHM, Behan PO and Doyle D (1982) Association of myasthenia gravis and polymyositis with neoplasia, infection and autoimmune disorders. *Acta Neuropathol* **57**, 221–229.

Block JA (1998) Hydroxychloroquine and retinal safety. *Lancet* **351**, 771.

Bloom BJ, Tucker LB, Miller LC *et al* (1995) Von Willebrand factor in juvenile dermatomyositis. *J Rheumatol* **22**, 30–35.

Bohan A and Peter JB (1975) Polymyositis and dermatomyositis. *N Engl J Med* **292**, 343–347.

Bohan A, Peter JB, Bohrman RL *et al* (1973) A computer assisted analysis of 153 patients with polymyositis and dermatomyositis. *Medicine* **56**, 255–286.

Bondeson J, Veress B, Lindroth Y *et al* (1998) Polymyositis associated with asymptomatic primary biliary cirrhosis. *Clin Exp Rheumatol* **16**, 172–174.

Brook I (1996) Pyomyositis in children caused by anaerobic bacteria. *J Pediatr Surg* **31**, 394–396.

Brumback RA and Staton RD (1983) Muscle granulomas after injection (letter). *Muscle Nerve* **6**, 387.

Caccamo DV, Keene CY, Durham J *et al* (1993) Fulminant rhabdomyolysis in a patient with dermatomyositis. *Neurology* **43**, 844–845.

Caldwell CJ, Swash M, Van Der Walt JD *et al* (1995) Focal myositis: A clinicopathological study. *Neuromusc Disord* **4**, 317–321.

Callen AM, Pachman LM, Hayford JR *et al* (1994) Intermittent high-dose intravenous methylprednisolone (IV pulse) therapy prevents calcinosis and shortens disease course in juvenile dermatomyositis. *Arthritis Rheum* **37**, R10.

Callen JF (1987) Dermatomyositis. *Neurol Clin* **5**, 379–403.

Carpenter S (1996) Inclusion body myositis, a review. *J Neuropath Exp Neurol* **55**, 1105–1114.

Carpenter S, Karpati G (1984) *Pathology of Skeletal Muscle*, pp 559–571. Edinburgh, Churchill Livingstone.

Carpenter S and Karpati G (1992) Coexistence of polymyositis (PM) with mitochondrial myopathy (MM). *Neurology* **42**, (Suppl), 388.

Carroll GJ, Will RK, Peter JB *et al* (1987) Penicillamine induced polymyositis and dermatomyositis. *J Rheumatol* **14**, 995–1001.

Cherin P, Herson S, Wechsler B *et al* (1991) Efficacy of intravenous gammaglobulin therapy in chronic refractory polymyositis and dermatomyositis: An open study with 20 adult patients. *Am J Med* **91**, 162–168.

Cherin P, Piette JC, Wechsler B *et al* (1994) Intravenous gamma globulin as first line therapy in polymyositis and dermatomyositis: An open study in 11 adult patients. *J Rheumatol* **21**, 1092–1097.

Chou S-M (1967) Myxovirus-like structures in a case of human chronic polymyositis. *Science* **158**, 1453–1455.

Cranney A, Markman S, Lach B *et al* (1997) Polymyositis in a patient with thymoma and T-cell lymphocytosis. *J Rheumatol* **24**, 1413–1416.

Crowson AN and Magro CM (1996) The role of microvascular injury in the pathogenesis of cutaneous lesions of dermatomyositis. *Hum Pathol* **27**, 15–19.

da Rocha G, Pinheiro C, Goldenberg J *et al* (1992) Juvenile dermatomyositis and pregnancy: Report and literature review. *J Rheumatol* **19**, 1798–1801.

Dahan V, Geny M and Frey G (1984) Association d'une polymyosite et d'une thyroidite auto-immune. *Presse Med* **13**, 563.

Dalakas MC (1991) Polymyositis, dermatomyositis and inclusion body myositis. *N Engl J Med* **325**, 1487–1498.

Dalakas MC, Illa I, Dambrosia JM *et al* (1993) A controlled trial of high-dose intravenous immune globulin infusions as treatment for dermatomyositis. *N Engl J Med* **329**, 1993–2000.

Dalakas MC, and Sivakumar K (1996) The immunopathologic and inflammatory differences between dermatomyositis, polymyositis and sporadic inclusion body myositis. *Curr Opin Neurol* **9**, 235–239.

Dalakas MC, Sonies B, Dambrosia J *et al* (1997) Treatment of inclusion body myositis with IVIG: a double blind placebo-controlled study. *Neurology* **48**, 712–716.

de Bleecker JL and Engel AG (1994) Expression of cell adhesion molecules in inflammatory myopathies and Duchenne dystrophy. *J Neuropathol Exp Neurol* **53**, 369–376.

Deodhar AA, Bruce MG, Krohn KD *et al* (1997) A case of secondary Sjögren's syndrome with a swollen thigh. *Ann Rheum Dis* **56**, 162–164.

de Visser M, Emslie-Smith AM and Engel AG (1989) Early ultrastructural alterations in adult dermatomyositis. Capillary abnormalities precede other structural changes in muscle. *J Neurol Sci* **94**, 181–192.

Dewberry RG, Schneider BF, Cale WF *et al* (1993) Sarcoid myopathy presenting with diaphragm weakness. *Muscle Nerve* **16**, 832–835.

Dietzman DE, Schaller JG, Ray CG *et al* (1976) Acute myositis associated with influenza B infection. *Pediatrs* **57**, 255–258.

Douglas AC, Macleod JG and Matthews JD (1973) Symptomatic sarcoidosis of skeletal muscle. *J Neurol Neurosurg Psychiat* **36**, 1034–1040.

Drake LA, Dinehart SM, Farmer ER *et al* (1996) Guidelines of care for dermatomyositis: American Academy of Dermatology. *J Am Acad Dermatol* **34**, 824–829.

Editorial (1983) The hypereosinophilic syndrome. *Lancet* **1**, 1417–1418.

Emslie-Smith AM and Engel AG (1990) Microvascular changes in early and advanced dermatomyositis: A quantitative study. *Ann Neurol* **27**, 343–356.

Emslie-Smith AM and Engel AG (1991) Necrotizing myopathy with pipestem capillaries, deposition of the complement membrane attack complex (MAC) and minimal cellular infiltration. *Neurology* **41**, 936–939.

Engel AG (1986) Duchenne dystrophy. In: Engel AG and Banker BQ (eds) *Myology*, pp 1185–1240. New York: McGraw-Hill.

Engel AG, Hohlfeld R and Banker BQ (1994) The polymyositis and dermatomyositis syndromes. In: Engel AG and Franzini-Armstrong C (eds) *Myology*, 2ed, pp 1335–1383. New York: McGraw-Hill.

Espino-Montoro A, Medina M, Martin-Martin J *et al* (1997) Idiopathic eosinophilic myositis associated with vasculitis and symmetrical polyneuropathy. *Brit J Rheumatol* **36**, 276–279.

Euwer RI and Sontheimer RD (1991) Amyopathic dermatomyositis (dermatomyositis sine myositis). *J Am Acad Dermatol* **24**, 959–966.

Fauci AS, Harley JB and Roberts WC (1982) The idiopathic hypereosinophilic syndrome: Clinical, pathophysiologic and therapeutic considerations. *Ann Intern Med* **97**, 78–92.

Feldman BM, Reichlin M, Laxer RM *et al* (1996) Clinical significance of specific auto-antibodies in juvenile dermatomyositis. *J Rheumatol* **23**, 1794–1797.

Flaisler F, Blin D, Asencio G *et al* (1993) Focal myositis. A localized form of polymyositis? *J Rheumatol* **20**, 1414–1416.

Fonseca GA, Baca S and Altman RD (1993) Acute myositis and dermatitis as the initial presentation of sarcoidosis. *Clin Exp Rheumatol* **11**, 553–556.

Gamboa F, Sanchez-Burson J, Gomez-Mateos J *et al* (1993) Bacterial pyomyositis due to *Streptococcus pneumoniae* in a previously healthy man. *Scand J Rheumatol* **24**, 396.

Garcia-Consuegra J, Moralis C, Gonzales J *et al* (1995) Relapsing focal myositis: A case report. *Clin Exp Rheum* **13**, 395–397.

Garlepp MJ (1996) Genetics of the idiopathic inflammatory myopathies. *Curr Opin Rheumatol* **8**, 514–520.

Garlepp MJ, Laing B, Zilko PJ *et al* (1994) HLA associations with inclusion body myositis. *Clin Exp Immunol* **98**, 40–45.

Giordano N, Senesi M, Mattii G *et al* (1997) Polymyositis associated with simvastitin. *Lancet* **349**, 1600–1601.

Gonzalez-Gay MA, Sanchez-Andrade A, Cereijo MJ *et al* (1993) Pyomyositis and septic arthritis from *Fusobacterium nucleatum* in a nonimmunocompromised adult. *J Rheumatol* **20**, 518–520.

Gordon BA, Martinez S and Collins AJ (1995) Pyomyositis. Characteristics at CT and MR imaging. *Radiology* **197**, 279–286.

Griggs R, Mendell J and Miller R (1994) *Evaluation and Treatment of Myopathies*. Philadelphia: FA Davis.

Griggs RC, Askanas V, DiMauro S *et al* (1995) Inclusion body myositis and myopathies. *Ann Neurol* **38**, 705–713.

Grove DI (1988) Parasitic and fungal infections of muscle. In: Mastaglia FL (ed) *Inflammatory Diseases of Muscle*, pp 164–184. Oxford: Blackwell Scientific Publications.

Gutierrez G, Dagnino R and Mintz G (1984) Polymyositis (dermatomyositis) and pregnancy. *Arthritis Rheum* **27**, 291–294.

Hassel B, Gilhus NE, Aarli JA *et al* (1992) Fulminant myasthenia gravis and polymyositis after thymectomy for thymoma. *Acta Neurol Scand* **85**, 63–65.

Haupt HM and Hutchins GM (1982) The heart and cardiac conduction system in polymyositis-dermatomyositis: A clinicopathologic study of 16 autopsied patients. *Am J Cardiol* **50**, 998–1006.

Hennekam RCM, Hiemstra I, Jennekens FGI *et al* (1990) Juvenile dermatomyositis in first cousins. *N Engl J Med* **23**, 199.

Hiketa T, Matsumoto Y, Ohashi M *et al* (1992) Juvenile dermatomyositis: A statistical study of 114 patients with dermatomyositis. *J Dermatol* **19**, 470–476.

Hochberg MC, Feldman D and Stevens MB (1986) Adult onset polymyositis/dermatomyositis: An analysis of clinical and laboratory features and survival in 76 patients with a review of the literature. *Sem Arthritis Rheum* **15**, 168–178.

Hohlfeld R, Engel AG and Goebels N (1997) Cellular immune mechanisms in inflammatory myopathies. *Curr Opin Rheumatol* **9**, 520–526.

Jeandel C, Perret C, Blain H *et al* (1994) Rhabdomyolysis with acute renal failure due to *Borrelia burgdorferi*. *J Int Med* **235**, 191–192.

Jennekens FGI, Kater L and Baart de la Faille H (1995) Dermatomyositis, polymyositis and inclusion body myositis. In: Kater L and Baart de la Faille H (eds) *Multi-Systemic Autoimmune Diseases*, pp 241–265. Amsterdam: Elsevier.

Job CK (1994) Pathology of leprosy. In: Hastings RC (ed) *Leprosy*, 2ed, pp 193–224. Edinburgh: Churchill Livingstone.

Joffe MM, Love LA, Leff RL *et al* (1993) Drug therapy of the idiopathic inflammatory myopathies: Predictors of response to prednisolone, azathioprine and methotrexate and a comparison of their efficacy. *Am J Med* **94**, 379–387.

Jongen PJ, ter Laak HJ and Stadhouders AM (1995) Rimmed vacuoles and filamentous inclusions in neuromuscular disorders. *Neuromusc Disord* **5**, 31–38.

Kaipainen-Seppanen O and Savolainen A (1996) Incidence of chronic juvenile rheumatic diseases in Finland during 1980–1990. *Clin Exp Rheumatol* **14**, 441–444.

Kasteler JS and Callen JP (1997) Low-dose methotrexate administered weekly is an effective corticosteroid-sparing agent for the treatment of the cutaneous manifestations of dermatomyositis. *J Am Acad Dermatol* **36**, 67–71.

Kavanagh GM, Colaco MB and Kennedy CTC (1993) Juvenile dermatomyositis associated with partial lipoatrophy. *J Am Acad Dermatol* **28**, 348–351.

Kaufman LD, Kephart GM, Seidman RJ *et al* (1993) The spectrum of eosinophilic myositis. *Arthritis Rheum* **36**, 1014–1023.

Kissel JT, Mendell JR and Rammohan KW (1986) Microvascular deposition of complement membrane attack complex in dermatomyositis. *N Engl J Med* **314**, 329–334.

Kissel JT, Halterman RK, Rammohan KW *et al* (1991) The relationship of complement-mediated microvascularity to the histologic features and clinical duration of disease in dermatomyositis. *Arch Neurol* **48**, 26–30.

Koh ET, Scow A and Ong B (1993) Adult onset polymyositis/dermatomyositis: Clinical and laboratory features in 75 patients. *Ann Rheum Dis* **52**, 857–861.

Laxer RM and Feldman BM (1997) General and local scleroderma in children and dermatomyositis and associated syndromes. *Curr Opin Rheumatol* **9**, 458–464.

Lee W, Zimmerman B and Lally EV (1997) Relapse of polymyositis after prolonged remission. *J Rheumatol* **24**, 1641–1644.

Leaute-Labreze C, Perel Y and Taieb A (1995) Childhood dermatomyositis associated with hepatocarcinoma. *N Engl J Med* **333**, 1083.

Leff RL, Love LA, Miller FW *et al* (1992) Viruses in idiopathic inflammatory myopathies: Absence of candidate viral genomes in muscle. *Lancet* **339**, 1192–1195.

Leff RL, Miller FW and Hicks *et al* (1993) The treatment of inclusion body myositis: A review and a randomized prospective trial of immunosuppressive therapy. *Medicine* **72**, 225–235.

Lennon VA, Krijzer TJ, Griesman GE *et al* (1995) Calcium channel antibodies in the Lambert-Eaton syndrome and other paraneoplastic syndrome. *N Engl J Med* **332**, 1467–1474.

Leon-Monzon M and Dalakas MC (1992) Absence of persistent infection with enteroviruses in muscles of patients with inflammatory myopathies. *Ann Neurol* **32**, 219–222.

Lindberg C, Persson LI, Bjorkander J *et al* (1994) Inclusion body myositis: Clinical, morphological, physiological and laboratory findings in 18 cases. *Acta Neurol Scand* **89**, 123–131.

Louwerse ES, Weverling GJ, Bossuyt PMM *et al* (1995) Randomized double-blind controlled trial of acetylcysteine in amyotrophic lateral sclerosis. *Arch Neurol* **52**, 559–564.

Lotz BP, Engel AG, Nishino H *et al* (1989) Inclusion body myositis. Observations in 40 patients. *Brain* **112**, 727–747.

Luciano CA and Dalakas MC (1997) Inclusion body myositis: No evidence for a neurogenic component. *Neurology* **48**, 29–33.

Macchioni P, Boiard L, Meliconi R *et al* (1995) Immunohistochemical analysis of an additional case of focal myositis. *Clin Exp Rheumatol* **13**, 753–757.

Maddison PJ and Jablonska S (1995) Overlap syndromes. In: Kater L and Baart de la Faille H (eds) *Multi-Systemic Autoimmune Diseases*, pp 227–240. Amsterdam: Elsevier.

Manchul LA, Jin A, Pritchard KI *et al* (1985) The frequency of malignant neoplasm in patients with polymyositis-dermatomyositis. *Arch Intern Med* **145**, 1835–1839.

Marie I, Cardon T, Hachulla E *et al* (1998) Magnetic resonance imaging in focal myositis. *J Rheumatol* **25**, 378–382.

Mastaglia FL and Ojeda VJ (1985a) Inflammatory myopathies: Part 1. *Ann Neurol* **17**, 215–227.

Mastaglia FL and Ojeda VJ (1985b) Inflammatory myopathies: Part 2. *Ann Neurol* **17**, 317–323.

Mastaglia FL and Walton JN (1992) Inflammatory myopathies. In: Mastaglia FL and Walton JN (eds) *Skeletal Muscle Pathology*, 2ed, pp 453–491. Edinburgh: Churchill Livingstone.

Mastaglia FL, Phillips BA and Zilko P (1997) Treatment of inflammatory myopathies. *Muscle Nerve* **20**, 651–664.

Maugars YM, Berthelot JMM, Abbas AA *et al* (1996) Long-term prognosis of 69 patients with dermatomyositis or polymyositis. *Clin Exp Rheumatol* **14**, 263–274.

Mease PJ, Ochs HD and Wedgewood RJ (1981) Successful treatment of echovirus meningo-encephalitis and myositis-fascitis with intravenous immuno globulin therapy in a patient with X-linked agammaglobulinaemia. *N Engl J Med* **304**, 1278–1281.

Medsger TA Jr, Dawson WN and Masi AT (1970) The epidemiology of polymyositis. *Am J Med* **48**, 715–723.

Mendell JR and Florence J (1990) Manual muscle testing. *Muscle Nerve* (Suppl) S16–S20.

Mendell JR, Sahenk Z, Gales T *et al* (1991) Amyoid filaments in inclusion body myositis: Novel findings provide insight into nature of filaments. *Arch Neurol* **48**, 1229–1234.

Mendell JR, Garcha TS and Kissel JT (1996) The immunopathogenetic role of complement in human muscle disease. *Curr Opin Neurol* **9**, 226–234.

Mierau R, Dick T, Bartz-Barronella P *et al* (1996) Strong association of dermatomyositis specific Mi-2 autoantibodies with a tryptophan at position 9 of the HLA-DR β chain. *Arthritis Rheum* **39**, 868–876.

Miller FW (1993) Myositis-specific autoantibodies: Touchstones for understanding the inflammatory myopathies. *JAMA* **270**, 1846–1849.

Miller RG and Kiprov D (1984) Polymyositis and benign gammopathy: A new syndrome? (abstract). *Neurology* **34** (Suppl 1), 191.

Miller FW, Leitman SF, Cronin ME *et al* (1992) Controlled trial of plasma exchange and leukapheresis in polymyositis and dermatomyositis. *N Engl J Med* **326**, 1380–1384.

Mozaffar T, Lopate G, Pestronk A (1998) Clinical correlates of granuloma in muscle. *J Neurol* **245**, 519–524.

Mrak RE (1982) Muscle granulomas following intramuscular injection. *Muscle Nerve* **5**, 637.

Munsat TL (1986) Facioscapulohumeral dystrophy and the scapuloperoneal syndrome. In: Engel AG, Banker BQ (eds) *Myology*, pp 1251–1266. New York: McGraw-Hill.

Muzio A, Guglielmo G, Feliciani C *et al* (1997) Inflammatory myopathy after intravenous streptokinase. *Muscle Nerve* **20**, 619–621.

Nagar H and Bar-Ziv Y (1993) Focal eosinophilic myositis: Unusual cause of a tumour on the chest wall. *Eur J Surg* **159**, 187–188.

Nishikai M, Ohya K, Kosaka M *et al* (1998) Anti-Jo-1 antibodies in polymyositis and dermatomyositis: Evaluation by ELISA using recombinant fusion protein Jo-1 as antigen. *Brit J Rheumatol* **37**, 357–361.

Norris AL (1989) Juvenile dermatomyositis. *Med Clin N Amer* **73**, 1193–1209.

Oldfors A, Larsson N-G, Lindberg C *et al* (1993) Mitochondrial DNA deletions in inclusion body myositis. *Brain* **116**, 325–336.

Otero C and Dalakas MC (1992) Is there dermatomyositis (DM) without myositis? *Neurology* **43**, (Suppl) 388.

Pachman LM (1995) Imperfect indications of disease activity in juvenile dermatomyositis. *J Rheumatol* **22**, 193–196.

Pachman LM (1986) Juvenile dermatomyositis. *Paed Clin N Amer* **33**, 1097–1117.

Pachman LM, Hayford JR, Hochberg MC *et al* (1997) New onset juvenile dermatomyositis. Comparison with a healthy cohort and children with juvenile rheumatoid arthritis. *Arthritis Rheum* **40**, 1526–1533.

Pachman LM, Hayford JR, Chung A *et al* (1998) Juvenile dermatomyositis at diagnosis: Clinical characteristics of 79 children. *J Rheumatol* **25**, 1198–1204.

Papapetropoulos T, Kanellakopoulos N, Tsibri E *et al* (1998) Polymyositis and pregnancy: report of a case with three pregnancies. *J Neurol Neurosurg Psychiat* **64**, 406.

Park JH, Olsen NJ, King L Jr *et al* (1995) Use of magnetic resonance imaging and P-31 magnetic resonance spectroscopy to detect and quantify muscle dysfunction in the amyopathic and myopathic variants of dermatomyositis. *Arthritis Rheum* **38**, 68–77.

Parker P, Chao NJ, Ben-Ezra J *et al* (1996) Polymyositis as a manifestation of chronic graft-versus-host disease. *Medicine* **75**, 279–285.

Parker PM, Openshaw H and Forman SJ (1997) Myositis associated with graft-versus-host disease. *Curr Opin Rheumatol* **9**, 513–519.

Pegoraro E, Mancias P, Swerdlow SH *et al* (1996) Congenital muscular dystrophy with primary laminin alpha2 (merosin) deficiency presenting as inflammatory myopathy. *Ann Neurol* **40**, 782–791.

Plotz PH (1989) Current concepts in the idiopathic inflammatory myopathies: Polymyositis, dermatomyositis and related disorders. *Ann Intern Med* **111**, 143–157.

Plotz PH (1995) Myositis: Immunologic contributions to understanding cause, pathogenesis and therapy. *Ann Int Med* **122**, 715–724.

Pringle CE and Dewar CL (1997) Respiratory muscle involvement in severe sarcoid myositis. *Muscle Nerve* **20**, 379–381.

Provost TT and Kater L (1995) Guidelines for the clinical application of immunologic laboratory investigations. In: Kater L and Baart de la Faille H (eds) *Multisystem Autoimmune Diseases: An Integrated Approach*, pp 61–84. Amsterdam: Elsevier.

Reed AM, Pachman LM and Ober C (1991) Molecular genetic studies of major histocompatibility complex genes in children with juvenile dermatomyositis: Increased risk associated with HLA-DQA1*0501. Hum Immunol **32**, 235–240.

Reimers CD and Finkenstaedt M (1997) Muscle imaging in inflammatory myopathies. *Curr Opin Rheumatol* **9**, 475–485.

Reimers CD, de Koning J, Neubert U *et al* (1993) *Borrelia burgdorferi* myositis: Report of eight patients. *J Neurol* **240**, 278–283.

Reimers CD, Schedel H, Fleckenstein JL *et al* (1994) Magnetic resonance imaging of skeletal muscles in idiopathic inflammatory myopathies of adults. *J Neurol* **241**, 306–314.

Rider LG (1995) Childhood myositis: Newly recognized diversity. In: Plotz PH (moderator) *Myositis: Immunologic Contributions to Understanding Cause, Pathogenesis And Therapy*. Ann Intern Med **122**, 715–724.

Riminton DS, Chambers ST, Parkin PJ *et al* (1993) Inclusion body myositis presenting solely as dysphagia. *Neurology* **43**, 1241–1243.

Rockerbie NH, Woo TY, Callen JP *et al* (1989) Cutaneous changes of dermatomyositis precede muscle weakness. *J Am Acad Dermatol* **20**, 629–632.

Robinson LR (1991) AAEM Case report polymyositis. *Muscle Nerve* **14**, 310–315.

Roddy SM, Ashwal S, Peckham N *et al* (1986) Infantile myositis: A case diagnosed in the neonatal period. *Pediatr Neurol* **2**, 241–244.

Roux S, Seelig H-P and Meyer O (1998) Significance of Mi-2 autoantibodies in polymyositis and dermatomyositis. *J Rheumatol* **25**, 395–396.

Rowland LP, Lisak RL, Schotland DL *et al* (1973) Myasthenic myopathy and thymoma. *Neurology* **23**, 282–288.

Rugiero M, Koffman B and Dalakas MC (1995) Association of inclusion body myositis with autoimmune diseases and autoantibodies (abstract). *Ann Neurol* **38**, 333.

Sansome A and Dubowitz V (1995) Intravenous immunoglobulin in juvenile dermatomyositis – four year review of nine cases. *Arch Dis Child* **72**, 24–28.

Schwartzman WA, Lamperts MW, Kennedy CA *et al* (1991) Staphylococcal pyomyositis in patients infected with the human immunodeficiency virus. *Am J Med* **90**, 595–600.

Scott IU and Siatkowski RM (1997) Idiopathic orbital myositis. *Curr Opin Rheumatol* **9**, 496–535.

See Y, Martin K, Rooney M *et al* (1997) Severe juvenile dermatomyositis complicated by pancreatitis. *Brit J Rheumatol* **36**, 912–916.

Seelig HP, Moosbrugger I, Ehrfeld H *et al* (1995) The major dermatomyositis specific Mi-2 autoantigen is a presumed helicase involved in transcriptional activities. *Arthritis Rheum* **38**, 1389–1399.

Sekul EA, Chow C and Dalakas MC (1997) Magnetic resonance imaging of the forearm as a diagnostic aid in patients with sporadic inclusion body myositis. *Neurology* **48**, 863–866.

Serratrice G, Pelissier MD, Roux H *et al* (1990) Fasciitis, perimyositis, myositis, polymyositis and eosinophilia. *Muscle Nerve* **13**, 385–395.

Sherry DD, Haas JE and Milstein JM (1993) Childhood polymyositis as paraneoplastic phenomenon. *Pediatr Neurol* **9**, 155–156.

Shulman IE (1975) Diffuse fasciitis with eosinophilia: A new syndrome. *Transactions of the Association of American Physicians* **88**, 70–86.

Sigurgeirsson B, Lindelof B, Edhag O *et al* (1992) Risk of cancer in patients with dermatomyositis or polymyositis. A population-based study. *N Engl J Med* **326**, 363–367.

Singh U and Scheid WM (1996) Infectious etiologies of rhabdomyolysis: Three case reports and review. *Clin Infect Dis* **22**, 642–649.

Singsen BH, Bernstein BH, Kornreich HK *et al* (1977) Mixed connective tissue disease in childhood. A clinical and serologic survey. *J Pediatr* **90**, 893–900.

Sivakumar K, Semino-Mora C and Dalakas MC (1997) An inflammatory familiar inclusion body myositis with autoimmune features and a phenotype identical to sporadic inclusion body myositis. *Brain* **120**, 653–661.

Smith AG, Blaivas M, Russell JW *et al* (1997) Clinical and pathological features of focal myositis. Abstract. *Ann Neurol* **42**, 414.

Sonies BC (1997) Evaluation and treatment of speech and swallowing disorders associated myopathies. *Curr Opin Rheumatol* **9**, 486–495.

Spector SA, Koffman BM, Feuerstein IM *et al* (1997) Safety and efficacy of strength training in patients with sporadic inclusion body myositis. *Muscle Nerve* **20**, 1242–1248.

Spuler S, Engel AG (1997) SMI-3 immunoreactivity in inclusion body myositis. *Ann Neurol* **42**, 185.

Stommel EW and Parsonnet J (1993) Another case of polymyositis after ciguatera toxin exposure. *Arch Neurol* **50**, 571.

Stonecipher MR, Jorizzo JL, White WL *et al* (1993) Cutaneous changes of dermatomyositis in patients with normal muscle enzymes: Dermatomyositis sine myositis? *J Am Acad Dermatol* **28**, 95–96.

Swartz M, Silver R (1984) D-penicillamine induced polymyositis in juvenile chronic arthritis: report of a case. *J Rheumatol* **11**, 250–251.

Symmons DPM, Sills JA and Davis SM (1995) The incidence of juvenile dermatomyositis. Results from a nation-wide study. *Brit J Rheumatol* **34**, 732–736.

Tanimoto K, Nakano K, Kano S *et al* (1995) Classification criteria for polymyositis and dermatomyositis. *J Rheumatol* **22**, 668–674.

Targoff IN (1998) Polymyositis and dermatomyositis in adults. In: Maddison PJ, Iserberg DA, Woo P *et al* (eds) *Oxford Textbook of Rheumatology*, 2ed, pp 1249–1287. Oxford: Oxford University Press.

Targoff IN (1995) Humoral autoimmunity in myositis: The myositis-specific-autoantibodies. In: Plotz PH (moderator) *Myositis: Immunologic Contributions to Understanding Cause, Pathogenesis and Therapy*. *Ann Int Med* **122**, 715–724.

Targoff IN, Miller FW, Medsger TA *et al* (1997) Classification criteria for the idiopathic myopathies. *Curr Opin Rheumatol* **9**, 527–535.

Tazelaar HD, Viggiano RW, Pickersgill J *et al* (1990) Interstitial lung disease in polymyositis and dermatomyositis: Clinical features and prognosis as correlated with histologic findings. *Am Rev Resp Dis* **141**, 727–733.

Telerman-Toppet N, Wittek M, Bacq M *et al* (1982) Benign monoclonal gammopathy and relapsing polymyositis. *Muscle Nerve* **5**, 490–491.

Uthman I, Vazquez-Abad D and Senecal JL (1996) Distinctive features of idiopathic inflammatory myopathies in French Canadians. *Sem Arthritis Rheum* **26**, 447–458.

van der Kooi AJ, Ginjaar HB, Busch HFM *et al* (1998) Limb girdle muscular dystrophy: A pathological and immunohistochemical re-evaluation. *Muscle Nerve* **21**, 584–590.

van der Meulen MFG, Hoogendijk JE, Jansen GH *et al* (1998a) Absence of characteristic features in two patients with inclusion body myositis. *J Neurol Neurosurg Psychiat* **64**, 396–401.

van der Meulen MFG, Hoogendijk JE, Wokke JHJ *et al* (1998b) Pulsed high-dose dexamethason therapy for myositis; An uncontrolled pilot study. Abstract. *J Neurol* **245**, 414.

van Rossum MAJ, Hiemstra I, Rijkers GT *et al* (1994) Juvenile dermato/polymyositis: A retrospective analysis of 33 cases with special focus on initial CPK levels. *Clin Ex Rheumatol* **12**, 339–342.

Varga J and Kähäri VM (1997) Eosinophilia-myalgia syndrome, eosinophilic fasciitis and related fibrosing disorders. *Curr Opin Rheumatol* **9**, 562–570.

Varga J, Heimann-Patterson T, Munoz S *et al* (1993) Myopathy with mitochondrial alterations in patients with primary biliary cirrhosis and mitochondrial antibodies. *Arthritis Rheum* **36**, 1468–1475.

Vazquez-Abad D and Rothfield NF (1996) Sensitivity and specificity of anti-Jo-1 antibodies in autoimmune diseases with myositis. *Arthritis Rheum* **39**, 292–296.

Verschuuren JJ, Badrising UA, Wintzen AR *et al* (1997) Inclusion body myositis. In: Emery AEH (ed) *Diagnostic Criteria for Neuromuscular Disorders*, 2nd ed, pp 81–84. London: Royal Society of Medicine Press.

Voll C, Ang LC, Sibley J *et al* (1993) Polymyositis with plasma cell infiltrate in essential mixed cryo-globulinaemia. *J Neurol Neurosurg Psychiat* **56**, 317–318.

Warner CL, Fayad PB and Heffner RH (1991) Legionella myositis. *Neurology* **41**, 751–752.

Whitaker JN and Engel WK (1972) Vascular deposits of immunoglobulin and complement in idiopathic inflammatory myopathy. *N Engl J Med* **286**, 333–338.

Whitmore E, Watson R, Rosenshein NB *et al* (1996) Dermatomyositis sine myositis: Association with malignancy. *J Rheumatol* **23**, 101–105.

Whitmore SE, Rosenshein NB and Provost TT (1994) Ovarian cancer in patients with dermatomyositis. *Medicine* **73**, 153–160.

Weitoft T (1997) Occurrence of polymyositis in the county of Gävleborg, Sweden. *Scand J Rheumatol* **26**, 104–106.

Wintzen AR, Bots GTAM, de Bakker HM *et al* (1988) Dysphagia in inclusion body myositis. *J Neurol Neurosurg Psychiat* **51**, 1542–1545.

Yeo LMW, Swaby DSA, Situnayake RD *et al* (1995) Irreversible visual loss in dermatomyositis. *Brit J Rheumatol* **34**, 1179–1181.

Ytterberg SR (1996) Infectious agents associated with myopathies. *Curr Opin Rheumatol* **8**, 507–513.

Yunis EJ and Samaha FJ (1971) Inclusion body myositis. *Lab Invest* **25**, 240–248.

Zantos D, Zhang Y, Felson D *et al* (1994) The overall and temporal association of cancer with polymyositis and dermatomyositis. *J Rheumatol* **21**, 1855–1859.

7

Systemic Lupus Erythematosus

INTRODUCTION

SLE is a complex, multisystemic auto-immune disease of uncertain origin with variable clinical presentation and variable course. A multitude of circulating antibodies is often present, and some of them are specific for SLE. There is not one simple criterion for the diagnosis; instead, a panel of clinical and laboratory characteristics is decisive. As known from previous reviews, a surprising number of psychiatrical and neurological disorders may complicate the disease (Johnson and Richardson, 1968; Feinglass et al., 1976; Futrell et al., 1992; Schur, 1996). This chapter intends to cover all the manifestations of SLE in the nervous system and the skeletal musculature. The first part contains a short introduction to the disease. The second part deals with the psychiatrical and neurological manifestations.

SHORT GENERAL DESCRIPTION OF SLE

EPIDEMIOLOGY

Figures for prevalence of SLE disease vary from approximately 20 to 50/100 000, and vary for incidence from 2 to 7/100 000/year (Schur, 1996; Baart de la Faille and Kater, 1995; Johnson et al., 1995; McCarthy et al., 1995; Felson, 1997; Rothfield, 1997). A substantial number of patients escape diagnosis (Johnson et al., 1996). The incidence and prevalence were found to be much higher in Afro-Caribbean, Afro-American, and Asian groups than in Caucasians, at least in the USA and the UK (McCarthy et al., 1995; Johnson et al., 1995). It is not clear whether this is fully due to genetic factors or to socio-economic circumstances in part (Hopkinson, 1992). SLE affects predominantly females in their reproductive years (female:male ratio for adults is about 9:1). In childhood, the preponderance of affected females in comparison to males is less striking than in adults (ratio 3:1). The onset of SLE in approximately 15% of patients is between 5 and 16 years (mean age at onset 12–13 years).

AETIOLOGY AND PATHOGENESIS

As already stated, the origin is still unknown, but genetic, immunological, hormonal and environmental factors all play a role (see Baart de la Faille and Kater, 1995; Schur, 1996; Rothfield, 1997). The concordance of SLE in monozygotic twins is high. Various subgroups of patients have been identified in which genetic molecular defects are associated with disease expression (Duits *et al.*, 1995; Salmon *et al.*, 1996). Among first degree relatives, the frequency of SLE, auto-antibodies, and T-suppressor cell defects is increased. The increased prevalence of SLE in females during their reproductive years and in patients suffering from Klinefelter's syndrome suggests a role for hormonal factors. Sunlight may induce onset of clinical symptoms or may cause exacerbation of the disease. This is explainable by the induction of apoptosis of keratinocytes by ultraviolet irradiation and the release of auto-antigens from these keratinocytes. The latter gives rise to activation of both T- and B-cells (Casciola *et al.*, 1994).

Why and how all these different defects arise and interact in causing the clinical manifestations of SLE is not easy to establish. Several or all of the following factors play a role in the mechanisms underlying SLE: auto-antibodies cross-reacting with different tissue components, immune complexes, deficiency of complement components, abnormal handling of immune complexes, polyclonal B-cell activation, deficient activity of T-suppressor cells, activation of other T-cells, and abnormal cytokine production (see Baart de la Faille and Kater, 1995; Kater *et al.*, 1995).

PATHOLOGY

SLE is above all a disease of vessels, mainly small vessels (Johnson and Richardson, 1968). Sometimes inflammatory cells, mainly lymphocytes, are infiltrated in the vessel walls. In other cases, endothelial cells are swollen and proliferated, fibrin is deposited, or there is fibrinoid or hyalin degeneration, fibroblast proliferation, or fibrosis and thrombosis.

The mechanisms underlying these processes are far from clear. Immune complex deposition, including complexes which contain antibodies to DNA, plays a role in inducing the vasculitic lesions. Upregulation of adhesion molecules on endothelial cell surfaces, the counterparts of the adhesion molecules of neutrophilic granulocytes, and increased adhesiveness of leukocytes may lead to occlusion ('leuko-occlusion') of small vessels (Belmont *et al.*, 1996). Endothelial cell activation can also give rise to expression of membrane–associated, coagulation proteins that may become the target of antiphospholipid (APL) antibodies and thereby lead to thrombosis. The role of APL antibodies will be mentioned at several places in this chapter and will be discussed *in extenso* in Chapter 8.

CLINICAL MANIFESTATIONS

Nearly all body organs can be affected, albeit not all of them with the same frequency or to the same extent. The prevalence and characteristics of the clinical and laboratory features of the disease were assessed in a large prospective study of 1000 patients (Cervera *et al.*, 1993). Unless otherwise stated the percentages given in the following are from that study.

At onset and during exacerbations, patients often experience malaise and develop fever. During the course of the disease, the clinical picture may become very complex with symptoms from a variable number of organs.

Arthritis
This is the most frequent manifestation at onset (49% of patients) and one of the most frequent during the course of the disease (84%). Arthritis in SLE differs from rheumatoid arthritis (RA) by rarely causing any irreversible changes (as Jaccoud's arthropathy), by being transient and sometimes asymmetrical, by not causing significant destruction of cartilage and bone, and by not having any preference for the cervical spine. All small and large joints of the limbs may become affected. Affected joints are painful, especially during movements, and joints and periarticular tissue tend to swell by effusion of fluid.

Skin lesions
These occur during the course of the disease in approximately 85–90% of patients. At onset, a rash in butterfly distribution is present on the face in approximately 50% of patients, and widespread lesions may appear elsewhere, either acute or subacute, predominantly in sun-exposed skin (Fig. 7.1). The lesions are erythematous at the edge, may be slightly scaly, tend to be annular in shape, and leave no scars. In some cases, the lesions are erythemato-papular. A discoid lesion consisting of an erythematous plaque raised at the periphery, spreading outward with a central depressed area of hyperkeratosis leaving atrophic scar-like tissue when healing, may be the sole manifestation of the disease for a long time (Fig. 7.2). A wide range of other skin lesions may develop: a maculo-papular eruption resembling a drug-eruption, alopecia, vasculitic skin lesions with periungual erythema or ulcerations, livedo reticularis, periorbital oedema, bullae, petechiae or ecchymosis, panniculitis, and others. Oral ulcers are common and appear at exacerbation of the disease; they are localized on the palatum and on the buccal, nasal, pharyngeal, and laryngeal mucosa. Erythematous and discoid lesions can occur also in the oral cavity.

Nephropathy
This is a frequent and serious complication, occurring in 16% from onset of the disease and in 39% (Cervera *et al.*, 1993) to 50% (our view) during the course of the disease. The onset is mostly insidious and the course chronic, but an acute onset and a rapid progressive course occur occasionally (Churg and Sobin, 1982). Hypertension of renal origin and endstage uraemia may cause neurological disorders.

Serositis
Pericarditis and pleuritis may each be present at onset (17%), and occur in approximately 40–60% during the course of the disease. Pericarditis is often mild or subclinical, but can be life threatening. It causes precordial, retrosternal, or substernal pain. Pain is aggravated by coughing, swallowing, and twisting or bending. Pleuritis can cause unilateral or bilateral chest pain. Abdominal serositis has been documented also (Miller *et al.*, 1984).

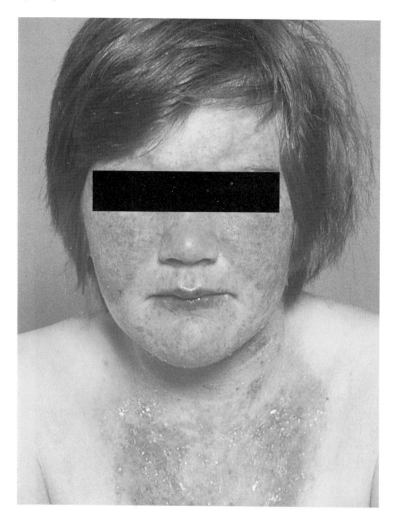

Figure 7.1 Malar and photosensitive dermatitis in a patient with acute SLE. [From Baart de la Faille and Kater (1995), with permission.]

Vasculitis, vasculopathy and vasospasm

The tendency to atherosclerosis seems to be increased. This has been concluded on the basis of post-mortem investigations of coronary vessels and laboratory studies of SLE sera. The raised tendency is likely to be due to the disease itself, to the medication (corticosteroids!), or both and may explain, in part, the increased frequency of vessel occlusion in SLE. APL antibodies are also associated with an increased tendency to arterial and venous occlusions and are frequent in patients with SLE (Love and Santoro, 1990; Derksen and Stephens, 1995; see also Chapter 8).

Vasculitis is generally considered to be due to deposition of immune complexes on endothelial cells and subsequent attraction of inflammatory cells. The vessel walls are damaged and this in turn can lead to thrombosis and obstruction of the

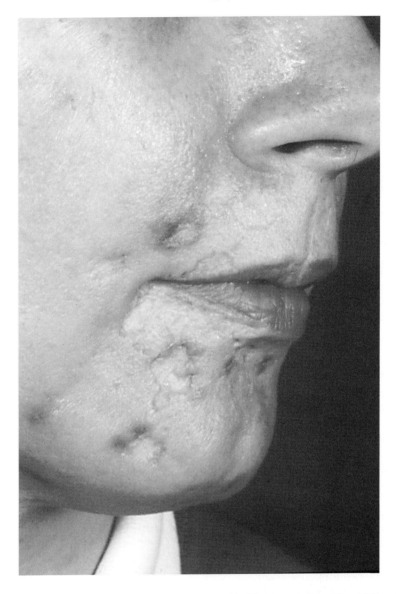

Figure 7.2 Deep atrophic patches on the chin; 'wolf'. (Courtesy of Dr. Harold Baart de la Faille.)

vessel lumina. The prevalence of arteritis has been overestimated in the past due to confusion with other forms of vasculopathy.

Raynaud's phenomenon (attacks of pallor due to vasospasm in the fingers and toes at exposure to cold or emotional stimuli) occurs in approximately 40% of patients with SLE. Exposure of digits to the cold causes, in occasional patients, vasospasm also in the lungs or heart, and this may then lead to symptoms of dyspnoea and angina (Kallenberg and Callen, 1995).

Lungs
Pulmonary embolism is associated with recurrent deep venous thrombosis (DVT). Recurrent thromboembolism can lead to pulmonary hypertension. 'Interstitial lung disease' is pathologically characterized by interstitial fibrosis and inflammation. Patients complain about non-productive cough and shortness of breath at exertion. The prevalence of this complication in SLE is low (3%). Some patients are dyspnoic due to diaphragmatic weakness of uncertain origin.

Heart
SLE can affect all layers of the heart, including the coronary arteries. It is important to distinguish primary SLE effects from secondary manifestations, *e.g.* those due to atherosclerosis, hypertension, and infective endocarditis. Pericarditis is the most common cardial manifestation of SLE and has already been mentioned under *serositis*. Libman-Sachs endocarditis is the classic cardiac lesion in SLE and consists of single vegetations – or conglomerates of vegetations – that adhere to the endocardium, mostly at the mitral valves. Other valvular abnormalities, such as aortic and mitral insufficiency occur as well. The frequency of coronary heart disease is increased (see also Chapter 8).

Haematologic disorders
Auto-immune haemolytic anaemia, drug-induced haemolytic anaemia, drug-induced normochromic anaemia, pernicious anaemia, and non-immune mediated anaemias related to chronic disease occur, all together, in approximately 70% of SLE patients. Leukocytopenia (predominantly lymphocytopenia) is also frequent (prevalence 65%) but not very severe: leukocyte counts of less than 2000/mm^3 are rare. The figures on the prevalence of thrombocytopenia vary from 7–52%.

Psychiatrical, neurological and muscular disorders
These will be dealt with in the second part of this chapter.

Other organs
The gastrointestinal tract does not escape from SLE. Abdominal pain, nausea and diarrhoea are common complaints, especially in children, and are due to gastritis or enteritis and to mesenterial arteritis or arteriopathy. Pancreatitis occurs only in few patients, but hepatomegaly is frequent (prevalence 30%) and is usually attributed to fatty infiltration or to congestion. Lymph node enlargement occurs in 50% of patients at some stage in the disease. Salivary gland enlargement is described in 8% and is associated to concommittant Sjögren's syndrome (see Chapter 11). Conjunctivitis and episcleritis are the most frequent ocular manifestations and occur in approximately 15%. Retinopathy is much less common and presents as microangiopathy with cotton wool spots or bleeding or as vasculitis. Stillbirth and spontaneous abortion are common in active untreated stages of the disease and in patients with APL antibodies. Neonatal lupus including congenital heartblock has been documented and is associated with the presence of Ro/SS-A antibodies (see Chapter 3).

DIAGNOSIS

There is, as already stated in the introduction, not one simple clinical or laboratory criterion for the diagnosis of SLE. However, consensus has been obtained on classification criteria and on the number of these criteria required for the diagnosis (Table 7.1; see Kater and Provost, 1995). Classification criteria are meant primarily to obtain homogeneous groups for different types of studies and not for diagnostic purposes in individual cases. They have not been developed for diagnosing individual patients, and for this purpose they lack sensitivity.

Two of the 11 SLE criteria concern auto-antibodies. Antinuclear antibody (ANA) titres are nearly always raised in SLE (> 98%), but the specificity of this phenomenon is low. Raised ANA titres are often present in Sjögren's syndrome, scleroderma, and dermatomyositis (DM) and polymyositis (PM), and occur in up to 10% of controls also. The magnitude of the titre has no predictive value. Anti-double-stranded DNA (anti-dsDNA) antibodies occur in 40% of SLE patients and are SLE specific if demonstrated by the appropriate assays (see Chapter 3). Anti-Smith (anti-Sm) antibodies are directed against ribonuclear protein and are not found in any other disease. They are present in 20% of patients. False-positive serological tests for syphilis are due to the presence of anticardiolipin antibodies (see Chapter 8). A person may be considered to suffer from SLE, if any four or more of the 11 criteria are present serially or simultaneously.

SLE ACTIVITY

Several systems have been developed to quantify the activity of SLE in the individual patient (Kater and Provost, 1995). Systemic Lupus Activity Measure (SLAM) and SLE Disease Activity Index (SLEDAI) are validated activity scores. They are reliable and not too difficult to complete. There is no unanimity on which of the two systems is most sensitive to change in disease activity (Gladman *et al.*, 1992; Bootsma *et al.*, 1996).

TREATMENT

Antimalarials, corticosteroids, cytotoxic agents (such as azathioprine, methotrexate, and cyclophosphamide), immunoglobulins, and plasma exchange are all used for therapy of SLE. Though most of these drugs or methods have not been sufficiently evaluated in intervention studies, no-one doubts that immunosuppression is better than placebo. A long series of other therapeutic strategies is under investigation at present; none of these has been accepted for clinical use yet. For a short review of all forms of immuno-therapy we refer to Chapter 4.

Therapy of vessel occlusion in SLE should aim at reperfusion first and at prevention of recurrence secondly. Prospective intervention studies on strategies for fostering reperfusion or secondary prevention in SLE have not been performed. There is no evidence that immunosuppression is effective for these purposes (Khamashta *et al.*, 1995; see Chapter 8, *Course and Therapy*). The method currently available for advancement of reperfusion by thrombolysis is not entirely without possibilities, but it is still largely in the stage of research, at least as far as the CNS is concerned (see Chapter 2, *Treatment of Ischaemic Stroke*). For secondary prevention of vascular events, at present it seems that one may have to choose between effective

Table 7.1 Classification criteria for systemic lupus erythematosus.

Criterion	Definition
Malar rash	Fixed erythema, flat or raised, over the malar eminencies, tending to spare the nasolabial folds
Discoid rash	Erythematous raised patches with adherent keratotic scaling and follicular plugging; atrophic scarring may occur in older lesions
Photosensitivity	Skin rash as a result of unusual reaction to sunlight, by patient history or physician observation
Oral ulcers, oral or nasopharyngeal ulceration	Usually painless, observed by a physician
Arthritis	Non-erosive arthritis involving 2 or more peripheral joints, characterized by tenderness, swelling or effusion
Serositis	Pleuritis – convincing history of pleuritic pain or rub heard by a physician or evidence of pleural effusion, or Pericarditis – documented by ECG or rub or evidence of pericardial effusion
Renal disorder	Persistent proteinuria greater than 0.5 g per day or greater than 3+ if quantification is not performed, or Cellular casts – may be red cell, haemoglobulin, granular, tubular or mixed.
Neurological disorder	Seizures – in the absence of offending drugs or known metabolic derangements, e.g. uraemia, ketoacidosis, or electrolyte imbalance, or Psychosis – in the absence of offending drugs or known metabolic derangements, e.g. uraemia, ketoacidosis, or electrolyte imbalance
Haematological disorder	Haemolytic anaemia – with reticulosis, or Leukopenia – less than 4000/mm^3 on 2 or more occasions, or Lymphopenia – less than 1500/mm^3 on two or more occasions, or Thrombocytopenia – less than 100 000/mm^3 in the absence of offending drugs
Immunological disorder	Positive LE cell preparation, or Anti-DNA: antibody to native DNA in abnormal titre, or Anti-Sm: presence of antibody to Sm nuclear antigen, or False-positive serological test for syphilis known to be positive for at least 6 months and confirmed by treponema pallidum immobilization or fluorescent treponemal antibody absorption test
Antinuclear antibody	An abnormal titre of antinuclear antibody by immunofluorescence or an equivalent assay at any point in time and in the absence of drugs known to be associated with 'drug-induced lupus' syndrome

For the purpose of identifying patients in clinical studies, a person shall be said to have systemic lupus erythematosus if any 4 or more of the 11 criteria are present, serially or simultaneously, during any interval of observation.
From Tan *et al.* (1982), with permission.

prevention of occlusions with a risk of bleeding as a drawback, or not fully-effective prevention without the risk on bleeding (Hylek *et al.*, 1996; The Stroke Prevention In Reversible Ischemia Trial, 1997; see also Chapter 8, *Course and Therapy*). In this mine-field of therapeutic uncertainties, the responsible physician has to find his or her way.

PROGNOSIS

Present data point to a 10-year survival of 85% for adults and a 20-year survival of 68% (Abu-Shakra *et al.*, 1995a; Tucker *et al.*, 1995). There is an almost five-fold increased risk of death for patients with SLE compared to the general population (Abu-Shakra *et al.*, 1995a). Risk factors for mortality are renal damage, seizures, thrombocytopenia, lung involvement, age over 50 years at diagnosis, and disease activity index (SLEDAI) equal or higher than 20 at onset of the disease (Abu-Shakra *et al.*, 1995b; Ward *et al.*, 1996). Outcome is partly dependent on potentially modifi-able psychosocial factors, such as self-efficacy for disease management (Karlson *et al.*, 1997). Onset of SLE in children is generally more severe than in adults and requires more aggressive therapy. However, survival of children at 10 years after onset is at least as good as in adults or even slightly better (Tucker *et al.*, 1995). Overall, the number of organs involved in the disease increases during its course. Treatment-free remissions are not exceptional (Drenkard *et al.*, 1996; Euler *et al.*, 1994).

PSYCHIATRY AND NEUROLOGY (TABLE 2)

INTRODUCTION

Figures on the prevalence of nervous system involvement in SLE differ from 18 to 65% (Futrell *et al.*, 1992; Sibley *et al.*, 1992; Hochberg and Petri, 1993). This wide range is because some studies are limited to hospitalized patients or include a number of patient years in each case, while others are purely cross-sectional and concern a cohort of sequentially examined outpatients. Figures on the incidence or prevalence of dif-ferent psychiatrical or neurological manifestations are not available. From series of patients published by different centres, it appears, however, that 'behavourial disorders', headache, and seizures are the most frequent syndromes or symptoms. Stroke and neuro-infections occur only in a minority of patients. In addition, there is a long list of more or less rare CNS manifestations (Table 7.2). Some of these have been described in tens of patients or even larger numbers (*e.g.* chorea, transverse myelitis) and others in only one (acute amnesia) or several (Parkinsonism). Peripheral neuropathies are less frequent than CNS manifestations and do not dominate the clinical picture. Among the rarely occurring disorders of terminal nerve fibres and neuromuscular junctions, myasthenia gravis (MG) is most frequent. Lambert-Eaton myasthenic syndrome (LEMS) and acquired neuromyotonia have only been described in few patients. Myositis occurs in a small minority of SLE patients. Orbital myositis and Brown's syndrome are rarities. Futrell *et al.* (1992) did a combined retrospective and prospective study of 91 patients and found CNS disease in 65%: 14 (15%) had strokes; 22 had seizures of which five were focal in onset; 31(!) had behavourial disorders (depression, suicide attempts, disorientation, confusion,

Table 7.2 Psychiatrical and neurological complications in SLE with estimated frequencies

Category	Manifestations	Estimated frequency*
Psychiatrical	Depression	++++
	Cognitive impairment	+++
	Dementia	+
	Organic brain syndrome, delirium	++/+++
	Schizophrenia-like psychosis	++/+++
Neurological-CNS	Headache/migraine	++++
	Seizures	+++
	TIAs and stroke	++/+++
	Cerebral vasculitis	+
	Encephalopathy due to small vessel disease	++
	Multifocal leukoencephalopathy	+
	Cerebral venous thrombosis	++
	Idiopathic intracranial hypertension	++
	Acute amnesia	+
	Chorea and ballism	++/+++
	Parkinsonism	+
	Optic neuritis/neuropathy	++
	Inappropriate secretion of antidiuretic hormone	+
	INO**, gaze paralysis, nystagmus	++
	Cranial nerve palsies	++
	Cerebellar syndromes	+
	Transverse myelitis/myelopathy	++
	Neuro-infections	++
Neurological-PNS	Sensomotor polyneuropathy (PN)	++/+++
	Acute inflammatory PN	+
	Chronic inflammatory PN	+
	Mononeuritis multiplex	+
	Clinical symptoms of autonomic neuropathy	+
Neurological-terminal motor nerves and neuromuscular junctions	Myasthenia gravis	++
	Lambert-Eaton myasthenic syndrome	+
	Acquired neuromyotonia	+
Neurological – muscles	Inflammatory polymyositis	++/+++
	Inclusion body myositis	+
	Orbital myositis	+
	Brown's syndrome	+

*Estimated frequency: ++++, among the most frequent neuro-psychiatrical manifestations in SLE; +++, occurring in a minority of patients with SLE; ++, described in tens of patients or in an even larger number; + described in few patients.
**INO, internuclear ophthalmoplegia.

hallucinations); and nine had headache. Sibley *et al.* (1992) reviewed the charts of all the definite cases of SLE they had seen since 1975; both outpatient and hospital records were included. Headache, personality change, depression, neurosis, and peripheral neuropathy were excluded from analysis. SLE-related CNS events were found in 18% (48 cases) of the patients: seizures in 18, brainstem dysfunction in 12, psychosis in 11, organic brain syndrome in 11, and stroke in seven.

Nervous system disorders develop in most patients months or years after SLE has been diagnosed, but virtually every neurological and psychiatrical manifestation of SLE may be the first and only symptom or sign of the disease (Miguel *et al.*, 1994; Tola *et al.*, 1992; Mitsias and Levine, 1994). Overall, the frequency of CNS involvement and the type of CNS disorders are not different in children and adults. It may be, however, that some CNS disorders, especially chorea and psychosis, occur more frequently in children (Parikh *et al.*, 1995; Steinlin *et al.*, 1995; see also this Chapter, *Chorea*).

PATHOLOGY AND PATHOGENESIS OF PSYCHIATRICAL AND NEUROLOGICAL MANIFESTATIONS

Changes observed by macroscopic and microscopic investigations of the brain primarily concern the vascular system. Secondly they concern the brain tissue itself. By far the most frequent – and in most cases the most widespread – disorder is the vasculopathy (abnormal vessel walls, no inflammatory cell infiltrate) of small vessels, predominantly arterioles and capillaries (Hanly *et al.*, 1992; Bruyn, 1995; see also this Chapter, *Pathology*, p 209). Some of these abnormal or obstructed vessels are surrounded by small haemorrhages or infarcts. The sizes of the infarcts vary in diameter from 200 μm to 1.5 mm. Some of them are even smaller and are little more than microglia nodules. It seems possible that some of the sensory or mixed sensomotor polyneuropathies of SLE are also due to small vessel vasculopathy. Small vessel vasculitis with inflammatory cells in the vessel walls occurs much less often than small vessel vasculopathy. Thrombotic occlusions of large vessels and large vessel periarteritis nodosa-like vasculitis are relatively uncommon (Devinsky *et al.*, 1988; Johnson and Richardson, 1968).

The question is whether all neurological and psychiatrical manifestations can be considered as consequences of ischaemia. Most authors feel that this is unlikely. Diffuse loss of neurones, as for instance documented by Kuroe *et al.* (1994), is not easily explainable by ischaemia, and fully reversible conditions such as depression and psychosis are more likely to be due to disturbances at the level of synapses than to multiple small infarcts. It is conceivable that brain function becomes compromised by antibodies or cytokines that are synthesized in the CNS compartment or that leak through damaged small vessels into the neuropil.

Still another point is whether the psychiatrical and neurological manifestations are due directly to an SLE-dependent process. Headache, mild disorders of cognition, and mood disorders may be expressions of inability to cope with the disease. Some disorders are iatrogenic in origin.

LABORATORY INVESTIGATIONS: THE CEREBROSPINAL FLUID

In a patient with SLE, a slight to moderate raise of the protein content of the cerebrospinal fluid (CSF) and a moderate degree of pleocytosis are compatible with involvement of the brain or spinal cord. However, similar slight changes may be found in some forms of meningitis complicating SLE, *e.g.* cryptococcus meningitis (see this Chapter, *Neuroinfections*).

In patients with CNS involvement, the intrathecal synthesis of immunoglobulins may be increased (Golombek *et al.*, 1986; Long *et al.*, 1990; Jongen *et al.*, 1990). There is also evidence for increased synthesis of C4 in the CNS compartment, possibly by astrocytes or microglia cells (Jongen *et al.*, 1990). DNA auto-antibodies are present in some cases, but titres are not high (Winfield *et al.*, 1978). Antineuronal antibodies have been demonstrated in the CSF (Bluestein *et al.*, 1981; Golombek *et al.*, 1986), and there is evidence for intrathecal synthesis of antibodies (Mevorach *et al.*, 1994). Schizozawa *et al.* (1992) demonstrated increased levels of interferon alpha in the CSF of five of six patients with lupus psychosis but not in other SLE patients. The cytokines interleukine-1 and interleukine-6 are increased in the CSF of patients with neurological manifestations (Alcocer-Varela *et al.*, 1992; Hirohata and Miyamoto, 1990). All these findings point to immune activation within the CNS. It is still largely unknown how they interact and contribute to CNS disease.

COMPUTED TOMOGRAPHY (CT) AND MAGNETIC RESONANCE IMAGING (MRI) OF THE CNS

Changes revealed by CT and MRI comprise cerebral atrophy, small punctate lesions of unknown significance, diffuse white matter changes, small and large infarcts, haemorrhages, calcification of the basal ganglia, evidence of disruption of the blood-brain barrier, and oedema (Kaye *et al.*, 1992; Miller *et al.*, 1992; Isshi *et al.*, 1994; Jarek *et al.*, 1994; Gieron *et al.*, 1995; Gonzales-Crespo *et al.*, 1995; Chinn *et al.*, 1997). MRI is in general more sensitive than CT. CT and MRI are not very informative when only psychiatrical manifestations are present. In some patients with acute or subacute onset of a CNS syndrome, CT and MRI initially reveal no abnormality and changes may become apparent only at repeat investigations.

Small punctate lesions
Patients with and without clinical signs of CNS involvement may present multiple small punctate lesions of increased signal intensity at T2-weighted images (Gonzales-Crespo *et al.*, 1995; Chinn *et al.*, 1997). Such lesions are located preferentially in the periventricular and subcortical white matter, but they also occur in the basal ganglia, thalamus, brainstem, and cerebellum (Gonzales-Crespo *et al.*, 1995). It is suggested that such lesions represent perivascular spaces without nerve fibres and with gliosis or small infarcts (Stimmler *et al.*, 1993). Similar lesions are found in healthy elderly people (see Pantoni and Garcia, 1995).

Diffuse white matter changes
Diffuse white matter changes, confluent white matter lesions, or leukoaraiosis have been described in SLE (Kaye *et al.*, 1992; Isshi *et al.*, 1994). Leukoaraiosis (from the Greek *leuko* meaning white and *araiosis* meaning rarefaction) is characterized on CT scans by confluent areas of hypodensity of the white matter in the cerebral hemispheres and on MRI by confluent areas of increased signal density at T2-weighted images. Leukoaraiosis due to SLE small-vessel disease is likely to be related histologically to perivascular loss of myelin and axons (Kaye *et al.*, 1992; Pantoni and Garcia, 1995). Patients with these changes may show some degree of subcortical dementia, urinary incontinence, and gait abnormalities (see Chapter 2, *White Matter Lesions*). Multifocal leukoencephalopathy, primarily in the hemispheres but to a lesser extent also in the brainstem and spinal cord, has been described in a few cases

of SLE. It is the diagnostic label for a demyelinative disorder caused by an opportunistic infection of oligodendroglia by the JC strain of papovavirus (see this
Chapter, *Neuroinfections*, and Chapter 2 *White Matter Lesions of Viral Origin*).

Cerebral atrophy
Cerebral atrophy develops in 37–71% of SLE patients and is not sufficiently
explained (Carette *et al.*, 1982). To some degree it might be an effect of corticosteroid
medication, but Chinn *et al.* (1997) found no support for this contention.

Disruption of blood-brain barrier in patients with vasculitis or vasculopathy
Gadolinium MRI may demonstrate swelling and enhancement of affected parts in
the CNS (optic system, myelum), presumably due to disruption of the blood-brain
barrier. These changes are attributed to small vessel vasculopathy or vasculitis
(Sklar *et al.*, 1996).

Calcifications
Calcification in the basal ganglia and other locations is well known from several
disorders (mitochondrial encephalopathy, hypoparathyroidism, etc) and has been
described in SLE (Garcia-Rayo, 1994; Raymond *et al.*, 1996).

POSITRON EMISSION COMPUTED TOMOGRAPHY (PET) AND SINGLE PHOTON EMISSION COMPUTERIZED TOMOGRAPHY (SPECT)

PET has been applied in a small series of patients. It may reveal a deficit in cerebral
metabolism in patients with psychiatric SLE. When neurological and psychiatrical
manifestations are absent, PET is reported to be normal as well (Stoppe *et al.*, 1990;
Carbotte *et al.*, 1992). PET is expensive and not easily accessible for diagnosis or
evaluation.

SPECT is less expensive, in many centres easily accessible, and has been demonstrated to provide additional information to CT scans (Szer *et al.*, 1993; Kovacs *et al.*,
1995; Kodama *et al.*, 1995). SPECT shows hypoperfusion of the frontal lobes and
some other locations in patients with florid psychiatrical manifestations, without
any other evidence of CNS involvement and with normal CT scans. Hypoperfusion
has also been demonstrated in patients without CNS manifestations who shortly
after SPECT developed psychiatrical illness. This would indicate that SPECT might
have predictive value. Results in control SLE patients without CNS manifestations
and psychiatric patients without SLE are at present not sufficiently available.

CLINICAL FEATURES OF CNS INVOLVEMENT

Depression
Depression is by far the most frequent psychiatrical disorder in SLE. Attempts to
trace it back to organic brain disease due to SLE or to a disorder in adjustment have
not led to definite conclusions (Miguell *et al.*, 1994; Hay *et al.*, 1992; Utset *et al.*, 1994).
Severe depressions are likely to be of an organic origin.

The classification of depressions in the Diagnostic and Statistical Manual of
Mental Disorders, fourth edition (DSM-IV, American Psychiatric Association, 1994),
is based on differences in severity and aetiology, not on differences in symptoms.
Psychological symptoms of mild depressions (low mood, lack of interest in daily

events, pessimistic thinking, loss of self-esteem, neglect of dress and grooming) are more intense in severe depressions. Biological symptoms (sleep disturbance, loss of appetite and weight, loss of libido, amenorrhoea) are prominent in severe depressions and absent or in the background in mild depressions (Gelder *et al.*, 1996).

Diagnosis and management. The psychiatrical interview and observation of behaviour are the main diagnostic instruments. Laboratory tests for depression are not available yet. Consultation of a psychiatrist is required for classification of the type of depression and advice for management. SLE activity should be examined to establish whether the psychiatrical manifestations are related to an increase of severity in the disease processes (see this Chapter, *SLE Activity*). If SLE activity has increased approximately concomitantly with onset of depression, (more vigorous) immunosuppression should be considered.

From the viewpoint of management of depression, the first point is to decide whether the patient can stay at home. *i.e.* whether he/she is looked after sufficiently and what the risk is of suicide attempts (Matsukawa *et al.*, 1994; Gelder *et al.*, 1996). Once this is clear, and dealt with accordingly, a drug has to be chosen. Tricyclic antidepressants probably exert the strongest antidepressive effect and therefore are indicated in severe depressions. The tricyclic antidepressant of first choice is amitryptiline (dose at onset 1 tablet of 10 mg, increasing slowly up to 6 tablets of 25 mg). Its main drawbacks are the long delay until the antidepressive effect becomes manifest (weeks), the anticholinergic side effects, and cardiac toxicity. Drugs belonging to the category of serotonine specific re-uptake inhibitors (SSRIs) have less side effects and are less risky in case of overdose (fluvoxamine, 100 mg at night; fluoxetine 20 mg in the morning; paroxetine 20 mg at breakfast; trazodon 150 mg at night before going to bed). SSRIs inhibit cytochrome P450 enzyme in the liver and can thus be responsible for an elevation of serum levels of other drugs (*e.g.* anticoagulants or antiepileptics). Depressed patients are in need of regular control and psychic support.

Cognitive impairment
Cognitive impairment is not rare (see Table 7.2) and may be present when SLE has caused damage to the CNS. This was established in several studies and was only to be expected (Denburg *et al.*, 1987; Hanly *et al.*, 1992a; Hay *et al.*, 1992). In addition, some degree of cognitive deficit has been demonstrated in groups of non-brain damaged SLE patients and in individual patients without obvious brain involvement (Denburg *et al.*, 1987; Hanly *et al.*, 1992b; Ginsburg *et al.*, 1992; Kozora *et al.*, 1996). Four explanations have been offered for this observation. It has been suggested that subclinical cognitive impairment may be the only manifestation of mild involvement of the brain in SLE (Carbotte *et al.*, 1995a). In favour of this explanation is that imaging of the brain of patients without obvious CNS manifestations has revealed definite changes in some cases (see this Chapter, pages 219–230). The second explanation is based on the findings of Kozora *et al* (1996). These authors found a similar degree of cognitive impairment in a group of carefully selected SLE patients without CNS involvement as in a group of matched patients with RA. They considered that mild cognitive impairment could be related to factors shared by different inflammatory connective tissue disease (ICTDs), such as inflammation or pain. The two final explanations are a deleterious effect of drugs, such as corticosteroids, and of psychiatrical disorders, such as depression or emotional distress.

The potential effects of these factors are not denied, but most authors feel that they have sufficiently been ruled out as explanations for the cognitive impairment under discussion here (see Carbotte *et al.*, 1995b).

The consequences of mild cognitive dysfunction in SLE for daily life have not been sufficiently analysed as of yet. Another question is whether mild cognitive impairment will prove to be the first step towards significant cognitive dysfunction. Repeat examinations over a period of five years do not point in this direction (Hanley *et al.*, 1994; Hanley *et al.*, 1997). The effect of SLE on global intellectual functioning in children and adolescents does not seem severe, at least in short term (Wyckoff *et al.*, 1995).

Diagnosis and management. Neuropsychological investigation is required to diagnose cognitive impairment. In patients without CNS manifestations, demonstration of cognitive impairment is indicated only for research purposes. In patients with CNS manifestations, revealing the presence and the degree of cognitive deficit completes assessment of the patient's condition and may be required for social rehabilitation in some cases.

Dementia

Dementia in SLE is rare (see Table 7.2). In publications on psychiatrical manifestations, the cause of dementia often is not specified. One presumes, however, that most cases will be due to multiple infarcts or diffuse white matter changes (see this Chapter, *Encephalopathy* and *CT and MRI of the CNS*).

Dementia is, according to DSM-IV, characterized by deficit in multiple cognitive domains, including the domain of memory. The cognitive deficits should be severe enough to cause problems in occupational or social functioning and should represent a decline from a previously higher level of functioning.

Diagnosis and management. A neuropsychological investigation is indicated for confirmation of the diagnosis, for establishing the cognitive domains that are affected, and for assessment of the degree of impairment. Metabolic derangements (*e.g.* serum electrolyte abnormalities) may induce a reversible form of dementia and therefore should be excluded. Multiple infarcts and white matter disease are potential causes of dementia in SLE and can be demonstrated or excluded by CT scannning or MRI.

Management of dementia should aim at improvement of function, relief of distress, and support of the family. Improvement of functional ability can be attained by adapting and simplifying the living conditions of the patient. Relief of anxiety or agitation may require medication, for instance benzodiazepine or haloperidol.

Organic brain syndrome and delirium

Many authors use the expression organic brain syndrome (OBS) somewhat loosely when the designation delirium seems not, or not yet, justified. OBS or delirium in SLE are ominous syndromes and not very rare (see Table 7.2). They develop usually during a flare-up of SLE, within a period of hours or a day, and point to a rapidly evolving cerebral process that requires immediate medical attention.

Features of OBS are one or more of the following: reduced consciousness and disturbances in orientation, perception, memory, and other intellectual functions. The DSM-IV criteria for delirium due to a general medical condition are presented in Table 7.3.

Table 7.3 Diagnostic criteria for delirium due to a general medical condition

– Disturbance of consciousness (*i.e.* reduced clarity of awareness of the environment) with reduced ability to focus, sustain, or shift attention.

– A change in cognition (such as memory deficit, disorientation, language disturbance) or the development of a perceptual disturbance that is not better accounted for by a pre-existing, established, or evolving dementia.

– The disturbance develops over a short period of time (usually hours to days) and tends to fluctuate during the course of the day.

– There is evidence from the history, physical examination, or laboratory findings that the disturbance is caused by the direct physiological consequences of a general medical condition.

From The American Psychiatric Association, DSM-IV (1994), with permission.

A delirious patient does not fully realize what is going on in his environment and misinterprets events. Orientation in time and place is disturbed. Visual hallucinations are often present but are not always easily distinguished from misinterpretations of actual events. A delirious patient is often agitated and anxious. Delirium may be drug induced or drug related, for example caused by a psychotropic drug with anticholinergic side effects or by withdrawal of alcohol. The pathogenesis of OBS and delirium is not known, even though these disorders are often surmised to be manifestations of a 'diffuse brain disorder'. Dependent on the underlying cause, OBS and delirium can be fully reversible, indicating that they may be due to neuronal dysfunction. The reduced level of consciousness points to involvement of the reticular system in the brain stem or to a more widespread dysfunction of cortical neurones (see Chapter 2, *Coma and Delirium*).

Diagnosis and management. OBS and delirium are diagnosed by interviewing and observing the patient. It is noteworthy that patients with SLE in a state of delirium have seizures sometimes. The differential diagnosis should include a drug-induced condition and encephalopathy due to small vessel vasculitis or vasculopathy.

The management of delirious conditions requires adherence to a few principles (Gelder *et al.*, 1996). (1) prevent accidents, (2) explain to the patient what is happening to him and tell him that he will be better, (3) use drugs to calm him down and to help him sleep at night. For calming down the patient, haloperidol is the best choice because it does not cause drowsiness and has no cardiac and hypotensive side effects (see Chapter 2 for tardive dyskinesia as side effect of neuroleptics). One can best start with 2–5 mg haloperidol/day, the effective daily dose being between 3 and 15 mg/day. The first dose can be given by intramuscular injection. In patients with seizures, haloperidol is not necessarily the first choice because seizures are a rare side effect! Diazepam is an alternative. It acts as an anxiolyticum and has a sedative effect, and therefore may help patients to sleep. In addition, it raises the threshold for seizures, but its drawback is a slight depressant effect on consciousness and respiration. The doses at onset may vary between 5 to 20 mg.

Schizophrenia-like psychosis

DSM-IV does not have one definition for all forms of psychosis. The criteria for a psychotic disorder due to a general medical condition are given in Table 7.4.

Table 7.4 Diagnostic criteria for psychotic disorders due to general medical conditions

– Prominent hallucinations or delusions.

– There is evidence from the history, physical examination, or laboratory findings that the disturbance is the direct physiological consequence of a general medical condition.

– The disturbance is not better accounted for by another mental disorder.

– The disorder does not occur exclusively during the course of a delirium.

From The American Psychiatric Association, DSM-IV (1994), with permission.

Psychotic episodes in SLE are not very rare (see Table 7.2) and tend to recur. Steinlin *et al.* (1995) reported that, of their 11 children with psychoses due to SLE, three had three psychotic episodes, four had two episodes, and another 4 had one episode.

Delusions (*i.e.* false beliefs maintained despite evidence to the contrary) in this form of psychosis are mostly persecutory. Psychotic periods, when adequately treated, need not last long; in some patients, however, it may take days, weeks or even months before a normal sense of reality is restored. Once this is achieved, patients demonstrate no residual abnormalities, which is in contrast to patients suffering from schizophrenia. The two main differential diagnostic considerations for SLE psychosis are delirium and psychosis due to corticosteroids. Psychosis differs from delirium in two essential aspects: cognition is intact and consciousness is preserved. Psychotic patients deny reality, but this is not due to cognitive impairment or lack of clarity of consciousness. Corticosteroids evoke in a few patients a psychotic syndrome, usually with paranoid symptoms (Kershner and Wang-Cheng, 1989; Rogers and Kelly, 1993; see Chapter 4, *Side Effects of Corticosteroids*).

Diagnosis and management. Schizophrenia-like psychosis is diagnosed on the basis of clinical criteria, taking the description given above into consideration and using the psychiatrical interview and observation of the patient as main diagnostic instruments. Laboratory tests to confirm the diagnosis are not available yet. The contention of Bonfa *et al.* (1987) that in 90% of patients lupus psychosis is associated with the presence of anti-ribosomal P protein antibodies in serum is not generally supported (Teh and Isenberg, 1994; Isshi and Hirohata, 1996; Press *et al.*, 1996). Authors agree, however, that psychotic patients with serum anti-ribosomal P protein are likely to suffer from SLE. The SLE disease activity, as expressed in clinical and laboratory features, should be examined. However, schizophrenia-like psychosis, unlike delirium, has not been found to be clearly related to a flare-up of SLE.

Immunosuppression is not known to exert an anti-psychotic effect and is justified only for treatment of increased activity of SLE or other associated signs of SLE disease activity. Haloperidol is the drug of first choice for symptomatic treatment of psychosis (Gelder *et al.*, 1996). Haloperidol is not less effective than most other antipsychotic drugs and has relatively few side effects (see Chapter 2 for tardive dyskinesia as side-effect of haloperidol and other neuroleptics). The daily dose should be between 5 and 15 mg. The patient and his/her relatives should be informed that complete recovery from psychotic behaviour is to be expected.

Headache

Complaints about a severe headache of recent onset, with or without other neurological symptoms, have to be taken very seriously. Often, they are the first manifestation of a severe CNS syndrome. Other, more chronic or intermittent forms of
headache are frequent in SLE, though it is not confirmed that the incidence is higher
than in controls. In three prospective studies, the percentage of SLE patients with
headache amounted to 28, 42 and 68% respectively (Grigor *et al.*, 1978; Anzola *et al.*,
1988; Vazquez-Cruz *et al.*, 1990). Headache developed, in the large majority of the
patients, after onset of SLE. In approximately 50% of the patients, headache was
classified as vascular, mostly common migraine (no aura). The other 50% had mus-
cle-contraction type headaches, and these were considered a reaction to the underlying disease. Thirty two percent of 71 Greek patients with SLE declared in
interviews that they had at least one headache episode every two weeks. In a large
control group of healthy Greek males, this percentage was 30%; the data from these
controls was obtained by questionnaires. The authors concluded that they could not
confirm the suggested relation between SLE and headache (Sfikakis *et al.*, 1998).
Headache has been reported frequently in small series of SLE patients with
ischaemic events. Eighteen of 30 patients (60%) with SLE, cerebrovascular disease,
and proven occlusion of one or more cerebral arteries complained of unspecified
headache (Mitsias and Levine, 1994). Toubi *et al.* (1995) reported that 41 of 56
patients (73%) with cerebral or retinal ischaemic manifestations had 'severe
migraine'. These percentages are much higher than in non-SLE induced cerebral
ischaemic events (Koudstaal *et al.*, 1991). It is clear that more evidence is needed
before the suggestion can be accepted that chronic headache or a form of migraine
may be evoked by SLE-induced cerebral vasculopathy.

Diagnosis and treatment. A severe headache of recent onset without any neurological
abnormalities at examination is reason for a full diagnostic investigation. Diagnosis
of more chronic forms of headache is based on anamnestic data. On its own,
migraine is not sufficient reason for more vigorous immunosuppression. Migraine
is treated with aspecific drugs (paracetamol, naproxen) or with specific anti-
migraine medication (sumatriptan). When attacks occur frequently (more than
twice a month), prophylactic treatment (propanolol, metoprolol, natriumvalproate,
pizotifene) should be considered.

Epilepsy

Since the landmark studies of Johnson and Richardson (1968) and Feinglass *et al.*
(1976), epilepsy in SLE has attracted relatively little interest. Since then, only the
terminology for different types of seizures has changed. Seizures are suggested to
be mostly secondary generalized or partial. Status epilepticus has been described
in several patients (Johnson and Richardson, 1968; Gieron *et al.*, 1995). Seizures
may occur before SLE has been diagnosed (Brinciotti *et al.*, 1993) and during all
stages of the disease. Seizures can occur only once, only in one period, in several
periods, or recurrently for some time. There are many descriptions in the literature
of patients in whom seizures are the first manifestation of a turn for the worse in a
CNS disorder. This is the reason why some authors have used the expression 'terminal convulsions' (Johnson and Richardson, 1968). Often, CT scans or MRI show
abnormalities only at repeat investigations after a few days. Epilepsy in SLE, not
secondary to another identified cause, has been reported to be associated with

high titres of anticardiolipin antibodies (ACAs) (Liou *et al.*, 1996; Herranz *et al.*, 1994).

Diagnosis and treatment. An unexpected epileptic fit in a patient who is not regularly treated for epilepsy should always cause a high degree of suspicion because it may be a manifestation of a sometimes rapidly evolving CNS syndrome. Therefore, it requires a full neurological evaluation, including brain imaging and electro-encephalography. Examination of the CSF is indicated to exclude neuro-infections (see this Chapter *Neuro-infections*). When seizures recur or when a more complex CNS syndrome develops, repeat brain imaging may be worthwhile. A seizure in a patient with SLE should always be treated. At present, carbamazepine is the drug of first choice for partial or secondary generalized seizures; most seizures in SLE belong to this category (see Chapter 2, *Epilepsy* for definitions of the major cate-gories of epilepsy). There is always a risk on a convulsive epileptic status, and in brain disorders of recent onset, status epilepticus is often difficult to control and potentially life-threatening. The management of status epilepticus is described in the section on epilepsy in Chapter 2.

Transient ischaemic attacks (TIAs) and stroke

In every review of large series of SLE patients, TIAs and stroke are among the neu-rological complications (Fig. 7.3 and Fig. 7.4) (Futrell and Millikan, 1989; Kitagawa *et al.*, 1990; Toubi *et al.*, 1995). The study of Futrell and Millikan (1989) may serve as an example. These authors reported on 91 SLE patients who had been under control for an average period of 7 years. Seven patients had been treated for TIAs, 13 for strokes due to CT-confirmed infarcts, and one for stroke due to cerebral haemor-rhage. Nine of these patients had multiple infarcts. The mean age at first stroke was 40 years! Mitsias and Levine (1994) collected from the literature data on 30 patients (mean age 35 years) with one or several infarcts due to angiography-proven large vessel occlusion. The reason why angiography was performed in these patients was not commented upon, but it may have been used because of the young age of the patients. The authors analysed the factors that determined the increased risk of occlusion of large vessels in SLE. Two factors were suggested to be primarily responsible: a hypercoagulable state and cardiogenic embolism. A third factor, angiopathy, was considered of less importance. The hypercoagulable state was con-sidered to be due, in part, to the presence of APL antibodies; at least 17% of the patients were positive for LAC and 57% for ACA (see Chapter 8). It should be recalled that APL antibodies occur in 10–50% of SLE patients, according to different authors (Derksen and Stephens, 1995; Love and Santoro, 1990). These antibodies do not explain, therefore, (all) large vessel occlusions in SLE. Protein S or C, antithrom-bin, and plasminogen had not been determined in the patients studied by Mitsias and Levine (1994) (see this Chapter, *Venous Sinus Obstruction*). Cardiogenic embolism was another important factor. Valvular lesions and valvular or ventricu-lar vegetations predisposing to embolism were present in 5 of the 30 cases of Mitsias and Levine (1994). APL antibodies are held responsible for these vegetations by some authors (Hughes, 1993), but this is disputed (see Chapter 8). A high frequency of valvular abnormalities was also discovered in a retrospective investigation of autopsy material (Devinsky *et al.*, 1988). The incidence of vasculitis of cerebral and extracerebral vessels was low (see this Chapter, *Vasculitis*).

In addition to the factors now reviewed, premature arteriosclerosis and hyper-

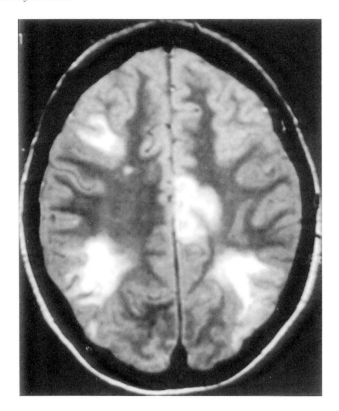

Figure 7.3 Multiple infarcts shown on axial T2-Wi (PD) MRI. Three watershed infarcts and one arteria cerebri anterior infarct, cortical and subcortical, in acute stage in a patient with SLE and antiphospholipid antibodies. (Courtesy of Dr. Lino Ramos.)

tension could also be important. Prolonged treatment with high doses of corticosteroids may cause an atherogenic serum lipid profile, and this predisposes to arteriosclerosis, to cerebral vessel occlusion, and to ischaemic heart disease with risk of cardiogenic emboli. Hypertension is another risk factor for cerebral vessel disorders. The prevalence of hypertension may be higher in SLE than in a control population, due to SLE nephritis or corticosteroid medication. It is of interest that two patients in the series of Mitsias and Levine (1994) had evidence of cervical artery dissection. Case histories have been published on aortic dissection in SLE.

Diagnosis and management. Diagnosis of cerebral haemorrhage or cerebral vessel occlusion is based on findings at neurological examination and on imaging of the brain and extra– and intracranial vessels. SLE activity should be assessed and an attempt should be made to discover factors responsible for haemorrhage (thrombocytopenia) or vessel occlusion (Table 7.5).

Treatment aims at limitation of cerebral damage and prevention of new occlusions or renewed haemorrhage. Immunosuppression is indicated only in patients with increased SLE activity. The measures that should be taken in ischaemic stroke and intracranial haemorrhage are described in Chapter 2.

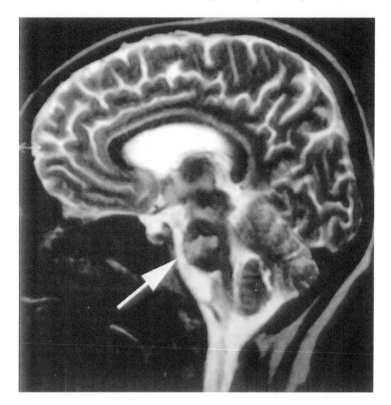

Figure 7.4 Brainstem infarcts in pons (arrow), transition pons-mesencephalon, and thalamus in a patient with SLE and antiphospholipid antibodies. MRI T2-Wi (TSE) image. (Courtesy of Dr. Lino Ramos.)

Cerebral vasculitis

There is no denying that vasculitis of cerebral vessels occurs in SLE, but it is a lot less than vasculitis of the skin (Drenkard *et al.*, 1997). The number of patients reported with cerebral vasculitis is small, but it is correctly pointed out that the required diagnostic techniques – angiography and histology of cerebral vessels –

Table 7.5 Factors predisposing to arterial occlusion in SLE

Angiopathy	Arteriosclerosis
	Vasculitis
	Dissection
Cardiopathy	Endocarditis
	Myocardial infarcts
	Valvular vegetations
Circulation	Atherogenic serum lipid profile
	APL antibodies
	Hypertension

often have not been applied in the past (Weiner and Allen, 1991). The neurological changes in patients with medium or large vessel vasculitis are of two kinds. In some patients, progressive neurological signs from one or both sides of the brain develop more or less rapidly, and angiography shows narrowing and ectasia of cerebral vessels (see also Chapter 5, *Vasculitis Confined to The Nervous System*). In other patients, vasculitis is responsible for aneurysmatic haemorrhages in the subarachnoid space or intracerebral (Fody *et al.*, 1980). The aneurysms are typically multiple and often develop near bifurcations (Liem *et al.*, 1996). Small vessel vasculitis occurs also, as is exemplified by several case histories (Suzuki *et al.*, 1990; Smith *et al.*, 1994; see below, *Encephalopathy due to Small Vessel Disease*).

Diagnosis and management. MRI angiography is an elegant technique used to visualize the characteristic changes of medium or large vessel vasculitis, but it is less sensitive than conventional angiography. Even with conventional arteriography not all patients are diagnosed (see Chapter 5, *Cerebral Arteritis*). Once the diagnosis has been established, aggressive immunosuppressive therapy with intravenous pulse doses of cyclophosphamide in combination with daily oral prednisone is indicated (see Chapter 4 for guidelines). CNS small vessel vasculitis can only be distinguished from small vessel vasculopathy by histological investigation of biopsy material (see below).

Encephalopathy due to small vessel disease

Occasional patients with SLE develop an acute, subacute, or more chronic life-threatening encephalopathic condition with few if any localizing neurological signs (Kaye *et al.*, 1992; Isshi *et al.*, 1994; Mitchell, 1994; Wise *et al.*, 1995). When onset is acute or subacute, headache is often the first symptom. Patients may demonstrate intellectual impairment and may become depressed, agitated, or delirious. They may also have seizures. Drowsiness or even coma may develop. At any stage during this process, progression may halt and improvement may follow. In some patients, however, the course is downhill and fatal despite every possible intervention. Imaging of the brain may initially reveal no changes at all or may provide evidence of oedema (Fig. 7.5) or diffuse white matter changes.

Diagnosis and management. Diagnosis is difficult because small vessels can only be examined under the microscope and not by angiography. The main diagnostic techniques are (1) assessment of SLE disease activity, (2) imaging of the brain to rule out other conditions, (3) examination of the CSF, which may reveal pleiocytosis, and a raised protein content, and (4) brain biopsy, in some cases. The condition should be treated by vigorous immunosuppression. Many authors will choose intravenous pulse doses either of methylprednisolone or cyclophosphamide for this purpose (see Chapter 4 for guidelines).

Cerebral venous thrombosis (CVT)

Cerebral venous thrombosis in SLE was rarely reported in the past, but it is now easier to diagnose due to improved imaging techniques (Vidailhet *et al.*, 1990; Laversuch *et al.*, 1995; Steinlin *et al.*, 1995; Flussner *et al.*, 1996). Early diagnosis and treatment are important because they increase the chance of full recovery (Uziel *et al.*, 1995). CVT usually develops when SLE is in an active stage, and may be the first manifestation of the disease, just as all other neurological manifestations. The clini-

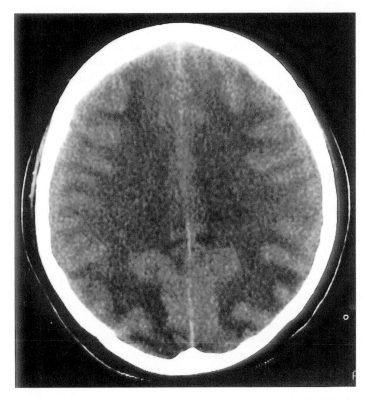

Figure 7.5 CT scan showing brain oedema of a patient with SLE and antiphospholipid antibodies, who was admitted for increasing headache, seizures, and coma. Flow in dural sinuses was patent. At a later stage she developed infarcts in watershed areas. (Courtesy of Dr. Lino Ramos.)

cal symptoms of CVT and the currently preferred treatment are discussed in Chapter 2. Risk factors for CVT are nephrotic syndrome and activated protein C resistance (Brey and Coull, 1996). Some authors stress that APL antibodies enhance the chance of CVT (Hughes, 1993a; see also Chapter 8). It is not entirely clear how nephrotic syndrome increases the risk of arterial and venous thrombosis. Decrease of fibrinolysis may be one factor and loss of protein S into the urine another. Protein S, when not bound to C4b-binding protein, is a co-factor to protein C, and together these proteins strongly inhibit coagulation by degrading procoagulant factors (Lloyd *et al.*, 1993; van Kuijck *et al.*, 1994; Laversuch *et al.*, 1995; Simmonds *et al.*, 1998). A young girl with SLE and acquired protein S deficiency who developed central retinal vein thrombosis has been reported (Prince *et al.*, 1995).

Diagnosis and management. Severe headache that does not respond to analgesic drugs may be the first and only manifestation of CVT and should make one aware of the possibility of this diagnosis (Uziel *et al.*, 1995). The association of headache with papilloedema and infarcts or haemorrhages is in support of the diagnosis. CVT is best visualised by MRI venography. Treatment should comprise administration of low-molecular-weight heparin for 3 weeks, followed by warfarin in combination with corticosteroids and/or cytotoxic agents to decrease SLE activity, if enhanced (Einhäupl *et al.*, 1991; Uziel *et al.*, 1995; de Bruyn *et al.*, 1996). See Chapter 2 for a more extensive description of diagnosis and management of CVT.

Idiopathic intracranial hypertension (IIH)

IIH is a rare manifestation in SLE and is diagnosed when three conditions are met: intracranial pressure should be raised (cerebrospinal fluid or CSF pressure > 200 mm Hg); the cellular and biochemical composition of the CSF should show only minor abnormalities or be normal; and hydrocephalus, intracranial mass lesion, and cerebral sinus thrombosis (CST) should be excluded. The best method to demonstrate or exclude venous sinus thrombosis is MRI venography (Padeh and Passwell, 1996). Patients complain about headache, blurred vision, or diplopia and may show one or more of the following at neurological examination: papilloedema, decreased visual acuity, unilateral or bilateral abducens nerve palsy, palsy of other ocular nerves and even facial palsy (Green *et al.*, 1995). The scalp veins may be dilated (Karahalios *et al.*, 1996). It has been suggested that increased cerebral venous pressure underlies most or all cases of IIH (King *et al.*, 1995; Karahalios *et al.*, 1996). Among the causes for raised intracranial venous pressure are obstruction of intracranial venous sinuses by thrombosis or partial thrombosis, defective absorption of CSF through arachnoid villi due to inflammation, extracranial or intracranial venous stenosis, and raised central venous pressure. The data from Green *et al.* (1995) show that, in a majority of the IIH patients with SLE, evidence for a hypercoagulable state was present (see this Chapter, *CVT*).

For the differential diagnosis it is important to know that chronic cryptococcal meningitis may cause raised intracranial pressure and only very minor changes in the composition of the CSF (pseudotumour syndrome) (Cremer *et al.*, 1997). Cryptococcal meningitis is a rare complication in the immunocompromised SLE patient (see Zimmerman *et al.*, 1992).

Diagnosis and treatment. IIH is diagnosed when the clinical findings are compatible with this diagnosis, when CSF pressure is raised, and when MRI provides no evidence for sinus thrombosis. Treatment with corticosteroids and cytostatic agents has been successful in some cases. There is a report of a patient who received intravenous immunoglobulins and recovered. Anticoagulants and diuretics have been attempted in others (Green *et al.*, 1995). If CSF pressure remains high, despite these treatments, measures should be taken to preserve visual acuity. The preferred method is CSF shunting, but optic nerve sheath decompression has also been performed (Corbett *et al.*, 1988; Tang, 1990).

Acute amnesia

Sudden onset of permanent or transient global amnesia is rare (see Table 7.2). Schnider *et al.* (1995) reported on sudden onset of permanent global amnesia and six months thereafter generalized seizures in a 55-year-old man who appeared to fulfil the criteria for SLE (Tan *et al.*, 1982). Antibodies against phospholipids and anti-neuronal antibodies were not present. MRI, 10 days after onset of amnesia, showed the hippocampi to be discretely swollen with blurring of cortical structures. This was not seen at all 3 and 10 months after onset. Global amnesia persisted despite immunotherapy.

Chorea

There are one or several cases of chorea in almost every large series of patients with SLE. Its prevalence in a cohort of 1000 patients augmented, however, to no more than 1% (Cervera *et al.*, 1993). Bruyn and Padberg (1984) collected a series of 51 definite cases from the literature and summarized the main clinical features:

1. Patients were relatively young. Of six males in this series, no-one was older than 20. The mean age of the 45 female patients at the time chorea developed was 19. In the study of Cervera *et al.* (1993), the mean age of onset of SLE was 29.
2. Chorea was transient: it disappeared within days or months in most patients, but in occasional patients it took three years before it was gone.
3. In most cases, the distribution was symmetrical and in a minority (14 of 51) asymmetrical. One would expect some degree of asymmetry when a vascular cause would be decisive.
4. In approximately 50% of the patients, chorea was associated with other neurological manifestations.

In another group of 12 patients, six with definite SLE (Tan *et al.*, 1982) and six with lupus-like symptoms, nine had antiphospholipid antibodies (Asherson *et al.*, 1987). MR imaging in five patients with CNS lupus and chorea revealed high signal intensity on T1-weighted MR images in the striatum. In one case this was presumably due to a vascular insult (see Kashihara *et al.*, 1998). Post-mortem investigations of the brain in 10 cases revealed vascular changes in the basal ganglia of two (see Bruyn and Padberg, 1984). In a more recent and more detailed neuropathological study of one patient, multiple small infarcts or microinfarcts were seen throughout the cerebral and cerebellar cortices and to some degree also in the cerebral white matter, the putamen, caudate nucleus, and globus pallidus (Kuroe *et al.*, 1994). Histology of the putamen revealed widespread neuronal loss, probably more loss of large neurones than of small neurones. It was felt that the infarcts could not explain the widespread neuronal loss in the putamen and that a role for an auto-antibody had to be considered.

Diagnosis and management. Diagnosis is based on clinical inspection and is supported in some cases by MRI changes in the striatum. In case of increased SLE activity, immunosuppression is indicated either with corticosteroids or a combination of corticosteroids and a cytotoxic agent (Cervera *et al.*, 1997). Immunosuppression is not required for chorea, as this has mostly a favourable prognosis anyway. If brain imaging reveals striatal infarction, measures to prevent recurrence of vascular events should be considered (see Chapter 2, *Therapy of Ischaemic Stroke*). Patients should move and walk as little as possible since activity promotes chorea. A low daily dose of haloperidol has a beneficial effect on the abnormal movements (see Chapter 2 for haloperidol–induced tardive dyskinesia).

Ballism

Ballistic movements are coarser than those in chorea and are due to contractions in more proximal limb muscles. Ballism is presumed to be caused by lesions in the nucleus subthalamicus and has been described in two SLE patients. In both cases, the ballistic movements were restricted to one side of the body. A vascular origin was deemed likely in view of the acute onset in one case and the presence of multiple cerebral infarcts in the other (Tam *et al.*, 1995; Thompson, 1976). In most respects, management is similar as in chorea. Measures to prevent recurrence of vascular events should be considered (see Chapter 2, *Therapy of Ischaemic Stroke*).

Akinetic mutism and Parkinson's syndrome

There are several case reports on akinetic mutism and Parkinson's syndrome in patients with SLE (Shahar *et al.*, 1996; Miyoshi *et al.*, 1993; Yancey *et al.*, 1981). In two adolescent girls, SPECT showed impaired cerebral blood flow in the basal ganglia region. The girls were treated with dopamine agonists, which was followed by complete to partial improvement (Shahar *et al.*, 1996). In a 30-year-old Japanese woman, Parkinson's syndrome developed (with akinesia, cogwheel muscle rigidity, mask-like expression, and impairment of speech) after she had recovered first from transverse myelitis and thereafter from delirium. MRI of the brain and spinal cord did not reveal any changes. The CSF was examined twice and showed only slight pleocytosis. The Parkinson's syndrome disappeared following treatment with cyclophosphamide and corticosteroids. The authors suggest an immune-mediated origin of the Parkinson's syndrome in their patient and in other cases (Osawa *et al.*, 1997).

Optic neuritis and neuropathy

A marked and usually rapid, but not acute, decrease of visual acuity may occur in one or both eyes (see Table 7.2) (Simeon-Aznar *et al.*, 1992; Barruat *et al.*, 1994; Kira and Goto, 1994; Cordeiro *et al.*, 1994; Eckstein *et al.*, 1995; Keane, 1995). Some patients complain about pain when moving the affected eye. At fundoscopy, the optic papil is often prominent or swollen. Gadolinium MRI may demonstrate enhancement and swelling of the optic nerves, chiasma, or optic tracts, which is commonly interpreted as pointing to disruption of the blood-brain barrier and extravasation of fluid (Sklar *et al.*, 1996). These MRI changes are not seen in all reported patients, perhaps because they are evanescent. The clinical features are compatible with optic neuritis but do not rule out an ischaemic origin either due to vasculitis or vasculopathy or to a heterogeneous origin (see Chapter 2, *Optic Neuritis*). Optic neuritis may precede other signs of SLE for months or even years (Kira and Goto, 1994). It can be the only symptom of CNS involvement in SLE (Eckstein *et al.*, 1995) or may occur in combination with other neurological changes or lesions (Simeon-Aznar *et al.*, 1992). The association with transverse myelitis seems particularly frequent (Simeon-Aznar *et al.*, 1992; Kira and Goto, 1994; Cordeiro *et al.*, 1994).

Diagnosis and management. Diagnosis is based on ophthalmological and neurological examinations and on imaging of the optic system. Whether immunotherapy really achieves more than creating a risk of side effects is questionable (see however, the effect of pulse doses of methylprednisolone in optic neuritis, Chapter 2, *Optic Neuritis*). In our view, increasing the chance of recovery merits taking pulse doses of methylprednisolone, particularly as the associated risks with this form of treatment are limited (see Chapter 4, for side effects). The choice should be submitted to the patient. Success of treatment is reported in some patients but not in all. In these latter cases, the optic papil becomes white and atrophic (Cordeiro *et al.*, 1994).

Inappropriate secretion of antidiuretic hormone

A clinical syndrome of inappropriate secretion of antidiuretic hormone has been observed in a few patients with SLE (see Table 7.2). Patients present with oedema, weight gain, hyponatremia, and elevated levels of antidiuretic hormone. The nature of the defect in the hypothalamo-pituitary axis is not known. A patient reported by Ben Hmida *et al.* (1992) reacted favourably to intravenous administration of a bolus of cyclophosphamide, repeated once after one month, with oral prednisone 1.5 mg/kg daily.

Internuclear ophthalmoplegia, horizontal gaze paralysis, nystagmus and Horner syndrome

Eye movement disorders are not very rare (see Table 7.2). Internuclear ophthalmoplegia (INO) is due to a lesion of the fasciculus longitudinalis superior. This fasciculus runs from pons to mesencephalon in the dorsal and medial part of the brainstem, and it co-ordinates horizontal eye movements. A lesion of one of the fascicles impedes horizontal gazing: adduction of the ipsilateral eye is impossible and the abducting eye usually shows a coarse gaze-directed nystagmus. Multiple sclerosis (MS) is the most frequent and best known cause of INOs. Unilateral and bilateral INOs do occur in SLE however, but are probably not due to demyelination but to ischaemia or infarctions in one or both fasciculi (Jackson *et al.*, 1986; Keane, 1995). Pontine infarcts may cause horizontal gaze paralysis to the ipsilateral side. Downbeat or upbeat vertical nystagmus due to lesions in the medulla oblongata or mesencephalon and Horner's syndrome also have been reported (Keane, 1995). All these eye movement impediments usually do not occur on their own, but in combination with other signs of brainstem dysfunction.

Diagnosis and management. A small infarct in the brainstem, presumably due to vasculopathy or vasculitis, may be visualized in some cases by either CT scan or MRI. Beneficial effects have been reported in some cases of intravenous pulse doses of methylprednisolone or cyclophosphamide (Jackson *et al.*, 1986).

Cranial nerve palsies

The nerves that are most frequently reported as affected are the VIth, VIIth and IIIrd nerve, in that order (Johnson and Richardson, 1968; Feinglass *et al.*, 1976; Muniain *et al.*, 1992; Friedman *et al.*, 1995; Keane, 1995). There are several causes for cranial nerve disorders in SLE: brainstem ischaemia, nerve ischaemia, meningitis, Guillain-Barré syndrome, and raised intracranial pressure. Transverse sinus thrombosis can be the cause of isolated, single, or multiple cranial nerve palsies, particularly of nn. VIII, VII and VI (Kuehnen *et al.*, 1998). A fissura orbitalis superior syndrome with involvement of the IIIrd and IVth nerve and of the ophthalmicus branch of the Vth nerve was reported in one case, and diplopia due to orbital pseudotumour and myositis was reported in a number of cases (see Keane, 1995). Ptosis without any other clinical sign is not that rare and is not always well explained. Sensory trigeminus neuropathy, an inflammatory disorder of the ganglion Gasseri, has been described in few patients (Hughes, 1993a), and occurs much more frequently in systemic sclerosis, Sjögren's syndrome, or overlap syndromes than in SLE (see Chapters 2 and 11). Left recurrent laryngeal palsy is usually associated with pulmonary hypertension and is surmised to be caused by compression of the nerve by the enlarged pulmonary artery. Right recurrent laryngeal nerve palsy has also been observed (Espana *et al.*, 1990; Gordon and Dunn, 1990). Palsy of the XIIth cranial nerve is rare in SLE (Chan *et al.*, 1989).

Diagnosis and management. Diagnosis is based on neurological examination and other associated examinations dependent on the nature of associated signs. Treatment in most cases involves immunosuppression.

Cerebellar disorders

In the more recent literature, case reports on at least seven patients with cerebellar ataxia were published (Singh *et al.*, 1988; Shimomura *et al.*, 1993; Smith *et al.*, 1994; Al-Arfaq and Naddaf, 1995). It appears that cerebellar ataxia may develop subacutely and that it can be asymmetrical. Signs of involvement of the nearby brainstem structures are often present. Imaging of the brain reveals either infarcts or no changes at all. Immunosuppression may be beneficial in some cases (Singh *et al.*, 1988). In other patients, cerebellar ataxia develops more gradually and becomes chronic. In one such case, imaging of the brain showed cerebellar atrophy (Al-Arfaq and Naddaf, 1995). In another case, specific antibodies against human Purkinje's cells were discovered in serum (Shimomura *et al.*, 1993). Selective and severe loss of Purkinje's cells was discovered in the brain of a patient who had suffered from chorea (Kuroe *et al.*, 1994).

Myelopathy or transverse myelitis

Myelopathy, or transverse myelitis (TM) as it is called by different authors, is a rare but well known complication in SLE (Andrianakos *et al.*, 1975; Warren and Kredich, 1984; Propper and Bucknall, 1989; Chan *et al.*, 1995; Lopez Dupla *et al.*, 1995) (Table 7.6). If it is the presenting symptom, other clinical and laboratory manifestations of SLE are usually also present (see however, Kira and Goto, 1994). TM develops acutely or subacutely, usually within a few hours, but can take up to 48 hours. A more protracted course has also been reported (see also Chapter 2). The first symptoms are numbness, paraesthesia and weakness of the lower limbs, back pain, urinary retention, and faecal incontinence. In most cases, an upper border of sensory disturbance is found, and a complete or incomplete spinal cord syndrome may develop with paraplegia or quadriplegia. MRI reveals either swelling of part or all of the cord with increased signal intensity at T2-weighted images (Boumpas *et al.*, 1990; Baca *et al.*, 1996; Mok *et al.*, 1998a) or intramedullary lesions with increased signal intensities on T2-weighted images (Simeon-Aznar, 1992 *et al.*; Harisdangkul

Table 7.6 Transverse myelitis in SLE

Age	10–65
Relation to SLE	In all stages
Time until nadir	Less than 48 hours, seldom more slowly in months
Initial symptoms	Numbness, tingling, weakness of lower limbs, dorsal pain, inability to urinate
Signs	Paraparesis or quadriparesis, Babinski's, upper sensory level, urinary retention
MRI	Swelling of part of the cord or the whole cord with increased signal at T2-weighted images
Treatment	IV pulse doses cyclophosphamide and daily dose of prednisone
Prognosis	Full recovery in approximately 50%. Probably more favourable when treatment is vigorous and starts early

et al., 1995). In some cases, MRI does not demonstrate changes, perhaps because these are not apparent early after onset (within the first 3 or 4 days) (Austin *et al.*, 1992). CSF, when examined, reveals pleocytosis in some cases (mostly less than a few hundred white cells per mm³) and a slightly raised protein content (usually less than 1 g/l). Lavalle *et al.* (1990) found anticardiolipin antibodies in 11 of 12 cases of TM and suggested a relation. However, this suggestion needs confirmation from findings in a larger group before it can be accepted because between 10–50% of SLE patients have such antibodies (Love and Santoro, 1990; Derksen and Stephens, 1995). Mok *et al.* (1998a) found anticardiolipin antibodies in 5 of 10 cases, which was not significantly different from findings in their control SLE group (46%). Neuropathological findings in 12 autopsies, as summarized by Andrianakos *et al.* in 1975, revealed vasculitis in five cases; perivascular inflammation with necrosis or infarction in two cases; myelitis, infarction, and subacute degeneration in one case each; and subdural haematoma with myelum necrosis in 2 cases. The outcome of TM in SLE is variable. Harisdangkul *et al.* (1997) reported that four of seven patients died and that one other patient remained wheelchair-bound. The two patients who did well had been treated with high-dose intravenous pulse steroid within one week after onset. In a study of 10 cases, it appeared that four had recovered completely, three had residual spasticity, two kept some degree of weakness of the lower limbs, and one had remained paraplegic (Mok *et al.*, 1998a). One patient had been treated with intravenous high-dose methylprednisolone pulse dose within 24 hours after onset but did not respond well.

Diagnosis and management. Diagnosis is based on neurological examination and MRI. The effect of treatment with standard high-oral doses of corticosteroids has been disappointing in several patients. There are now, however, a number of case reports on favourable results of early and vigorous immunosuppression with intravenous methylprednisolone or cyclophospamide pulse therapy (Barile and Laval, 1992; Baca *et al.*, 1995; Harisdangkul *et al.*, 1995; Kater, 1997, not published) (see also Chapter 4). Confirmation of this effect in an intervention study would be desirable, but the rarity of TMs seems to prohibit such studies. In our view, treatment regimens with a reasonable chance of improving outcome and a limited risk of side effects, as in pulse treatments with methylprednisolone or cyclophosphamide, are worth trying. Treatment with anticoagulants has not been attempted. Relapse of TM has been described in several patients (Chan and Boey, 1996; Mok *et al.*, 1998a).

Neuroinfections
Two reasons for the increased infection rate and the frequency of opportunistic infections in SLE are dysregulation of the immune system and immunosuppressive drug treatment. The main examples of such unusual infections are cryptococcal meningitis, aspergillus meningitis, aspergillus and nocardia asteroides brain abscesses, listeria monocytogenes meningitis and toxoplasmosis encephalitis (see Hellman *et al.*, 1987; Iliopoulos and Tsokos, 1996).

Bacterial infections in SLE involve all the common bacteria. Herpes zoster is the leading viral infection and has apparently a relatively benign course in most cases (Manzi *et al.*, 1995), though herpes zoster myelitis in SLE is reported (Ebo *et al.*, 1996). A notorious but rare opportunistic viral infection is with the JC strain of papovavirus. It causes depletion of oligodendroglia cells, multifocal demyelination, and is clinically characterized by a progressive course and lethal outcome within a year or less (Newton *et al.*, 1986) (see Chapter 2, *White Matter Lesion of Viral Origin* for diagnostic methods and therapy).

Intracranial fungal infections (cryptococcus neoformans, aspergillosis) and nocardiosis are notoriously difficult to diagnose, and are often fatal (Zimmerman *et al.*, 1992; Lammens *et al.*, 1992; Katz *et al.*, 1996; Mok *et al.*, 1997; Mok *et al.*, 1998b). In fungal meningitis, usually cryptococcus neoformans, clinical symptoms and changes in the cell and protein content of the CSF are often only minimal. Futrell *et al.* (1992) had, in their series of 63 SLE patients with CNS involvement, 10 complete autopsies. One case had cytomegalovirus in the brain, another one aspergillus, and in a third case nocardia brain abscess was discovered. In a retrospective investigation of postmortem CNS tissue, eight of 37 SLE patients with CNS manifestations had evidence of infection: aseptic meningitis, aspergillar and candidal brain abscesses, viral meningo-encephalitis and bacterial meningitis (Devinsky *et al.*, 1988).

Diagnosis and management. When SLE patients present with CNS symptoms, one should always be aware of the possibility of opportunistic infections. Each causative agent has its own clinical and laboratory characteristics as is illustrated in the following examples (Christin and Sugar, 1997). *Cryptococcus neoformans* localizes preferentially in the CNS, and is visualized in the CSF by the Indian ink stain or it is cultured from CSF. Aspergillosis usually presents in the brain with multiple infarcts or a ruptured mycotic aneurysm. *Nocardia asteroides* resembles fungi in several respects but is a gram positive bacteria. It spreads from pulmonary lesions by way of the blood stream and causes brain abscesses. For each of these agents, antimycotic or antibacterial therapy is available.

CLINICAL FEATURES OF PERIPHERAL NERVE INVOLVEMENT

Epidemiology of peripheral neuropathies in SLE

Disorders of the peripheral nervous system (PNS) are less frequent than those of the CNS and may be incapacitating, but are in general not life-threatening. In a cross-sectional study, Straub *et al.* (1996) used standardized clinical tests and discovered evidence of sensomotor neuropathy in 6%. Omdal *et al.* (1991) used nerve conduction velocities as criterion for neuropathy. In a consecutive series of 33 patients with definite SLE, eight (24%) had polyneuropathy. Feinglass *et al.* (1976) found in a cohort of 122 hospitalized patients clinical signs of peripheral neuropathy in 15 (8%). Johnson and Richardson (1968) established the presence of peripheral neuropathy in two of 24 selected cases, on whom autopsy had been performed.

Different types of peripheral neuropathy

Feinglass *et al.* (1976) observed that their patients had one of three types of neuropathy: a sensory or mixed sensomotor symmetrical neuropathy with predominantly sensory features (nine patients); a Guillain-Barré-like syndrome (one patient); and an asymmetrical neuropathy suggestive of a mononeuritis multiplex (five patients). With slight additions, this classification of SLE neuropathies was confirmed by other authors in the following decades (Chalk *et al.*, 1993). The Guillain-Barré syndrome in SLE had all the classical features (Chanduri *et al.*, 1989; Lesprit *et al.*, 1996) and presented in some patients with ophthalmoplegia and ataxia, as in Miller-Fisher syndrome (Bingisser *et al.*, 1994; Hess *et al.*, 1990). Chronic inflammatory demyelinating neuropathy (CIDP) was observed also (Rechthand *et al.*, 1984; Sigal *et al.*, 1989). Mononeuropathy multiplex or polyneuropathy due to vasculitis was reported by Hughes *et al.* (1982) and others (Markusse *et al.*, 1991; Martinez-Taboada *et al.*, 1996). Peripheral neuropathy often became manifest during an active stage of the disease.

Tests for autonomic neuropathy, in a cross-sectional study, revealed pupillary abnormalities in 29% of SLE patients (*n*=31) and cardiovascular changes in 10% (Straub *et al.*, 1996). In another study with less strict criteria, 15 of 17 SLE patients had one or more abnormal cardiovascular tests (Lioté and Osterland, 1994). Clinical evidence of autonomic neuropathy was present in one of the patients of Lioté and Osterland (1994). Studies of heart rate variability demonstrated significant differences between groups of SLE patients and age- and sex-matched controls (Stein *et al.*, 1996; Lagana *et al.*, 1996). Clinical evidence of dysautonomia in these latter two studies was not found (Lagana *et al.*, 1996) or not reported (Stein *et al.*, 1996). At present, it seems justified to conclude that the autonomic nervous system is not spared in SLE. Patients with clinical symptoms of autonomic neuropathy seem rare however.

Histopathology of peripheral neuropathy in SLE
The pathological basis for sensory, or predominantly sensory, neuropathy was investigated by McCombe *et al.* in 1987. Sural nerve biopsies of four definite SLE patients with mixed, predominantly sensory, neuropathy showed acute and chronic axonal degeneration and loss of unmyelinated and myelinated nerve fibres. The vessels were described as showing evidence of vasculitis. However, according to Chalk *et al.* (1993), the epineurial arterioles often are only surrounded by lymphocytes and macrophages. They may show some intimal thickening, but no angionecrosis. This description by Chalk *et al.* (1993) fits in with our own observations. It suggests that the underlying pathology of the predominantly sensory polyneuropathies is heterogeneous: it is due to an inflammatory neuropathy in some cases and to vasculitis or vasculopathy in others. Necrotizing vasculitis was convincingly documented in a case of mononeuritis multiplex (Hughes *et al.*, 1982).

Diagnosis and management. Standard techniques are applied to diagnose peripheral neuropathies. The results of corticosteroid therapy of the sensory or predominantly sensory polyneuropathies are described as 'variable' (McCombe *et al.*, 1987). Combination of corticosteroids with one of the cytotoxic agents would seem indicated to improve results, but reports on this approach have not been published yet. Guillain-Barré syndrome has been demonstrated to react favourably to intravenous immunoglobulins in some patients (Lesprit *et al.*, 1996). Vasculitic neuropathy (see Chapter 5, *Vasculitic Neuropathy*) is well treatable with corticosteroids or a combination of corticosteroids and cyclosphosphamide (Hughes, 1982; Enevoldson and Wiles, 1991; Markusse *et al.*, 1991; Martinez-Taboada *et al.*, 1996).

DISORDERS OF NEUROMUSCULAR JUNCTIONS AND TERMINAL MOTOR NERVE FIBRES IN SLE

The association of SLE and myasthenia gravis (MG) is well established, and has now been described in at least 30 patients (Vaiopoulos *et al.*, 1994). What happens in many patients is as follows: first, MG becomes evident, for which thymectomy or thymomectomy is performed after some time. A variable time period then passes before SLE develops (Mevorach *et al.*, 1995; Rosman *et al.*, 1995). SLE after thymomectomy without MG also has been reported. Two case histories were published on Lambert-Eaton myasthenic syndrome (LEMS) in patients with SLE (Deodhar *et al.*, 1996; Hughes and Katirji, 1986). The reader is referred to Chapter 2 for a description of the different aspects of these diseases and for their management.

Acquired neuromyotonia is characterized clinically by muscle twitching, aching or cramps, and myotonia-like symptoms in some cases. The disease is due to antibodies against voltage-gated potassium channels in the axonal membrane of terminal motor nerve fibres. A patient with SLE who developed neuromyotonia was recently reported. She did not respond to the standard treatment with either carbamazepine or phenytoin (Magnani *et al.*, 1998). The condition is described in more detail in Chapter 2.

INFLAMMATORY MYOPATHY AND SLE

Orbital myositis
Orbital myositis is a rare but well-documented complication in SLE (Serop *et al.*, 1994; Davalos *et al.*, 1984; Evans and Lexow, 1978). Pain in the affected eye, blurred vision, watery discharge, diplopia, conjunctivitis, episcleritis, chemosis and proptosis, and limitation of eye movements belong, in a variable degree, to the features of this syndrome. Histological studies of this syndrome in patients with SLE have not been performed to the best of our knowledge.

Diagnosis and management. CT shows a striking enlargement of the extraocular muscles in the affected eye(s). The condition responds well to corticosteroids (see Chapter 6, *Orbital Myositis*).

Acquired Brown's syndrome
Patients with this syndrome complain about vertical diplopia on upward and inward gaze. Ophthalmological investigation shows that patients are unable to fully elevate the affected adducted eye. Upward and inward gaze may be associated with pain and in some patients a palpable click may be felt over the trochlea. Brown's syndrome is due to swelling of the posterior part of the superior oblique tendon. Acquired Brown's syndrome has been described in few patients with SLE (Alonso-Valdivielso *et al.*, 1993; McGaillard and Bell, 1993).

Diagnosis and management. On CT scans, swelling of the tendon of the obliquus inferior muscle has been observed in several cases. The syndrome may be spontaneously evanescent. It responds to a low dose of prednisone (20 mg daily). (See also Chapter 6).

Polymyositis and dermatomyositis
Data on the prevalence of polymyositis (PM) or dermatomyositis (DM) in SLE were gathered in the seventies and early eighties when criteria for the diagnosis of SLE had not been agreed upon yet. Muscle weakness due to inflammatory myopathy was found in 5–10% of the patients (see Layzer, 1985), but this is probably an exaggeration (Grigor *et al.*, 1978; Isenberg and Snaith, 1981; Tsokos *et al.*, 1981). Many patients with SLE complain about muscle pain but this is not due to myositis.

Foot *et al.* (1982) studied the features of lupus myositis in 11 patients. Weakness was mild or moderate, symmetrical, and more severe proximally than distally at the limbs. The lower limbs seemed more affected than the upper limbs. Some patients had symptoms of dysphagia. Garton and Isenberg (1997) concluded, on the basis of a comparative study, that weakness due to lupus myositis was not milder than in DM or PM.

Muscle biopsies show perivascular infiltrates without destruction of vessel walls, and degenerating and regenerating muscle fibres with abnormal variation in muscle fibre sizes. The inflammatory changes of the vessels in the muscle biopsies have been described, in turn, as perivascular infiltrates and as vasculitis or lymphocytic vasculitis (Pallis *et al.*, 1993; Lim *et al.*, 1994; Engel *et al.*, 1994). Perivascular mononuclear cell infiltrates have often been found in skeletal muscles of LE patients at autopsy (Lowman, 1951; Ropes, 1976). According to Engel *et al.* (1994), the changes are similar to those in idiopathic DM. Crowson and Magro (1996) compared vascular changes in the skin between DM and SLE. Four of 19 SLE biopsies showed significant endothelial injury and fibrin deposits of dermal small vessels. Immunohistochemistry revealed vascular deposition of the membrane attack complex (MAC) in three of these biopsies. The changes occurred in the setting of mononuclear cell vasculitis in one case.

Diagnosis and management. Lupus myositis is treated similarly to PM or DM. (See Chapter 6).

Inclusion body myositis (IBM)
IBM in SLE has been reported by several authors (Yood and Smith, 1985; Mikol and Engel, 1994) (see Chapter 6).

CONCLUSIONS

Psychiatrical and neurological manifestations in SLE are frequent, highly variable, often incapacitating, and sometimes life-threatening. SLE may present with these manifestations or they may complicate SLE months or years after onset. Incidence and prevalence of different neuropsychiatrical abnormalities are insufficiently known. Until not so long ago, the neuropsychiatrical manifestations were attributed mostly to vasculitis, but now it is clear that the role of inflammatory changes has been exaggerated and that other, not fully understood factors, are responsible for the vasculopathy in the nervous system. Although the number of drugs available for immunotherapy is considerable, there is much uncertainty about the best form of therapy for neuropsychiatrical manifestations because of the lack of intervention studies.

REFERENCES

Abu-Shakra M, Urowitz MB, Gladman DD *et al.* (1995a) Mortality studies in systemic lupus erythematosus. Results from a single center. I. Causes of death. *J Rheumatol* **22**, 1259–1264.
Abu-Shakra M, Urowitz MB, Gladman DD *et al.* (1995b) Mortality studies in systemic lupus erythematosus. Results from a single center. II. Predictor variables for mortality. *J Rheumatol* **22**, 1265–1270.

Al-Arfaq HF and Naddaf HO (1995) Cerebellar atrophy in systemic lupus erythematosus. *Lupus* **4**, 412–414.

Alcocer-Varela J, Aleman-Hoey D and Alarcon-Segovia D (1992) Interleukin-1 and interleukin-6 activities are increased in the cerebrospinal fluid of patients with CNS lupus erythematosus and correlate with local late T-cell activation markers. *Lupus* **1**, 111–117.

Alonso-Valdivielso JL, Alvarez Lario B, Alegre Lopez J *et al.* (1993) Acquired Brown's syndrome in a patient with systemic lupus erythematosus. *Ann Rheum Dis* **52**, 63–64.

American Psychiatric Association (1994) *Diagnostic and Statistical Manual of Mental Disorders*, 4th edn. Washington, DC: APA.

Andrianakos AA, Duffy J, Suzuki M *et al.* (1975) Transverse myelopathy in systemic lupus erythematosus. Report of three cases and review of the literature. *Ann Int Med* **83**, 616–624.

Anzola GP, Dalla Volta G and Balestrieri G (1988) Headache in patients with systemic lupus erythematosus: Clinical and theletermographic findings. *Arch Neurol* **45**, 1061–1062.

Asherson RA, Derksen RHWM, Nigel Harris E *et al.* (1987) Chorea in systemic lupus erythematosus and 'lupus-like' disease: Association with antiphospholipid antibodies. *Semin Arthritis Rheum* **16**, 253–259.

Austin SG, Zee CS and Waters C (1992) The role of magnetic resonance imaging in acute transverse myelitis. *Can J Neurol Sci* **19**, 508–511.

Baart de la Faille H and Kater L (1995) Guidelines for the clinical application of immunologic laboratory investigations. In: Kater L and Baart de la Faille H (eds) *Multi-systemic Auto-immune Diseases: An Integrated Approach*, pp 85–128. Amsterdam: Elsevier.

Baca V, Sanchez-Vaca G, Martinez-Muniz G (1996) Successful treatment of transverse myelitis in a child with lupus erythematosus. *Neuropaediatrics* **27**, 42–44.

Barile L and Lavalle C (1992) Transverse myelitis in systemic lupus erythematosus – the effect of IV pulse methylprednisolone and cyclophosphamide. *J Rheumatol* **19**, 370–372.

Barruat FX, Prado T, Strominger M *et al.* (1994) Complication neuro-ophthalmologique du lupus erythemateux disséminé. *Klin Monatschr Augenheilk* **204**, 403–406.

Belmont HM, Abramson SB and Lie JT (1996) Pathology and pathogenesis of vascular injury in systemic lupus erythematosus. *Arthritis Rheum* **39**, 9–21.

Ben Hmida M, Bunker D, Baumelou A *et al.* (1992) Inappropriate secretion of antidiuretic hormone (SIADH) in a patient with systemic lupus erythematosus (SLE): A case report. *Clin Nephrol* **37**, 34–35.

Bingisser R, Speich R, Fontana A *et al.* (1994) Lupus erythematosus and Miller-Fisher syndrome. *Arch Neurol* **51**, 828–830.

Bluestein HG, Williams GW and Steinberg AD (1981) Cerebrospinal fluid antibodies to neuronal cells: Association with neuropsychiatric manifestations of systemic lupus erythematosus. *Am J Med* **70**, 240–246.

Bonfa E, Golomber SJ, Kaufman LD *et al.* (1987) Association between lupus psychosis and anti-ribosomal P protein antibodies. *N Engl J Med* **317**, 265–271.

Bootsma H, Derksen RHWM, Spronk PE, *et al.* (1996) Sensitivity to change of lupus disease activity indices: A long-term prospective analysis of 3 clinical measures. Paper presented at the Annual American College of Rheumatology Meeting.

Boumpas DT, Patronas NJ, Dalakas MC *et al.* (1990) Acute transverse myelitis in systemic lupus erythematosus: Magnetic resonance imaging and review of the literature. *J Rheumatol* **17**, 89–92.

Brey RL and Coull BM (1996) Cerebral venous thrombosis. Role of activated Protein C resistance and Factor V gene mutation. *Stroke* **27**, 1719–1720.

Brinciotti M, Ferrucci G, Trasatti G *et al.* (1993) Reflex seizures as initial manifestations of systemic lupus erythematosus in childhood. *Lupus* **2**, 281–283.

Bruyn GAW (1995) Controversies in lupus: Nervous system involvement. *Ann Rheum Dis* **54**, 159–167.

Bruyn GA and Padberg G (1984) Chorea and systemic lupus erythematosus – a critical review. *Eur Neurol* **23**, 435–448.

Carbotte RM, Denburg SD, Denburg JA *et al.* (1992) Fluctuating cognitive abnormalities and cerebral glucose metabolism in neuropsychiatric systemic lupus erythematosus. *J Neurol Neurosurg Psychiat* **55**, 1054–1059.

Carbotte RM, Denburg SD and Denburg JA (1995a) Cognitive dysfunction in systemic lupus erythematosus is independent of active disease. *J Rheumatol* **22**, 863–867.

Carbotte RAM, Denburg SD and Denburg JA (1995b) Cognitive deficit associated with rheumatic diseases: Neuropsychological perspectives. *Arthritis Rheum* **38**, 1363–1374.

Carette S, Urowitz MB, Grosman H *et al.* (1982) Cranial computerized tomography in systemic lupus erythematosus. *J Rheumatol* **9**, 855–859.

Casciola-Rosen L, Anhalt G and Rosen A (1994) Autoantigens targeted in systemic lupus erythematosus are clustered in two populations of surface structures on apoptotic keratinocytes. *J Exp Med* **179**, 1317–1330.

Cervera R, Khamashata MA, Font J *et al.* (1993) Systemic lupus erythematosus: Clinical and immunologic patterns of disease expression in a cohort of 1000 patients. *Medicine* **72**, 113–124.

Cervera R, Asherson RA, Font J *et al.* (1997) Chorea in the antiphospholipid syndrome. *Medicine* **76**, 203–212.

Chalk CH, Dyck PJ and Conn DL (1993) Vasculitic neuropathy. In: Dyck PJ, Thomas PK, Griffin JW *et al.* (eds) *Peripheral Neuropathy*, 3rd edn, pp 1424–1436. Philadelphia: WB Saunders.

Chan KF and Boey ML (1996) Transverse myelopathy in SLE: Clinical features and functional outcomes. *Lupus* **5**, 294–299.

Chan K-F, Kong K-H, Boey M-L (1995). 'Great mimicry' in a patient with tetraparesis: a case report. *Arch Phys Med Rehab* **76**, 391–393.

Chan CN, Li E, Lai FM *et al.* (1989) An unusual case of systemic lupus erythematosus with isolated hypoglossal nerve palsy, fulminant acute pneumonitis and pulmonary amyloidosis. *Ann Rheum Dis* **48**, 236–239.

Chanduri KR, Taylor IK, Niverr RM *et al.* (1989) A case of systemic lupus erythematosus presenting as Guillain-Barré syndrome. *Br J Rheumatol* **28**, 440–442.

Chinn RJS, Wilkinson ID, Hall-Craggs MA *et al.* (1997) Magnetic resonance imaging of the brain and cerebral proton spectroscopy in patients with systemic lupus erythematosus. *Arthritis Rheum* **40**, 36–46.

Christin L and Sugar AM (1997) Fungal infections. In: Roos KL (ed) *Central Nervous System Infectious Diseases and Therapy*, pp 167–192. New York: Marcel Dekker Inc.

Churg J and Sobin LH (1982) Lupus nephritis. In: Churg J and Sobin LE (eds) *Renal Disease Classification And Atlas of Glomerular Diseases*, pp 127–132. Tokyo: Igaku-Shoin.

Corbett JJ, Nerad JA, Tse DT *et al.* (1988) Results of optic nerve sheath decompression for pseudotumor cerebri. The lateral orbitomy approach. *Arch Ophthalmol* **106**, 391–397.

Cordeiro MF, Lloyd ME, Spalton DJ *et al.* (1994) Ischaemic optic neuropathy, transverse myelitis, and epilepsy in an antiphospholipid positive patient with systemic lupus erythematosus. *J Neurol Neurosurg Psychiat* **57**, 1142–1143.

Cremer PD, Johnston IH and Halmagyi GM (1997) Pseudotumor cerebri syndrome due to cryptococcal meningitis. *J Neurol Neurosurg Psychiat* **62**, 96–98.

Crowson AN and Magro CM (1996) The role of microvascular injury in the pathogenesis of cutaneous lesions of dermatomyositis. *Hum Pathol* **27**, 15–19.

Davalos A, Matias-Guiu J, Cadina A *et al.* (1984) Painful ophthalmoplegia in systemic lupus erythematosus. *J Neurol Neurosurg Psychiat* **47**, 323–325.

de Bruyn SFTM, Stam J and Kapelle LJ for CVST Study Group (1996) Thunderclap as first symptom of cerebral venous sinus thrombosis. *Lancet* **348**, 1623–1625.

Denburg SD, Carbotte RM and Denburg JA (1987) Cognitive impairment in systemic lupus erythematosus: A neuropsychological study of individual and group deficits. *J Clin Exp Neuropsychol* **9**, 323–339.

Deodhar A, Norden J, So Y *et al.* (1996) The association of systemic lupus erythematosus and Lambert-Eaton myasthenic syndrome. *J Rheumatol* **23**, 1292–1294.

Derksen RHWM and Stephens CJM (1995) The antiphospolipid syndrome. In: Kater L and Baart de la Faille H (eds) *Multi-systemic Auto-Immune Diseases: An Integrated Approach*, pp 129–140. Amsterdam: Elsevier.

Devinsky O, Petito CK and Alonso DR (1988) Clinical and neuropathological findings in systemic lupus erythematosus: The role of vasculitis, heart emboli and thrombotic thrombocytopenic purpura. *Ann Neurol* **23**, 380–384.

Drenkard C, Villa AR, Garcia-Padilla C, Pérez-Vazquez ME *et al.* (1996) Remission of systematic lupus erythematosus. *Medicine* **75**, 88–98.

Drenkard C, Villa AR, Garcia-Padilla C *et al.* (1997) Vasculitis in systemic lupus erythematosus. *Lupus* **6**, 235–242.

Duits AJ, Bootsma H, Derksen RHWM *et al.* (1995) Skewed distribution of IgGFc receptor IIa (CD 32) polymorphism is associated with renal disease in systemic lupus erythematosus patients. *Arthritis Rheum* **39**, 1832–1836.

Ebo DG, De Clerck LS, Stevens WJ *et al.* (1996) Herpes zoster myelitis occurring during treatment for systemic lupus erythematosus. *J Rheumatol* **23**, 548–550.

Eckstein A, Kötter I and Wilhelm H (1995) Atypische optikus neuritis bei systemischem lupus erythematosus (SLE). *Klin Monatschr Augenheilk* **207**, 310–313.

Engel AG, Hohlfeld R and Banker BQ (1994) The polymyositis and dermatomyositis syndromes. In: Engel AG and Franzini-Armstrong G (eds) *Myology*, Vol 2, 2ed, pp 1335–1383. New York: McGraw-Hill.

Einhäupl KM, Villringer A, Meister W *et al.* (1991) Heparin treatment in sinus venous thrombosis. *Lancet* **338**, 597–600.

Enevoldson TP and Wiles CM (1991) Severe vasculitic neuropathy in systemic lupus erythematosus and response to cyclophosphamide. *J Neurol Neurosurg Psychiat* **54**, 468–469.

Espana A, Guttierez JM, Soria C *et al.* (1990) Recurrent laryngeal palsy in systemic lupus erythematosus. *Neurology* **40**, 1143–1144.

Evans OB and Lexow SS (1978) Painful ophthalmoplegia in systemic lupus erythematosus. *Ann Neurol* **4**, 584–585.

Euler H, Schroeder JO, Harten P *et al.* (1994) Treatment free remission in severe systemic lupus erythematosus following synchronisation of plasmapheresis and subsequent pulse cyclophosphamide. *Arthritis Rheum* **37**, 1784–1789.

Feinglass EJ, Arnett FC, Dorsch CA *et al.* (1976) Neuropsychiatric manifestations of systemic lupus erythematosus: Diagnosis, clinical spectrum, and relationship to other features of the disease. *Medicine* **55**, 323–339.

Felson DT (1997) Epidemiology of the rheumatic diseases. In: Koopman WJ (ed) *Arthritis and Allied Diseases*, 13ed, pp 3–34. Baltimore: Williams and Wilkins.

Flussner D, Abu-Shakra M, Baumgartner-Kleiner A *et al.* (1996) Superior sagittal sinus thrombosis in a patient with systemic lupus erythematosus. *Lupus* **5**, 334–336.

Fody EP, Netsky MG and Mark RE (1980) Subarachnoid spinal hemorrhage in a case of systemic lupus erythematosus. *Arch Neurol* **37**, 173–174.

Foot RA, Kimbrough SM and Stevens JC (1982) Lupus myositis. *Muscle Nerve* **5**, 65–68.

Friedman AS, Folkert V and Khan GA (1995) Recurrence of systemic lupus erythematosus in a hemodialysis patient presenting as unilateral abducens nerve palsy. *Clin Nephrol* **44**, 338–339.

Futrell N and Millikan C (1989). Frequency, etiology, and prevention of stroke in patients with systemic lupus erythematosus. *Stroke* **20**, 583–591.

Futrell N, Schultz LR and Millikan C (1992) Central nervous system disease in patients with systemic lupus erythematosus. *Neurology* **42**, 1649–1657.

Garcia-Rayo P, Gil Aguado A, Simon Merlo MJ *et al.* (1994) Massive cerebral calcifications in systemic lupus erythematosus: Report of an unusual case. *Lupus* **3**, 133–135.

Garton MJ and Isenberg DA (1997) Clinical features of lupus myositis versus idiopathic myositis: A review of 30 cases. *Brit J Rheumatol* **36**, 1067–1074.

Ginsburg KS, Wright EA, Larson MG *et al.* (1992) A controlled study of the prevalence of cognitive dysfunction in randomly selected patients with systemic lupus erythematosus. *Arthritis Rheum* **35**, 776–782.

Gelder M, Gath D, Meyou R *et al.* (1996) *Oxford Textbook of Psychiatry*, 3ed, Oxford: Oxford University Press.

Gieron MA, Khoromi S and Campos A (1995) MRI changes in the central nervous system in a child with lupus erythematosus. *Pediatr Radiol* **25**, 184–185.

Gladman DD, Goldsmith CH, Urowitz MB *et al.* (1992) Cross-cultural validation and reliability of three disease activity indices in SLE. *J Rheumatol* **19**, 608–611.

Golombek SJ, Graus F and Elkon KB (1986) Auto-antibodies in the cerebrospinal fluid of patients with systemic lupus erythematosus. *Arthritis Rheum* **29**, 1090–1097.

Gonzalez-Crespo MR, Blanco FJ, Ramos A *et al.* (1995) Magnetic resonance imaging of the brain in systemic lupus erythematosus. *Brit J Rheumatol* **34**, 1055–1060.

Gordon T and Dunn EC (1990) Systemic lupus erythematosus and right recurrent laryngeal nerve palsy. *Br J Rheumatol* **29**, 308–309.

Green L, Vinker S, Amital A *et al.* (1995) Pseudotumor cerebri in systemic lupus erythematosus. *Semin Arthritis Rheum* **25**, 103–108.

Grigor R, Edmonds J, Leukonia R *et al.* (1978) Systemic lupus erythematosus. A prospective analysis. *Ann Rheum Dis* **37**, 121–128.

Hanly JG, Fisk JD and Sherwood G *et al.* (1992a) Cognitive impairment in patients with systemic lupus erythematosus. *J Rheumatol* **19**, 562–567.

Hanly JG, Walsh NMG and Sangalang V (1992b) Brain pathology in systemic lupus erythematosus. *J Rheumatol* **19**, 732–741.

Hanly JG, Fisk JD, Sherwood G and Eastwood B (1994) Clinical course of cognitive dysfunction in systemic lupus erythematosus. *J Rheumatol* **21**, 1825–1831.

Hanly JG, Cassell K and Fisk JD (1997) Cognitive function in systemic lupus erythematosus: Results of a 5 year prospective study. *Arthritis Rheum* **40**, 1542–1543.

Harisdangkul V, Doorenbos D and Subramony SH (1995). Lupus transverse myelopathy better outcome with early recognition and aggressive high dose intravenous corticosteroid pulse treatment. *J Neurol* **242**, 326–331.

Hay EM, Black D, Huddy A *et al.* (1992) Psychiatric disorder and cognitive impairment in systemic lupus erythematosus. *Arthritis Rheum* **35**, 411–416.

Hellman DB, Petri M and Whiting-O'Keefe Q (1987) Fatal infections in systemic lupus erythematosus: The role of opportunistic organisms. *Medicine* **66**, 341–348.

Herranz MT, Rivier G, Khamashata MA *et al.* (1994) Association between antiphospholipid antibodies and epilepsy in patients with systemic lupus erythematosus. *Medicine* **4**, 568–571.

Hess DC, Awad E, Posas H *et al.* (1990) Miller-Fisher syndrome in systemic lupus erythematosus. *J Rheumatol* **17**, 1520–1522.

Hirohata S and Miyamoto T (1990) Elevated levels of interleukin-6 in cerebrospinal fluid from patients with systemic lupus erythematosus and central nervous system involvement. *Arthritis Rheum* **33**, 644–649.

Hochberg MC, Petri M (1993) Clinical features of systemic lupus erythematosus. *Current Opin Rheumatol* **5**, 575–586.

Hopkinson N (1992) Epidemiology of systemic lupus erythematosus. *Ann Rheum Dis* **51**, 1292–1294.

Hughes GRV (1993) The antiphospholipid syndrome: Ten years on. *Lancet* **342**, 341–344.

Hughes RAC (1993a) Diseases of the fifth cranial nerve. In: Dyck PJ, Thomas PK, Griffin JW *et al.* (eds) *Peripheral Neuropathy*, Vol 2, 3ed, pp 801–817. Philadelphia: WB Saunders.

Hughes RAC, Cameron JS, Hall SM *et al.* (1982) Multiple mononeuropathy as the initial presentation of systemic lupus erythematosus – nerve biopsy and response to plasma exchange. *J Neurol* **228**, 239–247.

Hughes RL and Katirji MB (1986) The Eaton-Lambert (myasthenic) syndrome in association with systemic lupus erythematosus. *Arch Neurol* **43**, 1186–1187.

Hylek EM, Skates SJ, Sheehan A *et al.* (1996) An analysis of the lowest effective intensity of prophylactic anticoagulation for patients with nonrheumatic atrial fibrillation. *N Engl J Med* **335**, 540–546.

Iliopoulos AG and Tsokos GC (1996) Immunopathogenesis and spectrum of infections in systemic lupus erythematosus. *Semin Arthritis Rheum* **25**, 316–336.

Isenberg DA and Snaith ML (1981) Muscle disease in systemic lupus erythematosus: A study of its nature, frequency and cause. *J Rheumatol* **8**, 917–924.

Isshi K and Hirohata S (1996) Association of anti-ribosomal P protein antibodies with neuropsychiatric systemic lupus erythematosus. *Arthritis Rheum* **39**, 1483–1490.

Isshi K, Hirohata S, Hashimoto T *et al.* (1994) Systemic lupus erythematosus presenting with diffuse low density lesions in the cerebral white matter on computed axial tomography scans: Its implication in the pathogenesis of diffuse central nervous system lupus. *J Rheumatol* **21**, 1758–1762.

Jackson G, Miller M, Littlejohn G *et al.* (1986) Bilateral internuclear ophthalmoplegia in systemic lupus erythematosus. *J Rheumatol* **13**, 1161–1162.

Jarek MJ, West SG, Baker MR *et al.* (1994) Magnetic resonance imaging in systemic lupus erythematosus without a history of neuropsychiatric lupus erythematosus. *Arthritis Rheum* **37**, 1609–1613.

Johnson AE, Gordon C, Palmer RG *et al.* (1995) The prevalence and incidence of systemic lupus erythematosus in Birmingham, England. *Arthritis Rheum* **38**, 551–558.

Johnson AE, Gordon C and Bacon PA (1996) Undiagnosed systemic lupus erythematosus in the community. *Lancet* **347**, 337–369.

Johnson RT and Richardson EP (1968) The neurological manifestations of systemic lupus erythematosus. *Medicine* **47**, 337–336.

Jongen PJH, Boerbooms AMT, Lamers KJB *et al.* (1990) CNS involvement in systemic lupus erythematosus: Intrathecal synthesis of the 4th component of complement. *Neurology* **40**, 1593–1596.

Kallenberg CGM and Callen JF (1995) Raynaud's phenomenon. In: Kater L and Baart de la Faille H (eds) *Multi-System Auto-immune Diseases*, pp 299–306. Amsterdam: Elsevier.

Kashihara K, Nakashima S, Kohira I *et al.* (1998) Hyperintense basal ganglia on T1-weighted MR images in a patient with central nervous system lupus and chorea. *Am J Neuroradiol* **19**, 284–286.

Karahalios DG, Rekate HL, Khayata MH *et al.* (1996) Elevated intracranial venous pressure as a universal mechanism in pseudotumor cerebri of varying etiologies. *Neurology* **46**, 198–202.

Karlson EW, Daltroy LH, Lew RA *et al.* (1997) The relationship of socioeconomic status, race and modifiable risk factors to outcomes in patients with systemic lupus erythematosus. *Arthritis Rheum* **40**, 47–56.

Kater L, Gmelig-Meyling FHJ, Derksen RHWM *et al.* (1995) Immunopathogenesis and therapy of systemic lupus erythematosus. *Clin Immunotherapy* **4**, 471–493.

Kater L and Provost TT (1995) Classification criteria, disease activity criteria and chronicity criteria. In: Kater L and Baart de la Faille H (eds) *Muli-Systemic Auto-Immune Diseases: An Integrated Approach*, pp 43–59. Amsterdam: Elsevier.

Katz A, Ehrenfeld M, Livneh A *et al.* (1996) Aspergillosis in systemic lupus erythematosus. *Semin Arthritis Rheum* **26**, 635–640.

Kaye BR, Neuwelt CM, London SS *et al.* (1992) Central nervous system systemic lupus erythematosus mimicking progressive multifocal leukoencephalopathy. *Ann Rheum Dis* **51**, 1152–1156.

Khamashta MA, Cuadrado MJ, Mujic F *et al.* (1995) The management of thrombosis in the antiphospholipid antibody syndrome. *N Engl J Med* **332**, 993–997.

Keane JR (1995) Eye movement abnormalities in systemic lupus erythematosus. *Arch Neurol* **52**, 1145–1149.

Kershner P and Wang-Cheng R (1989) Psychiatric side effects of steroid therapy. *Psychosomatics* **30**, 135–139.

King JO, Mitchell PJ, Thomson KR *et al.* (1995) Cerebral venography and manometry in idiopathic intracranial hypertension. *Neurology* **45**, 2224–2228.

Kira J and Goto J (1994) Recurrent opticomyelitis associated with anti-DNA antibody. *J Neurol Neurosurg Psychiat* **57**, 1124–1125.

Kitagawa Y, Gotoh F, Koto A *et al.* (1990) Stroke in systemic lupus erythematosus. *Stroke* **21**, 1533–1539.

Kodama K, Okada S, Hino T *et al.* (1995) Single photon emission computed tomography in systemic lupus erythematosus with psychiatric symptoms. *J Neurol Neurosurg Psychiat* **58**, 307–311.

Koudstaal PJ, van Gijn J, Kapelle LJ *et al.* (1991) Headache in transient or permanent cerebral ischaemia. *Stroke* **22**, 754–759.

Kovacs JAJ, Urowitz MB, Gladman DD *et al.* (1995) The use of single photon emission computerized tomography in neuropsychiatric SLE: A pilot study. *J Rheumatol* **22**, 1247–1253.

Kozora E, Thompson LL, West SG *et al.* (1996) Analysis of cognitive and psychological deficits in systemic lupus erythematosus patients without overt central nervous system disease. *Arthritis Rheum* **39**, 2035–2045.

Kuehnen J, Schwartz A, Neff W *et al.* (1998) Cranial nerve syndrome in thrombosis of the transverse/sigmoid sinuses. *Brain* **121**, 381–388.

Kuroe K, Kurahashi K, Nakano I *et al.* (1994) A neuropathological study of a case of lupus erythematosus with chorea. *J Neurol Sci* **123**, 59–63.

Lagana B, Tubani L, Maffeo N *et al.* (1996) Heart rate variability and cardiac autonomic function in systemic lupus erythematosus. *Lupus* **5**, 49–55.

Lammens M, Robberecht W, Waer M *et al.* (1992) Purulent meningitis due to aspergillosis in a patient with systemic lupus erythematosus. *Clin Neurol Neurosurg* **94**, 39–43.

Layzer RB (1985) *Neuromuscular Manifestations of Systemic Disease*, p 228. Philadelphia: FA Davis Company.

Lavalle C, Pizarro S, Drenkard C *et al.* (1990) Transverse myelitis: A manifestation of systemic lupus erythematosus strongly associated with antiphospholipid antibodies. *J Rheumatol* **17**, 34–37.

Laversuch CJ, Brown MM, Clifton A *et al.* (1995) Cerebral venous thrombosis and acquired protein S deficiency: An uncommon cause of headache in systemic lupus erythematosus. *Brit J Rheumatology* **34**, 572–575.

Lesprit P, Mouloud F, Bierling P *et al.* (1996) Prolonged remission of SLE associated polyradiculoneuropathy after a single course of intravenous immunoglobulin. *Scand J Rheumatol* **25**, 177–179.

Liem MD, Gzesh DJ and Flanders AE (1996) MRI and angiographic diagnosis of lupus cerebral vasculitis. *Neuroradiology* **38**, 134–136.

Lim KL, Abdul-Wahab R, Lowe J *et al.* (1994) Muscle biopsy abnormalities in systemic lupus erythematosus: Correlation with clinical and laboratory parameters. *Ann Rheum Dis* **53**, 178–182.

Lioté F and Osterland CK (1994) Autonomic neuropathy in systemic lupus erythematosus: Cardiovascular autonomic function assessment. *Ann Rheum Dis* **53**, 671–674.

Liou HH, Wang CR, Chen CJ *et al.* (1996) Elevated levels of anticardiolipin antibodies and epilepsy in lupus patients. *Lupus* **5**, 307–312.

Lloyd ME, D'Cruz D, McAlindon TE *et al.* (1993) Free protein S levels in systemic lupus erythematosus. *Arthritis Rheum* **36**, D 247.

Long AA, Denburg SD, Carbotte RM *et al.* (1990) Serum lymphocytotoxic antibodies and neurocognitive function in systemic lupus erythematosus. *Ann Rheum Dis* **49**, 249–253.

Lopez Dupla M, Khamashta MA, Sanchez AD *et al.* (1995) Transverse myelitis as a first manifestation of systemic lupus erythematosus: A case report. *Lupus* **4**, 239–242.

Lowman EW (1951) Muscle nerve and synovial changes in lupus erythematosus. *Ann Rheum Dis* **10**, 16–21.

Love PE and Santoro SA (1990) Antiphospholipid antibodies: Anticardiolipin and the lupus anticoagulant in systemic lupus erythematosus (SLE) and in non-SLE disorders. *Ann Intern Med* **112**, 682–698.

Magnani G, Nemni R, Leocani L *et al.* (1998) Neuromyotonia, systemic lupus erythematosus and acetylcholine-receptor antibodies. *J Neurol* **245**, 182–189.

Manzi S, Kuller LH, Kutzer J *et al.* (1995) Herpes zoster in systemic lupus erythematosus. *J Rheumatol* **22**, 1254–1258.

Markusse HM, Vroom ThM, Heurkend AHM *et al.* (1991) Polyneuropathy as initial manifestation of necrotizing vasculitis and gangrene in systemic lupus erythematosus. *Neth J Med* **38**, 204–208.

Martinez-Taboada VM, Blanco Alanso R, Armona J *et al.* (1996) Mononeuritis multiplex in systemic lupus erythematosus: Response to pulse intravenous cyclophosphamide. *Lupus* **5**, 74–76.

Matsukawa Y, Sawada S, Hayama T *et al.* (1994) Risk of suicide in depressive and psychotic patients. Analysis of 7 cases, 4 successful. *Lupus* **3**, 31–35.

McCarthy DJ, Manzi S, Medsger TA Jr *et al.* (1995) Incidence of systemic lupus erythematosus. *Arthritis Rheum* **38**, 1260–1270.

McCombe J, McLeod JG, Pollard JD *et al.* (1987) Peripheral sensorimotor and autonomic neuropathy associated with systemic lupus erythematosus. Clinical, pathological and immunological features. *Brain* **110**, 533–549.

McGaillard J and Bell AL (1993) Acquired Brown's syndrome in a patient with SLE. *Ann Rheum Dis* **52**, 385–386.

Mevorach D, Pertot S, Buchanan NMM *et al.* (1995) Appearance of systemic lupus erythematosus after thymectomy. *Lupus* **4**, 33–37.

Mevorach D, Raz E and Steiner I (1994) Evidence for intrathecal synthesis of antibodies in systemic lupus erythematosus with neurological involvement. *Lupus* **3**, 117–121.

Miguel EC, Pereira RMR, DeBranganca Pereira CA *et al.* (1994) Psychiatric manifestations of systemic lupus erythematosus: Clinical features, symptoms and signs of central nervous system activity in 43 patients. *Medicine* **73**, 224–232.

Mikol J and Engel AG (1994). Inclusion body myositis. In: Engel AG and Franzini-Armstrong C (eds) *Myology*, Vol 2, 2nd ed, pp 1384–1398. New York: McGraw-Hill.

Miller DH, Buchanan N, Barker G *et al.* (1992) Gadolinium-enhanced magnetic resonance imaging of the central nervous system in systemic lupus erythematosus. *J Neurol* **239**, 460–464.

Miller MH, Urowitz MB, Gladman DD *et al.* (1984) Chronic adhesive lupus serositis as a complication of systemic lupus erythematosus. Refractory chest pain and small bowel obstruction. *Arch Intern Med* **144**, 1863–1864.

Mitchell I (1994) Case presentations: Cerebral lupus. *Lancet* **343**, 579–580.

Mitsias P and Levine SR (1994) Large cerebral vessel occlusive disease in systemic lupus erythematosus. *Neurology* **44**, 385–393.

Miyoshi Y, Atsum T, Kitagawa H *et al.* (1993) Parkinson-like symptoms as a manifestation of systemic lupus erythematosus. *Lupus* **2**, 199–201.

Mok CC, Yuen KY and Lau CS (1997) Nocardiosis in systemic lupus erythematosus. *Sem Arthritis Rheum* **26**, 675–683.

Mok CC, Lau CS, Chan EYT *et al.* (1998a) Acute transverse myelopathy in systemic lupus erythematosus. *J Rheumatol* **25**, 467–473.

Mok CC, Lau CS and Yuen KY (1998b) Cryptococcal meningitis presenting concurrently with systemic lupus erythematosus. *Clin Exp Rheumatol* **16**, 169–171.

Muniain MA, Toyos FJ, Giron JM *et al.* (1992) Right recurrent laryngeal nerve palsy in a patient with lupus erythematosus. *Lupus* **1**, 407–408.

Newton P, Aldridge RD, Lessells AM *et al.* (1986) Progressive multifocal leukoencephalopathy complicating systemic lupus erythematosus. *Arthritis Rheum* **29**, 337–343.

Omdal R, Henriksen OA, Mellgren SI *et al.* (1991) Peripheral neuropathy in systemic lupus erythematosus. *Neurology* **41**, 808–811.

Osawa H, Yamabe H, Kaizuka M *et al.* (1997) Case report. Systemic lupus erythematosus associated with transverse myelitis and Parkinsonian symptoms. *Lupus* **6**, 613–615.

Padeh S and Passwell J (1996) Systemic lupus erythematosus presenting as idiopathic intracranial hypertension. *J Rheumatol* **23**, 1266–1268.

Pallis M, Robson DK, Haskard DO *et al.* (1993) Distribution of cell adhesion molecules in skeletal muscle from patients with systemic lupus erythematosus. *Ann Rheum Dis* **52**, 667–676.

Pantoni L and Garcia JH (1995) The significance of cerebral white matter abnormalities: 100 years after Binswanger's report. A review. *Stroke* **26**, 1293–1301.

Parikh S, Swaiman KF and Kim Y (1995) Neurologic characteristics of childhood lupus erythematosus. *Pediatric Neurology* **13**, 198–201.

Press J, Palayew K, Laxer RM *et al.* (1996) Antiribosomal P antibodies in pediatric patients with systemic lupus erythematosus and psychosis. *Arthritis Rheum* **39**, 671–676.

Prince HM, Thurlow PJ, Buchanan RC *et al.* (1995) Acquired protein S deficiency in a patient with systemic lupus erythematosus causing central retinal vein thrombosis. *J Clin Pathol* **48**, 387–389.

Propper DJ and Bucknall RC (1989) Acute transverse myelopathy complicating SLE. *Ann Rheum Dis* **48**, 512–515.

Raymond AA, Zariah AA, Samad SA *et al.* (1996) Brain calcifications in patients with cerebral lupus. *Lupus* **5**, 123–128.

Rechthand E, Cornblath DR, Stern BJ *et al.* (1984) Chronic inflammatory demyelinating polyneuropathy in systemic lupus erythematosus. *Neurology* **34**, 1375–1377.

Rogers MP, Kelly MJ (1993) Psychiatric aspects of lupus. In: Schur P (ed) *The Clinical Management of Systemic Lupus Erythematosus*, 2nd ed, pp 155–173. Philadelphia: Lippincott-Raven.

Ropes MP (1976) *Systemic Lupus Erythematosus*. Cambridge, MA: Harvard University Press. Cited in: Layzer RB (1985) *Neuromuscular Manifestations of Systemic Disease*, p 228. Philadelphia, FA Davis Company.

Rosman A, Atsumi T, Khamashta MA *et al.* (1995) Development of systemic lupus erythematosus after chemotherapy and radiotherapy for malignant thymoma. *Brit J Rheum* **34**, 1175–1176.

Rothfield NF (1997) Systemic lupus erythematosus: Clinical aspects and treatment. In: Koopman WJ (ed) *Arthritis and Allied Conditions*, 13ed, pp 1319–1345. Baltimore: Williams and Wilkins.

Salmon JE, Millard S, Schachter LA *et al.* (1996) FcGAMMARIIA alleles are heritable risk factors for lupus nephritis. *J Clin Invest* **97**, 1348–1354.

Schizozawa S, Kuzaki Y, Kim M *et al.* (1992) Interferon-alfa in lupus psychosis. *Arthritis Rheum* **35**, 417–422.

Schnider A, Gutbrod K, Ozdoba C *et al.* (1995) Very severe amnesia with acute onset after isolated hippocampal damage due to systemic lupus erythematosus. *J Neurol Neurosurg Psychiat* **59**, 644–645.

Schur PH (1996) Systemic lupus erythematosus. In: Bennett JC and Plum F (eds) *Cecil Textbook of Medicine*, pp 1475–1488. Philadelphia: WB Saunders Co.

Serop S, Vianna RNG, Claeys M *et al.* (1994) Orbital myositis secondary to systemic lupus erythematosus. *Acta Ophthalmologica* **72**, 520–523.

Sfikakis PP, Mitsikostas DD, Manoussakis MN *et al.* (1998) Headache in systemic lupus erythematosus: A controlled study. *Brit J Rheumatol* **37**, 300–303.

Shahar E, Lahat E, Goshen E *et al.* (1996) Extrapyramidal Parkinson's syndrome complicating systemic lupus erythematosus. *Ann Neurol* **40**, 336.

Shimomura T, Kuno N, Takenaka T *et al.* (1993) Purkinje cell antibodies in lupus ataxia. *Lancet* **342**, 375–376.

Sibley JT, Olszynski WP, Decoteau WE *et al.* (1992) The incidence and prognosis of central nervous system disease in systemic lupus erythematosus. *J Rheumatol* **19**, 47–52.

Sigal LH (1989) Chronic inflammatory polyneuropathy complicating SLE: Succesful treatment with monthly pulse oral cyclophosphamide. *J Rheumatol* **16**, 1518–1519.

Simeon-Aznar CP, Tolosa-Vilella C, Cuenca-Luque R *et al.* (1992) Transverse myelitis in systemic lupus erythematosus: Two cases with magnetic resonance imaging. *Br J Rheumatol* **31**, 555–558.

Simmonds RE, Ireland H, Lane DA *et al.* (1998) Clarification of the risk for venous thrombosis associated with hereditary protein S deficiency by investigation of a large kindred with a characterized gene defect. *Ann Intern Med* **128**, 8–14.

Singh HR, Prasad K, Kumar A *et al.* (1988) Cerebellar ataxia in systemic lupus erythematosus: Three case reports. *Ann Rheum Dis* **47**, 954–956.

Sklar EML, Schatz NJ, Glaser JS *et al.* (1996) MR of vasculitis-induced optic neuropathy. *AJNR* **17**, 121–128.

Smith RW, Ellison DW, Jenkins EA *et al.* (1994) Cerebellum and brainstem vasculopathy in systemic lupus erythematosus: Two clinico-pathological cases. *Ann Rheum Dis* **53**, 327–330.

Stein KS, McFarlane IC, Goldberg N *et al.* (1996) Heart rate variability in patients with systemic lupus erythematosus. *Lupus* **5**, 44–48.

Steinlin MI, Blaser SI, Gilday DL *et al.* (1995) Neurologic manifestations of pediatric systemic lupus erythematosus. *Pediatric Neurology* **13**, 191–197.

Stimmler MM, Coletti PM, Quismorio P *et al.* (1993) Magnetic resonance imaging of the brain in neuropsychiatric systemic lupus erythematosus. *Semin Arthritis Rheum* **22**, 335–349.

Stoppe G, Wildhagen K, Seidel JW *et al.* (1990) Positron emission tomography in neuropsychiatric lupus erythematosus. *Neurology* **40**, 304–308.

Straub RH, Zeuner M, Lock G *et al.* (1996) Autonomic and sensorimotor neuropathy in patients with systemic lupus erythematosus and systemic sclerosis. *J Rheumatol* **23**, 87–92.

Suzuki Y, Kitagawa Y, Matsuoka Y *et al.* (1990) Severe cerebral and systemic necrotizing vasculitis developing during pregnancy in a case of systemic lupus erythematosus. *J Rheumatol* **17**, 1408–1411.

Szer LS, Miller JH, Rawlings D *et al.* (1993) Cerebral perfusion in children with central nervous system manifestations of lupus detected by single photon emission computed tomography. *J Rheumatol* **20**, 2143–2148.

Tam LS, Cohen MG, Li EK (1995) Hemiballism in systemic lupus erythematosus: Possible association with antiphospholipid antibodies. *Lupus* **4**, 67–69.

Tan EM, Cohen AS, Fries JF *et al.* (1982) The 1982 revised criteria for the classification of systemic lupus erythematosus. *Arthritis Rheum* **25**, 1271–1277.

Tang LM ((1990) Ventriculoperitoneal shunt in cryptococcal meningitis with hydrocephalus. *Surg Neurol* **33**, 314–319.

Teh LS and Isenberg DA (1994) Antiribosomal P protein antibodies in systemic lupus erythematosus. A re-appraisal. *Arthritis Rheum* **37**, 307–315.

The Stroke Prevention In Reversible Ischemia Trial (SPIRIT) Study Group (1997) A randomized trial of anticoagulants versus aspirin after cerebral ischaemia of presumed arterial origin. *Ann Neurol* **42**, 857–865.

Thompson SW (1976) Ballistic movements of the arm in systemic lupus erythematosus. *Dis Nerv Syst* **37**, 331–332.

Tola MR, Granieri E, Caniatti L *et al.* (1992) Systemic lupus erythematosus presenting with neurological disorders. *J Neurol* **239**, 61–64.

Toubi E, Khamashta MA, Panarra A *et al.* (1995) Association of antiphospholipid antibodies with central nervous system disease in systemic lupus erythematosus. *Am J Med* **99**, 397–401.

Tsokos GC, Haralampos M, Moutsopoulos M *et al.* (1981) Muscle involvement in systemic lupus erythematosus. *JAMA* **246**, 766–769.

Tucker LB, Menon S, Schaller JG *et al.* (1995) Adult- and childhood-onset systemic lupus erythematosus: A comparison of onset, clinical features, serology, and outcome. *Brit J Rheumatol* **34**, 866–872.

Uziel Y, Laxer RM, Blaser S *et al.* (1995) Cerebral vein thrombosis in childhood systemic lupus erythematosus. *J Pediatr* **126**, 722–727.

Utset TO, Golden M, Siberry G *et al.* (1994) Depressive symptoms in patients with systemic lupus erythematosus: Association with central nervous system lupus and Sjögren's syndrome. *J Rheumatol* **21**, 2039–2045.

Vaiopoulos G, Sfikakis PP, Kapsimali V *et al.* (1994) The association of systemic lupus erythematosus and myasthenia gravis. *Postgrad Med J* **70**, 741–745.

van Kuijk MAP, Rotteveel JJ, van Oostrom CG *et al.* (1994) Neurological complications in children with protein C deficiency. *Neuropediatrics* **25**, 16–19.

Vazquez-Cruz J, Traboulssi H, Rodriquez-De La Serna A *et al.* (1990) A prospective study of chronic or recurrent headache in systemic lupus erythematosus. *Headache* **30**, 232–235.

Vidailhet M, Piette J-C, Wechsler B *et al.* (1990) Cerebral venous thrombosis in systemic lupus erythematosus. *Stroke* **21**, 1226–1231.

Ward MM, Pyun E and Studenski S (1996) Mortality risks associated with specific clinical manifestations of systemic lupus erythematosus. *Arch Intern Med* **156**, 1337–1344.

Warren RW and Kredich D (1984) Transverse myelitis and acute central nervous system manifestations of systemic lupus erythematosus. *Arthritis Rheumat* **27**, 1058–1060.

Weiner DK and Allen NB (1991) Large vessel vasculitis of the central nervous system in systemic lupus erythematosus: Report and review of the literature. *J Rheumatol* **18**, 748–751.

Winfield JB, Brunner CM and Koffler D (1978) Serologic studies in patients with systemic lupus erythematosus and central nervous system dysfunction. *Arthritis Rheum* **21**, 289–294.

Wise MP, Manford U and Davies UM (1995) Systemic lupus erythematosus presenting as fulminating cerebral lupus. *Lancet* **345**, 459–460.

Wyckoff DM, Miller LC, Tucker LB *et al.* (1995) Neuropsychological assessment of children and adolescents with systemic lupus erythematosus. *Lupus* **4**, 217–220.

Yancey CL, Doughty RD and Athreya BH (1981) Central nervous system involvement in childhood systemic lupus erythematosus. *Arthritis Rheum* **24**, 1389–1395.

Yood RA and Smith TW (1985) Inclusion body myositis and systemic lupus erythematosus. *J Rheumatol* **12**, 568–570.

Zimmerman B, Spiegel M and Lally EV (1992) Cryptococcal meningitis in systemic lupus erythematosus. *Sem Arthritis Rheum* **22**, 18–24.

8

Hughes' Syndrome (Antiphospholipid Antibody Syndrome)

INTRODUCTION

In about 20–30% of patients with SLE, abnormal clotting times are found in phospholipid-dependent coagulation assays. This abnormality cannot be corrected by addition of normal plasma, and it is phospholipid-dependent because it is inhibited when additional phospholipids are in the test system and accentuated when phospholipid concentrations are low (Brandt *et al.*, 1995). This phenomenon has been termed *lupus anticoagulant* (LAC), and is caused by immunoglobulins that retard the conversion of prothrombin into thrombin. LAC is peculiar *in vivo* because it is not associated with bleeding, (despite its *in vitro* anticoagulant activity) but with thrombosis (see Asherson *et al.*, 1989; Derksen and Stephens, 1995).

Patients with LAC often have a false-positive syphilis test. This observation has led to the discovery of an antibody against the phospholipid, cardiolipin, which is the major antigen in the standard test for syphilis (VDRL agent). Anticardiolipin antibodies (ACAs) are found in 10–30% of patients with SLE. LAC and ACA are closely related but not identical, and can be isolated separately from sera of SLE patients. Together, they form the antiphospholipid (APL) antibodies.

Over the years, there has been a continuous search for a role of the numerous antibodies in SLE patients. In 1983, Hughes described a syndrome that he observed in ACA positive SLE patients. It consisted of three 'seemingly unrelated' clinical features, namely recurrent venous thrombosis, CNS disease, and recurrent abortions. Some of the patients also had thrombocytopenia. There was some support in the literature for the existence of this clinical entity. Mueh *et al.* (1980) published a study about a group of 35 patients with lupus anticoagulant; 11 of whom previously had one or more thrombotic episodes and six of whom had thrombocytopenia. In another group of 31 patients, there were 18 thrombotic episodes, and nine of the 26 women of the group had one or more abortions previously (Boey *et al.*, 1983). Six years before Hughes (1983), Johansson *et al* (1977) described a peripheral vascular syndrome overlapping with SLE that had recurrent venous thrombosis, haemorrhagic capillary proliferation with circulating anticoagulants, and false-positive sero-reactions for syphilis. The pathology of the syndrome was almost exclusively thrombotic and involved large and small arteries and veins (Lie, 1989; Out *et al.*, 1991). In 1987, the first proposal for classification criteria for the *antiphospholipid antibody syndrome* (APL syndrome) was made. It was suggested that the diagnosis of APL syndrome would require the presence of at least one of the four clinical features just mentioned and of ACA (of class IgG or IgM), LAC or both (Harris, 1987). (Table 8.1). Though these proposed criteria have not been validated, they have been used in a multitude of publications on APL antibodies and APL syndrome (see below).

This chapter consists of two parts. First, a summary is given of the clinically interesting knowledge on antiphospholipid antibodies. Then the antiphospholipid antibody or Hughes' syndrome is described along with a relatively new entity, the *catastrophic antiphospholipid syndrome*.

Table 8.1 Proposed classification criteria for antiphospholipid syndrome

Clinical criterion	Laboratory criterion
Venous thrombosis	IgG class ACA[a] (moderate/high levels)
Arterial thrombosis	and/or IgM class ACA
Recurrent fetal loss	(moderate/high levels and/or
Thrombocytopenia	positive LAC[b] test

[a]Anticardiolipin antibodies; [b]Lupus anticoagulant
The diagnosis APL syndrome requires at least one clinical and one laboratory finding during the disease. Test for ACA or LAC should be positive on at least two occasions more than three months apart.
From Harris (1987), with permission.

THE ANTIPHOSPHOLIPID ANTIBODIES (APL ANTIBODIES)

The association of APL antibodies with a set of clinical features has stimulated research to identify the antigen targets of the antibodies and to clarify the presumed role of the APL antibodies in thrombotic processes.

ANTIGEN TARGETS

Recent investigations have shed a new and surprising light on the antigen targets of the APL antibodies. It appears that most of them are not directed against phospholipids, but against phospholipid–binding proteins or complexes of plasma proteins with phospholipids. The evidence for this view was introduced almost simultaneously for both ACA and LAC (see Roubey, 1996; Cabral and Alarcon-Segovia, 1997).

Purification of ACAs has allowed investigation into the binding of the antibodies to cardiolipin and has shown that binding does not take place when there is no plasma or serum. The factor in plasma that is required for binding appears to be a glycoprotein, called $\beta_2$glycoprotein I (β_2GPI), that circulates in low quantities in normal plasma. β_2GPI has a phospholipid–binding region in its 5th domain, and seems to bind weakly to membranes containing physiological concentrations of anionic phospholipids. Most of the antibodies, which until recently were considered to be antiphospholipids, appear to bind to phospholipid-free β_2GPI, when this antigen is presented at high-binding gamma-irradiated enzyme-linked immunosorbent assay (ELISA) plates. Whether the antibodies bind to the molecule under these specific circumstances because it is presented at a high density or because a neo-epitope is expressed on β_2GP1 after it binds either to phospholipids or to irradiated plates is still a matter of debate (see Roubey, 1996). It can not be ruled out however that some of the ACAs will prove eventually to bind to one or several proteins other than β_2GPI. There are probably also true APL antibodies that do not bind to β_2GPI nor any other protein.

LACs, defined as immunoglobulins that prolong a phospholipid-dependent coagulation test *in vitro*, are directed, in part, against phospholipid-bound human prothrombin as demonstrated by Bevers *et al.* (1991). Approximately 50–70% of patients with SLE or APL syndrome and lupus anticoagulants have auto-antibodies against prothrombin. Bevers *et al* (1991) showed also that LACs in sera of some patients (5 of 16 patients in their study) act as auto-antibodies to β_2GPI. In reverse, several authors have shown that some auto-antibodies against β_2GPI have LAC activity. It may be that some of the LACs are truly APL antibodies, but this is not clear yet (Roubey, 1996).

From this summary, it is evident that the APL antibodies are in fact a heterogenous group of antibodies against different phospholipid-binding proteins. There is the possibility that more of these proteins will be discovered. Research in progress concerns the question about whether some of the 'antiphospholipid antibodies' or related antibodies are directed against the protein C anticoagulant pathway (see Roubey, 1996). Depending on the target of the different antibodies and the processes that are disturbed, clinical signs are likely to vary. This can potentially explain why some patients have venous and others arterial thrombosis, or why some have only recurrent abortions. Now that the APL antibodies appear, for the most part, not to be directed against phospholipids, the justification of the term APL antibody syndrome is in question and renaming of the syndrome after Graham Hughes, who was one of the first to describe the syndrome, is proposed (Khamashta and Petri, 1996).

IS THERE A ROLE FOR 'ANTIPHOSPHOLIPID ANTIBODIES' IN
THROMBOTIC PROCESSES? LABORATORY EVIDENCE

The mechanisms that are proposed for APL antibody-mediated thrombosis are manifold, and they include inhibition of the protein C pathway and APL antibody-mediated enhancement of endothelial procoagulant activity (Roubey, 1996; Roubey and Hoffman, 1997). The mechanism underlying fetal loss is now probably closest to clarification. The death of fetuses is due to placental infarction, and is related to vasculopathy of the maternal placental arteriae. Annexin V is synthesized in placental syncytiotrophoblast and vascular endothelium and is expressed on the apical surfaces of these cells. It has a high affinity to anionic phospholipids and the capacity to displace coagulation factors from phospholipid surfaces. The amount of annexin V on the aforementioned cells is decreased in women with APL syndrome and recurrent abortion (Rand *et al.*, 1994). Reduction of annexin V on cells in contact with circulating blood might favour the occurrence of thrombosis. It has been shown that the amount of annexin V in cultured trophoblast and endothelial cells derived from the umbilical vein is significantly lower in cells that are exposed to IgG antibodies from patients with severe APL syndrome, than in similar non-exposed cells (Rand *et al.*, 1997).

The annexin V effect is probably not the only way in which APLs contribute to thrombosis, but at present it is one of the best studied mechanisms (Cowchock 1997).

PREVALENCE OF ANTIPHOSPHOLIPID ANTIBODIES IN THE HEALTHY POPULATION

Figures on the prevalence of APL antibodies in the healthy population are mostly derived from control groups. In different studies, the controls were selected from hospitalized patients, blood donors, spouses, relatives, friends, etc. The methods used to determine APL antibodies varied in the past, and though much was done to obtain standardization, one still has to reckon with discrepancies between laboratories (Peaceman *et al.*, 1992). At present, ACA are determined by ELISA. Detection of LAC requires a well-prepared (low plated concentration), test-plasma sample and is cumbersome, as its detection needs laborious screening and confirmative coagulation tests. Probably, this is the reason that, in many studies on associations between clinical manifestations and APL antibodies, LAC is not estimated. However, this hampers proper evaluation of the relevance of the APL antibodies, as LAC is a serological hallmark of the Hughes' syndrome and as results of LAC and ACA tests only partially overlap.

A much cited reference paper is a review of studies published before 1990 (mostly before 1989) by Love and Santoro (1990). According to this review, the prevalence of LAC in the 'healthy population' is estimated to be 2%, and the frequency of ACA in 'normal subjects' ranges from 0–7.5%, depending on the type of assay and the cut-off for positivity. Percentages in this range were also found in studies by the Antiphospholipid Antibodies in Stroke Study (APASS) Group (1993), Chakravarty *et al.* (1991), and others. Ginsberg *et al.* (1995) confirmed the low percentage for LAC but found ACA in 18% of their controls. Other groups found values of 12 and 8% for ACA (Bongard *et al.*, 1992; Metz *et al.*, 1998). The prevalence of APL antibodies seems to increase with age (Fields *et al.*, 1989). Titres of ACA in controls are often low.

PREVALENCE OF ANTIPHOSPHOLIPID ANTIBODIES IN PATIENTS WITH ISCHAEMIC STROKE OR VENOUS THROMBO-EMBOLISM

If APL antibodies are indeed mediators of thrombosis, then one expects that they are independent risk factors for arterial or venous thrombo-embolism. This notion has stimulated several groups to investigate APL antibodies in series of patients with ischaemic stroke and venous thrombosis or thrombo-embolism. Most of these studies are hampered by the fact that no antibody values are known from the period before thrombosis, which means that one cannot rule out the possibility that changes in antibody titres may be the consequence of thrombosis rather than the cause. One exception to this is the Physicians Health Study that was performed in the UK on more than 22 000 male physicians, who had to give plasma upon entry into the study. Physicians who had an ischaemic stroke, deep venous thrombosis, or pulmonary embolism during the five-year period after entry were identified. For these physicians, IgG ACA values were determined from the plasma samples that were obtained at entry. Unfortunately, there are no data on antibody levels after the ischaemic event. Controls were selected from the same population of male physicians and were matched for age and life-style variables. The mean ACA level in stroke patients did not differ significantly from controls. The ACA titre of patients with venous thrombosis or pulmonary embolism was, however, significantly higher than in their controls. Patients with the highest titres had venous thrombosis or embolism more often. Individuals with ACA titres above the 95th percentile had a relative risk for developing venous thrombosis or pulmonary embolism of 5.3 (Ginsburg *et al.*, 1992).

Now, there are results of several prospective investigations of APL antibodies in patients with venous thrombo-embolism or ischaemic stroke. Ginsberg *et al.* (1995) examined 256 consecutive patients referred to one centre for clinically suspected venous thrombo-embolism. There was a strong and statistically significant association (odds ratio 9.4) between the presence of LAC and venous thrombo-embolism. In contrast to Ginsburg *et al.* (1992), no significant association could be established of IgG ACA with venous thrombo-embolism. Metz *et al.* (1998) examined prospectively 379 ischaemic stroke patients referred to two centres, and 111 controls. 228 patients (!) did not fit the entry criteria, leaving 151 patients. No significant association could be established between ACA (IgG, IgM and IgA) and stroke, which is in agreement with the results of Ginsburg *et al.* (1992). The APASS Group (1993) examined ACA in 255 first ischaemic stroke patients and in a control group of 255 hospitalized non-stroke patients. A significant difference of ACA (IgG, IgM and IgA) in patients and controls was established (present in 9.7% of patients and in 4.3% of controls, adjusted odds ratio 2.31). LAC was not evaluated. The authors stressed that the strength of the association of ACA and stroke paralleled that of diabetes mellitus and stroke. Brey *et al.* (1990), in a prospective study, examined plasma for ACA (IgG and IgM) and LAC in 46 consecutive patients younger than 50 years who presented with TIAs or stroke and compared the results with an age and sex matched control group of 26 patients with other neurological diseases. Twenty one patients (45%) had LAC or ACA versus 2 controls who had ACA. A similar type of study was done by Nencini *et al.* (1992) with essentially the same result. A relatively high percentage of patients with LAC and/or ACA was also found in a series of 120 young adults with ischaemic stroke by Munts *et al.* (1998), thus confirming the results of the two previous groups.

From this short resumé, it is clear that an association of APL antibodies with venous thrombo-embolism and ischaemic stroke is likely, although there are also many conflicting results. Many investigations performed so far are incomplete because only data on ACA or IgG ACA were collected. The assumed association of APL antibodies and thrombo-embolic events is confirmed by the increased chance of recurrence of vessel occlusions in patients with APL antibodies (see this Chapter, *Course and Outcome*).

ANTIPHOSPHOLIPID ANTIBODIES IN SLE AND OTHER DISEASES

Though an increased prevalence of APL antibodies is not a feature only of SLE, the most attention, by far, has been given to this disease. Love and Santoro (1990), in their review of the literature from before 1990, found 29 studies on over 1000 patients with SLE compared to 1–4 studies on each of 6 other disorders (Table 8.2). The results are widely scattered in practically all of these diseases, and although the percentages are obviously highest for SLE, the differences with other diseases are less impressive than one perhaps surmises (see Table 8.2).

As ischaemic events are frequent in vasculitides, it is of interest to know the prevalence of APL antibodies in these disorders. Manna *et al* (1998) found ACAs in 17 of 33 patients with giant cell arteritis at the time of diagnosis and in 0 of 21 controls. After a mean period of steroid treatment of 11 months, the number of positive cases was less than half of the original. The authors could not establish a relation beween presence of ACAs and ischaemic events or any other clinical sign or laboratory parameter.

Table 8.2 Prevalence of LAC, ACA and APL antibodies in 6 disorders and in one drug-associated condition in percentages

	LAC	ACA	APL	Number of references
SLE	*6–71 mean 34	21–63 mean 44		29
Systemic sclerosis	N.A.	N.A.	0–25	2
Rheumatoid arthritis	N.A.	N.A.	4–49	3
Auto-immune diseases	N.A.	N.A.	9–55	3
Acute infections	N.A.	N.A.	32	1
GB syndrome	N.A.	N.A.	23	1
Chlorpromazine	N.A.	N.A.	37–77	4

*Range, in percentages. Abbreviations: N.A., not available LAC, lupus anticoagulants; ACA anticardiolipin antibodies; APL, antiphospholipid antibodies; GB, Guillain-Barré.
Data selected from Love and Santoro (1992).

PATHOLOGY

The vessel pathology of APL syndrome is described by Hughson *et al.* (1993 and 1995) as a thrombotic angiopathy. Small arteries contain fibrin thrombi or are obstructed by myointimal cells and fibrous and mucoid connective tissue. Other arteries contain organized cellular and fibrous occlusions and may become recanalized. Intimal proliferation with concentric cellular and fibrous hyperplasia develops in small arteries and is identical to what is seen in hypertensive vascular diseases.

An observation that is not fully explained concerns the presence of cellular inflammatory infiltrates in association with thrombosis or intimal hyperplasia. Hughson *et al.* (1995) noticed in an amputated lower limb of a patient with APL antibodies a thrombosed popliteal artery without fibrinoid necrosis but with intense infiltration of media and adventitia by neutrophils. Similar observations in tissue from limb and digit amputations have been reported by others (Alarcon-Segovia *et al.*, 1989; Praderio *et al.*, 1990; Goldberger *et al.*, 1992). Vasculitis in Hughes' syndrome is not very exceptional, and is commonly interpreted as coincidental rather than causal, due to the co-existence of SLE or lupus-like disease (Cervera *et al.*, 1995; Lie, 1996). APL antibodies in patients with different types of vasculitis occur often, and perhaps most frequently in giant cell arteritis (Norden *et al.*, 1995).

HUGHES' SYNDROME

SYMPTOMS AND SIGNS

In 1993, Hughes presented a state of the art study, which came ten years after his first description of a 'clinical syndrome with widespread arterial and venous thrombosis associated with antibodies against phospholipids' (Hughes, 1983). The methods used to delineate the clinical picture of the syndrome were, mainly, careful clinical observation of selected patients, of series of patients, and careful registration of associations with APL antibodies. Most studies had still been retrospective. Hughes' 1993 description is summarized in Box 8.1 and completed with data from Cervera *et al.* (1995).

Not everyone agrees with the ascription of all the disorders summarized in Box 8.1 to the APL syndrome. Cardiac valvular lesions and migraine serve as examples. Khamashta *et al.* (1990) established, in a series of 132 patients with APL antibodies and SLE, that valvular abnormalities were present in 22.7% of patients compared to 2.9% in controls. Valvular lesions were significantly more frequent in patients with APL antibodies than in those without, suggesting a relation between the two phenomena. A causative relation seemed likely, when APL antibodies were discovered in the heart valve lesions (Hojnik *et al.*, 1996). Other authors found, however, that the prevalence of valvular abnormalities in SLE patients with antibodies did not differ from the prevalence in patients without such antibodies (Roldan *et al.*, 1992; Gleason *et al.*, 1993; Roldan and Crawford, 1997). Tietjen *et al.* (1998) performed a large prospective study into the relation of ACAs (IgG, IgM and IgA) and different types of migraine. They did not discover any differences with controls and concluded that ACAs were not associated with migraine.

Hughes' syndrome has been recognized most frequently in patients with SLE or with lupus-like disease. This latter disorder is also probably SLE but does not – or not yet – fully comply with the classification criteria for the disease (Tan *et al.*, 1982). Love and Santoro (1990), on the basis of their large scale analysis of pre-1990 literature, found it difficult to support the notion that Hughes' syndrome, or at least the association of thrombosis and APL antibodies, occurred in the setting of other diseases also. The available literature did not allow definite conclusions because not enough cases were surveyed, the populations that were surveyed consisted of selected cases (often with disorders predisposing to thrombosis), and disease-matched antibody-negative controls were not usually examined. In patients using chlorpromazine and some other drugs, APL antibodies are frequent, but APL syndrome develops only in few of these cases (Love and Santoro, 1990; Lillicrap *et al.*, 1998).

Box 8.1 Clinical features of the APL syndrome

1. APL antibodies: either LAC antibodies or ACAs or both are present.
2. Venous thrombosis: deep vein thrombosis of the lower limbs is often recurrent or bilateral and accompanied by pulmonary embolism. Less frequently involved veins are the superior or inferior vena cava, renal and hepatic veins, and upper limb veins.
3. Neurological: TIAs, ischaemic stroke(s), encephalopathy, epilepsy, chorea, transverse myelopathy, migraine, multi-infarct dementia, venous sinus thrombosis.
3. Heart: myocardial infarction and cardiomyopathy due to multiple small vessel thrombosis in patients with APL antibodies or APL syndrome have been described in a small series and case reports. Valvular lesions include thickening and thrombotic vegetations.
4. Pulmonary: thrombo-embolic pulmonary hypertension is infrequent. Occlusion of a main pulmonary artery has been described.
5. Nephrological: renal artery thrombosis with malignant hypertension and renal infarction; microvascular renal thrombosis with proteinuria, renal failure and hypertension.
6. Gut: ischaemic lesions, thrombosis within the hepatic circulation.
7. Endocrinological: adrenal venous occlusion with Addison's syndrome.
7. Haematological: thrombocytopenia.
8. Dermatological: livedo reticularis, skin ulceration, skin necrosis that may be widespread and recurrent, digital gangrene.
9. Obstetrical: recurrent fetal loss, especially in the second trimester.

Data from Hughes (1993) and Cervera *et al* (1995).

PRIMARY HUGHES' SYNDROME OR PRIMARY ANTIPHOSPHOLIPID ANTIBODY SYNDROME (PAPS)

Hughes' syndrome in patients without SLE, lupus-like disease, or other obvious disorder, is labelled as primary (primary APL syndrome or PAPS). The first large series of such patients was published by Asherson *et al.* (1989). The authors presented data on 70 cases, selected in four European tertiary referral centres. Patients were included if they had a history of venous or arterial occlusions and multiple fetal loss, and if they had a positive test for either LAC, ACAs, or both. There was a 2:1 preponderance of females, and the ages varied from 21 to 59 years with a mean of 38. The clinical characteristics of the patients are presented in Table 8.3.

ANAs were present in 32 of 70 patients and antimitochondrial antibodies in 11 of 40. Coombs' positivity was present in 10, and 6 had cryoglobulinaemia. Organ-specific antibodies were not present, apart from antibodies to thyroid tissue. A minority of the patients had low complement levels and circulating immune complexes or positive rheumatoid factor (RF). Five patients had relatives with 'connective tissue disease', or familial clotting tendency. From these data, it would seem that patients with primary Hughes' syndrome, or at least those in this group, had an increased tendency to synthesis of auto-antibodies. Several patients who first presented as primary Hughes' syndrome but who were also ANA positive developed,

Table 8.3 Clinical characteristics of 70 patients with primary Hughes' syndrome (PAPS)

	Numbers of patients	Specification
Deep vein thrombosis	38	Bilateral or multiple 13, pulmonary embolism 18
Arterial thrombosis	31	Cerebral 15, coronary 5, pedal 5, other 6
Thrombocytopenia	32	
Recurrent fetal loss	24	2 abortions or more per patient
Livedo reticularis	14	
Avascular necrosis	2	Femoral head

Data selected from Asherson *et al* (1989).

within years, a lupus-like disorder, SLE, or Sjögren's syndrome (see Derksen *et al.*, 1996; Cabral and Alarcon-Segovia, 1996), indicating some kind of relation between primary Hughes' syndrome and other systemic auto-immune diseases. Asherson *et al.* (1989) did not address the question whether there are clinically similar patients who have no APL antibodies.

Differences between primary and secondary Hughes' syndrome have not been established (Alarcon-Segovia *et al.*, 1992) but have not been sufficiently excluded either (Ginsberg *et al.*, 1995).

THE NEUROLOGY OF HUGHES' SYNDROME

Already in 1983, Hughes stressed the frequency of CNS disease in the syndrome described by him. In nine clinical studies of SLE and some other auto-immune diseases reviewed by Love and Santoro (1990), neurological disorders occurred in 4–35% of 180 antibody-negative cases and in 14–70% of 135 antibody-positive cases. APL antibodies were more strongly associated with neurological disorders of vascular origin than with neuropsychiatrical disorders, especially psychosis. In other respects, there was no clear difference between the neurological disorders in the two groups (SLE patients, APL antibodies positive and negative). Inventories of neurological changes in APL positive patients were published by several authors (Briley *et al.*, 1989; Kushner, 1990; Levine *et al.*, 1990; Montalban *et al.*, 1991; Levine and Brey, 1996). Recurrent ischaemic stroke after an index cerebral ischaemic event is significantly more frequent in patients with APL antibodies than in others without these antibodies (Brey *et al.*, 1990; Nencini *et al.*, 1992; Levine *et al.*, 1995), particularly when IgG ACA titres are high (Levine *et al.*, 1995; Verro *et al.*, 1995).

Many other CNS manifestations have been suggested to be associated with APL antibodies on the basis of observations in small series of patients or even observations in single patients. Multi-infarct dementia in APL positive SLE has been documented (Asherson *et al.*, 1987; see Levine and Brey, 1996). Some patients with Sneddon's syndrome (livedo reticularis and cerebral infarcts) are APL antibody positive (Kalashnikova *et al.*, 1990). Epilepsy in SLE, not secondary to another identified cause, was reported in two studies to be associated with high titres of ACA (Herranz *et al.*, 1994; Liou *et al.*, 1996). In small series of patients with transverse myelitis and SLE, between 50–90% had ACAs (Lavalle *et al.*, 1990; Mok *et al.*, 1998). A review of 50 non-SLE patients with chorea and APL antibodies has been published (Cervera *et al.*, 1997). Briley *et al* (1989) suggested a relation between acute or subacute SLE encephalopathy (increasing headache, organic brain syndrome, seizures, and drowsiness or coma) and APL antibodies because of unusually high ACA titres in four patients (8–16 times normal). A chronic encephalopathic condition with transient cognitive disturbances and chorea in a young woman with LACs and a history of thrombophlebitis responded favourably to immunosuppressive treatment (Van Horn *et al.*, 1996). Venous sinus thrombosis in patients with APL antibodies has been described (see this Chapter, *Brain Imaging*). The prevalence of APL antibodies in migraine is not increased (Levine and Brey, 1996).

BRAIN IMAGING OF PATIENTS WITH NEUROLOGICAL DISORDERS AND APL ANTIBODIES

Abnormal CT or MRI of the brains of 59 SLE or non-SLE, APL positive patients showed the following features: large infarcts in 24 cases, hyperintense white matter foci in 19, and small cortical or lacunar infarcts in five (Provenzale *et al.*, 1996). The hyperintense white matter lesions differed from those that occur normally with aging by often being larger and more frequent. The pathological lesion underlying these hyperintense signals is, in many cases, perivascular axonal degeneration or demyelination. However, in the present situation, because of the lesions' unusually large size some of them were considered to be small infarcts. The surprise finding was dural sinus venous thrombosis in five cases, with APL antibodies as the only risk factor. Venous sinus thrombosis has been reported both in SLE and in APL positive patients, but may require more attention (Levine *et al.*, 1987; Mokri *et al.*, 1993; see also Chapters 2 and 7, *Cerebral Venous Thrombosis*). Provenzale *et al.* (1996) advise that APL antibodies should be determined in patients with unexplained venous sinus thrombosis. They also feel that venous sinus thrombosis should be in the differential diagnosis when a patient with APL antibodies develops focal neurological signs.

THE CATASTROPHIC ANTIPHOSPHOLIPID SYNDROME (CAS)

CAS differs from Hughes' syndrome by its rapid onset, multi-organ failure, widespread predominantly small vessel angiopathy and thrombosis, and often fatal outcome. It develops usually in patients who already have evidence of Hughes' syndrome. The first description of the syndrome dates from 1984, and up until now at least 33 patients have been reported (Asherson, 1992; Asherson and Piette, 1996; Chinnery *et al.*, 1997; Kane *et al.*, 1998).

The average age of patients suffering from CAS is approximately 30 years. Females are at least twice as frequently affected as males. The majority of the patients have SLE, lupus-like disease, RA, or Sjögren's syndrome, as well as a history of arterial or venous occlusion and APL antibodies. In a minority, there is evidence of Hughes' syndrome without associated inflammatory connective tissue disease (ICTD). Acutely, subacutely, or after a period of malaise, patients develop signs of dysfunction or lesions in several organs, including the kidneys, adrenals, liver and gut, heart and lungs, CNS, and the skin, thus causing a life threatening situation. Imaging of the brain and other organs and histological studies of biopsy or autopsy material have revealed widespread ischaemic lesions and non-inflammatory microthrombi and thrombosis. CNS manifestations include organic brain syndrome, seizures, stupor or coma, and hemiplegia and other evidence of focal lesions. Eight of 31 patients in the series described by Asherson and Piette (1996) had features of 'disseminated intravascular coagulation', fragments of red cells in blood smears, low fibrinogen levels, increased fibrinogen degradation products, increased prothrombin and thrombin times, and thrombocytopenia.

COURSE AND THERAPY

Patients with a history of arterial or venous thrombosis and APL antibodies run an increased risk of recurrence of thrombosis, as appears from retrospective (Rosove and Brewer, 1992; Derksen *et al.*, 1993; Khamashta *et al.*, 1995) and prospective studies (Brey *et al.*, 1990; Finazzi *et al.*, 1996). In a retrospective investigation of the course of 70 patients (69% women, mean age 45, ± 17 years), 33 were not treated and were followed for 161 patient years. During this period, these patients had 31 thrombotic recurrences (0.19 per patient year) (Rosove and Brewer, 1992). During 110.2 patient years of high-intensity treatment (INR ≥ 3), no recurrences were noted. Recurrences tended, in general, to be venous when the first event had also been venous (in 76% and 84% respectively, in two studies), and when the first event had been arterial, the chance that the subsequent event was also arterial was even higher (100% and 93%) (Rosove and Brewer, 1992; Khamashta *et al.*, 1995). Rosove and Brewer (1992) had 9 patients in their group with initial events in the carotid distribution; these patients had 15 recurrences and 14 of these were again in the carotid territory! In a multicentre prospective investigation over a five-year period of 360 consecutive patients referred for examination 'because of thrombotic history, diseases known to be related to the presence of APL antibodies or coagulation abnormalities,' previous thrombosis and high IgG ACA titres were found to be independent predictors of thrombosis (Finazzi *et al.*, 1996). The relative risk for recurrence of thrombo-embolic events in patients with previous thrombosis was 4.90, and in patients with high IgG ACA titres it was 3.66. LAC had no predictive significance. In a small prospective study of 21 APL antibody positive patients versus 25 patients without APL antibodies all of whom had ischaemic stroke or TIAs, the chance on recurrence during a mean follow up period of 1.2 years was higher in the APL antibody positive group (Brey *et al.*, 1990).

A retrospective study of attempts at secondary prevention of thrombotic events revealed that recurrences could not be prevented by aspirin (75 mg/day or more), and could only partially be prevented by low (international normalized ratio or INR < 2) or intermediate intensity (INR 2–3) warfarin treatment (Khamashta *et al.*, 1995). In the evaluation of the effect of aspirin, no difference was made between venous and arterial thrombosis. A randomized, prospective study comparing efficacy of aspirin and warfarin for prevention of recurrences of vascular events in patients with APL antibodies is underway (McCrae, 1996). With high-intensity anticoagulation (INR ≥ 3, or between 2.5 and 4) the chance on recurrence is very low or non-existent (Rosove and Brewer, 1992; Derksen *et al.*, 1993; Khamashta *et al.*, 1995). There is, however, a risk on bleeding, particularly at high-intensity coagulation, but this compares favourably, according to Khamashta *et al.* (1995), to the recurrence risk for thrombosis (risk on serious bleeding 0.017 per year). At cessation of warfarin therapy, the recurrence risk is high, particularly in the first 6 months (1.30

thrombotic events per year) (Khamashta *et al.*, 1995; see also Derksen *et al.*, 1993).

The bleeding risk for patients on long-term, high-intensity anticoagulation should not be underestimated. According to Hylek and Singer (1994), the risk of intracranial haemorrhage increases considerably at INRs of approximately 3.7–4.0. Individuals treated for an indefinite time are likely to undergo one or several major haemorhages, of which 1–7% will be intracranial (see McCrae, 1996). Results of the Stroke Prevention in Reversible Ischaemia Trial (1997) showed an annual incidence of serious bleedings in patients on high-intensity anticoagulation of 7% (INR 3–4.5). Some authors, on the basis of other retrospective studies, suggest that intermediate anticoagulant therapy (INR 2–3) is as effective in prevention of recurrent ischaemic events as high-intensity anticoagulant treatment in patients with APL antibodies (McCrae, 1996). Intermediate-intensity anticoagulation effectively prevents brain infarcts in patients with atrial fibrillation and in those at high risk for vascular events (Stroke Prevention in Atrial Fibrillation Investigators, 1996). As well, it is calculated to be associated with 1/3rd of the bleeding risk of high-intensity anticoagulation (The Stroke Prevention in Reversible Ischaemia trial, 1997). Observations of patients on low-intensity anticoagulation for atrial fibrillation suggest this form of prevention to be insufficient (Hylek *et al.*, 1996).

As long as results of prospective studies are not available for secondary prevention of CNS infarcts due to arterial occlusion, we prefer intermediate-intensity anticoagulation (INR 2–3), because aspirin and low-intensity anticoagulation are likely to be insufficiently effective and because of the high risk of serious bleeding with high-intensity anticoagulation. How long anticoagulation should be continued has not been established. We suggest that it should not be ceased as long as APL antibodies are present. Cerebral venous thrombosis may be treated as described in Chapter 2: heparin until the patient improves or at least until symptoms stabilize and then warfarin, adjusted to obtain INR between 2 and 3. The duration of treatment depends on the increased risk of recurrence; the best measure for this risk is probably the presence of APL antibodies.

There is no agreement about a standard treatment for CAS. Various schedules of immunosuppressive therapy with plasma exchange, corticosteroids and cytostatic agents, in combination with intravenous heparin have been attempted, but have, in many cases, not prevented a fatal outcome.

CONCLUSION

The data accumulated by Hughes and collaborators and many others are in support of the existence of a clinical syndrome that is characterized by venous and arterial occlusions and recurrent fetal loss. A definite delineation of the syndrome awaits the identification of a golden standard. APL antibodies are present in patients with Hughes' syndrome but this need not imply that there is a causal relation. Vessel occlusions may feature other diseases not commonly associated with APL antibodies, *e.g.* thrombotic thrombocytopenic purpura, disseminated intravascular coagulation, cryoglobulinaemia and others. Some patients with these latter disorders will have APL antibodies simply because these antibodies occur in approximately 0–8% of the population. Not all thrombotic events in SLE are associated with APL antibodies (Long *et al.*, 1991). Some thrombotic events unrelated to APL antibodies may conceivably develop by chance in patients with these antibodies. The possibility of venous sinus thrombosis should be considered in all patients with APL antibodies and cerebral disorders. APL antibodies are known to disappear in some cases, and control for the presence of LAC and ACA in patients with evidence of the Hughes' syndrome is therefore advisable (Norden *et al.*, 1995).

REFERENCES

Alarcon-Segovia D, Cardiel MH and Reyes E (1989) Antiphospholipid arterial vasculopathy. *J Rheumatol* **16**, 762–767.

Alarcon-Segovia D, Perez-Vasquez ME, Villa AR *et al* (1992) Preliminary classification criteria for the antiphospholipid syndrome within systemic lupus erythematosus. *Sem Arthritis Rheum* **21**, 275–286.

Alarcon-Segovia D, Mestanza M, Cabiedes J *et al* (1997) The antiphospholipid/cofactor syndromes. II. A variant in patients with systemic lupus erythematosus with antibodies to β_2-Glycoprotein I but no antibodies detectable in standard antiphospholipid assays. *J Rheumatol* **24**, 1545–1551.

Antiphospholipid Antibodies in Stroke Study (APASS) Group (1993) Anticardiolipin antibodies are an independent risk factor for first ischemic stroke. *Neurology* **43**, 2069–2073.

Asherson RA (1992) The catastrophic antiphospholipid antibody syndrome. *J Rheumatol* **19**, 508–512.

Asherson RA, Mercy D, Phillips G *et al* (1987) Recurrent stroke and multi-infarct dementia in systemic lupus erythematosus. Association with antiphospholipid antibodies. *Ann Rheum Dis* **25**, 221–227.

Asherson R, Khamashta MA, Ordi-Ros J *et al* (1989) The 'primary' antiphospholipid syndrome: Major clinical and serological features. *Medicine* **68**, 366–374.

Asherson RA and Piette J-C (1996) The catastrophic antiphospholipid syndrome 1996: Acute multi-organ failure associated with antiphospholipid antibodies: A review of 31 patients. *Lupus* **5**, 414–417.

Bevers EM, Galli M, Barbui T *et al* (1991) Lupus anticoagulant IgGs (LA) are not directed to phospholipids only but to a complex of lipid bound human prothrombin. *Thromb Haemost* **66**, 629–632.

Boey ML, Colaco CB, Gharavi AE *et al* (1983) Thrombosis in systemic lupus erythematosus: Striking association with the presence of circulating lupus anticoagulant. *Brit Med J* **287**, 1021–1023.

Bongard O, Reber G, Bounameaux H *et al* (1992) Anticardiolipin antibodies in acute venous thromboembolism. *Thromb Haemost* **67**, 724.

Brandt JT, Triplett DA, Alving B *et al* (1995) Criteria for the diagnosis of lupus anticoagulants: an update. *Thrombosis Haemostasis* **74**, 1185–1190.

Brey RL, Hart RG, Sherman DG *et al* (1990) Antiphospholipid antibodies and cerebral ischemia in young people. *Neurology* **40**, 1190–1196.

Briley DP, Coull BM and Goodnight SH (1989) Neurological disease associated with antiphospholipid antibodies. *Ann Neurol* **25**, 211–217.

Cabral AR and Alarcon-Segovia D (1996) Will some day PAPS fade into SLE? *Lupus* **5**, 4–5.

Cabral AR and Alarcon-Segovia D (1997) Autoantibodies in systemic lupus erythematosus. *Curr Opin Rheumatol* **9**, 387–392.

Chakravarty KK, Byron MA, Webley M *et al* (1991) Antibodies to cardiolipin in stroke; Association with mortality and functional recovery in patients with systemic lupus erythematosus. *Q J Med* **79**, 397–405.

Cervera R, Asherson RA and Lie JT (1995) Clinicopathologic correlations of the antiphospholipid syndrome. *Sem Arthritis Rheum* **24**, 262–272.

Cervera R, Asherson RA, Font J *et al* (1997) Chorea in the antiphospholipid syndrome. *Medicine* **76**, 203–212.

Chinnery PF, Shaw PJ, Ince PC *et al* (1997) Fulminant encephalopathy due to the catastrophic primary antiphospholipid syndrome. *J Neurol Neurosurg Psychiat* **62**, 300–301.

Cowchock S (1997) Autoantibodies and pregnancy loss. *N Engl J Med* **337**, 197–198.

Derksen RHWM, deGroot PHG, Kater L *et al* (1993) Patients with antiphospholipid antibodies and venous thrombosis should receive long-term anticoagulation. *Ann Rheum Dis* **52**, 689–692.

Derksen RHWM and Stephens CJM (1995) The antiphospholipid syndrome. In: Kater L and Baart de la Faille H (eds) *Multi-Systemic Auto-Immune Diseases*, pp 129–140. Amsterdam: Elsevier.

Derksen RHWM, Gmelig-Meyling FHJ and de Groot PhG (1996) Primary antiphospholipid syndrome evolving into systemic lupus erythematosus. *Lupus* **5**, 77–80.

Fields RA, Tourbeh H, Searles RP *et al* (1989) The prevalence of anticardiolipin antibodies in a healthy elderly population and its association with antinuclear antibodies. *J Rheumatol* **16**, 623–625.

Finazzi G, Brancaccio V, Moia M *et al* (1996) Natural history and risk factors for thrombosis in 360 patients with antiphospholipid antibodies: A four year prospective study from the Italian Registry. *Am J Med* **100**, 530–536.

Ginsberg JS, Wells PS, Brill-Edwards P *et al* (1995) Antiphospholipid antibodies and venous thromboembolism. *Blood* **86**, 3685–3691.

Ginsburg KS, Liang MH, Newcomer L *et al* (1992) Anticardiolipin antibodies and the risk for ischemic stroke and venous thrombosis. *Ann Intern Med* **117**, 997–1002.

Gleason CB, Stoddard MF, Wagner SG *et al* (1993) A comparison of cardiac valvular involvement in the primary antiphospholipid syndrome versus anticardiolipin negative systemic lupus erythematosus. *Am Heart J* **125**, 1123–1129.

Goldberger E, Elder RC, Schwartz RA *et al* (1992) Vasculitis in the antiphospholipid syndrome: A cause of ischemia responding to corticosteroids. *Arthritis Rheum* **35**, 569–572.

Harris EN (1987) Syndrome of the black swan. *Brit J Rheumatol* **26**, 324–326.

Herranz MT, Rivier G, Khamashta MA *et al* (1994) Association between antiphospholipid antibodies and epilepsy in patients with systemic lupus erythematosus. *Medicine* **73**, 568–571.

Hojnik M, George J, Ziporen L *et al* (1996) Heart valve involvement (Libman-Sacks endocarditis) in the antiphospholipid syndrome. *Circulation* **93**, 1579–1587.

Hughes GRV (1983) Thrombosis, abortion, cerebral disease and lupus anticoagulant. *Brit Med J* **287**, 1088–1098.

Hughes GRV (1993) The antiphospholipid syndrome: Ten years on. *Lancet* **342**, 341–344.

Hughson MD, McCarthy GA, Sholer CM *et al* (1993) Thrombotic cerebral arteriopathy in patients with the antiphospholipid syndrome. *Mod Pathol* **6**, 644–653.

Hughson MD, McCarthy GA and Brumback RA (1995) Spectrum of vascular pathology affecting patients with the antiphospholipid syndrome. *Human Pathol* **26**, 716–724.

Hylek EM and Singer DE (1994) Risk factors for intracranial hemorrhage in outpatients taking warfarin. *Ann Int Med* **118**, 511–520.

Hylek EM, Skates SJ, Sheehan *et al* (1996) An analysis of the lowest effective intensity of prophylactic anticoagulation for patients with nonrheumatic atrial fibrillation. *N Engl J Med* **335**, 540–546.

Johansson EA, Niemi KM and Mustakallio KK (1977) A peripheral vascular syndrome overlapping with systemic lupus erythematosus: Recurrent venous thrombosis and haemorrhagic capillary proliferation with circulating anticoagulants and false-positive seroreactions for syphilis. *Dermatologia* **155**, 257–263.

Kalashnikova LA, Nasonov EL, Kushekbaeva AE *et al* (1990) Anticardiolipin antibodies in Sneddon's syndrome. *Neurology* **40**, 464–447.

Kane D, McSweeney F, Swann N *et al* (1998) Catastrophic antiphospholipid antibody syndrome in primary systemic sclerosis. *J Rheumatol* **25**, 810–812.

Khamashta MA, Cervera R, Asherson RA *et al* (1990) Association of antibodies against phospholipids with heart valve disease in systemic lupus erythematosus. *Lancet* **335**, 1541–1544.

Khamashta MA, Cuadrado MJ, Mujic F *et al* (1995) The management of thrombosis in the antiphospholipid-antibody syndrome. *N Engl J Med* **332**, 993–997.

Khamashta M and Petri M (1996) Antiphospholipid antibodies hasten atheroma. *Lancet* **348**, 1088.

Kushner MJ (1990) Prospective study of anticardiolipin antibodies in stroke. *Stroke* **21**, 295–298.

Lavalle C, Pizarro S, Drenkard C *et al* (1990) Transverse myelitis: A manifestation of systemic lupus erythematosus strongly associated with antiphospholipid antibodies. *J Rheumatol* **17**, 34–37.

Levine SR, Kieran S, Puzio K *et al* (1987) Cerebral venous thrombosis with lupus anticoagulant. Report of two cases. *Stroke* **18**, 801–803.

Levine SR, Deegan MJ, Futrell N *et al* (1990) Cerebrovascular and neurologic disease associated with antiphospholipid antibodies: 48 cases. *Neurology* **40**, 1181–1189.

Levine SR Brey RL and Saweya RN (1995) Recurrent stroke and thrombo-occlusive events in the antiphospholipid syndrome. *Ann Neurol* **38**, 119–124.

Levine SR and Brey RL (1996) Neurological aspects of antiphospholipid syndrome. *Lupus* **5**, 347–353.

Lie JT (1989) Vasculopathy in the antiphospholipid syndrome: Thrombosis or vasculitis or both? *J Rheumatol* **16**, 713–715.

Lie JT (1996) Vasculopathy of the antiphospholipid syndromes revisited: Thrombosis is the culprit and vasculitis the consort. *Lupus* **5**, 368–371.

Lillicrap MS, Wright G and Jones AC (1998) Symptomatic antiphospholipid syndrome induced by chlorpromazine. *Brit J Rheumatol* **37**, 346–347.

Liou H-H, Wang C-R, Chen C-J *et al* (1996) Elevated levels of anticardiolipin antibodies and epilepsy in lupus patients. *Lupus* **5**, 307–312.

Long AA, Ginsberg JS, Brill-Edwards P *et al* (1991) The relationship of antiphospholipid antibodies to thromboembolic disease in systemic lupus erythematosus; A cross-sectional study. *Thromb Haemost* **66**, 520–524.

Love PE and Santoro SA (1990) Antiphospholipid antibodies: Anticardiolipin and the lupus anticoagulant in systemic lupus erythematosus (SLE) and in non-SLE disorders. Prevalence and clinical significance. *Ann Intern Med* **112**, 682–698.

Manna R, Latteri M, Cristano G *et al* (1998) Anticardiolipin antibodies in giant cell arteritis and polymyalgia rheumatica: A study of 40 cases. *Brit J Rheumatol* **37**, 208–210.

McCrae KR (1996) Antiphospholipid antibody associated thrombosis: A consensus for treatment? *Lupus* **5**, 560–570.

Metz LM, Edworthy S, Mydlarski R *et al* (1998) The frequency of phospholipid antibodies in an unselected stroke population. *Can J Neurol Sci* **25**, 64–69.

Mok CG, Lau CS, Chat EYT *et al* (1998) Acute transverse myelopathy in systemic lupus erythematosus. *J Rheumatol* **25**, 467–473.

Mokri B, Jack CR Jr and Petty GW (1993) Pseudotumor syndrome associated with cerebral venous sinus occlusion and antiphospholipid antibodies. *Stroke* **24**, 469–472.

Montalban J, Codina A, Ordi J *et al* (1991) Antiphospholipid antibodies in cerebral ischemia. *Stroke* **22**, 750–753.

Mueh JR, Herbst KD and Rapaport SI (1980) Thrombosis in patients with the lupus anticoagulant. *Ann Int Med* **92**, 156–159.

Munts AG, van Genderen PJJ, Dippel DWJ *et al* (1998) Coagulation disorders in young adults with acute cerebral ischaemia. *J Neurol* **245**, 21–25.

Nencini P, Baruffi MC, Abbate R *et al* (1992) Lupus anticoagulant and anticardiolipin antibodies in young adults with cerebral ischemia. *Stroke* **23**, 189–193.

Norden DK, Ostrov BE, Shafritz AB *et al* (1995) Vasculitis associated with antiphospholipid syndrome. *Sem Arthritis Rheum* **24**, 273–281.

Out HJ, Kooyman CD, Bruinse *et al* (1991) Histopathological findings in placentae from patients with intra-uterine fetal death and anti-phospholipid antibodies. *Europ J Obstet Gynaecol Reprod Med* **41**, 179–186.

Peaceman AM, Silver N, MacGregor SN *et al* (1992) Interlaboratory variation in antiphospholipid antibody testing. *Am J Obstet Gynaecol* **166**, 1780–1787.

Praderio L, D'Angelo A, Taccagni G *et al* (1990) Association of lupus anticoagulant with poly-arteritis nodosa: Report of a case. *Haematologia* **75**, 387–390.

Provenzale JM, Barboriak DP, Allen NB *et al* (1996) Patients with antiphospholipid antibodies: CT and MR findings of the brain. *AJR* **167**, 1573–1578.

Rand JH, Wu XX, Guller S *et al* (1994) Reduction of annexin-V (placental anticoagulant protein I) on placental villi of women with antiphospholipid antibodies and recurrent spontaneous abortion. *Am J Obstet Gynecol* **171**, 1566–1572.

Rand JH, Wu XX, Andree HAM *et al* (1997) Pregnancy loss in the antiphospholipid-antibody syndrome – a possible thrombogenic mechanism. *N Engl J Med* **337**, 154–160.

Roldan CA, Shively BK, Lau CC *et al* (1992) Systemic lupus erythematosus valve disease by trans-esophageal echocardiography and the role of antibodies. *J Am Coll Cardiol* **20**, 1127–1134.

Roldan CA and Crawford MH (1997) Valvular heart disease and systemic lupus erythematosus. Reply. *N Engl J Med* **336**, 1324–1325.

Rosove MH and Brewer PMC (1992) Antiphospholipid thrombosis: Clinical course after the first thrombotic event in 70 patients. *Ann Intern Med* **117**, 303–308.

Roubey RAS (1996) Immunology of the antiphospholipid antibody syndrome. *Arthritis Rheum* **39**, 1444–1454.

Roubey RAS and Hoffman M (1997) From antiphospholipid syndrome to antibody mediated thrombosis. *Lancet* **350**, 1491–1493.

Stroke Prevention in Atrial Fibrillation Investigators (1996) Adjusted-dose warfarin versus low-intensity, fixed-dose warfarin plus aspirin for high-risk patients with atrial fibrillation: Stroke prevention in atrial fibrillation III randomised clinical trial. *Lancet* **348**, 633–638.

Tan EM, Cohen AS, Fries JS *et al* (1982) The 1982 revised criteria for the classification of systemic lupus erythematosus. *Arthritis Rheum* **25**, 1271–1277.

The Stroke Prevention in Reversible Ischemia Trial (SPIRIT) Study Group (1997) A randomized trial of anticoagulation versus aspirin after cerebral ischemia of presumed arterial origin. *Ann Neurol* **42**, 857–865.

Tietjen GE, Day M, Norris L *et al* (1998) Role of anticardiolipin antibodies in young persons with migraine and transient neurologic events. A prospective study. *Neurology* **50**, 1433–1440.

Van Horn G, Arnett FC and Dimachkie MM (1996) Reversible dementia and chorea in a young woman with the lupus anticoagulant. *Neurology* **46**, 1599–1603.

Verro P, Levine SR and Tietjen GE (1995) Cerebrovascular ischemic events with high positive anti-cardiolipin antibodies. *Stroke* **26**, 160.

9

Rheumatoid Arthritis, Juvenile Chronic Arthritis, Adult Still's Disease, and Acute Rheumatic Fever

INTRODUCTION

In this chapter, we describe the neurological aspects of a group of disorders that are, in part, related to each other. Rheumatoid arthritis (RA) is the most frequent of these diseases. It is a chronic inflammatory disorder affecting primarily the synovial-lined joints. Rheumatic nodules, vasculitis, and various other extra-articular manifestations are essential components of this disease. The central nervous system (CNS) is rarely involved, but spinal disorders and peripheral neuropathy are not infrequent and muscular atrophy near affected joints develops in the majority of the patients. One of the juvenile chronic arthritides, seropositive polyarticular arthritis, is the equivalent of RA in adolescents. Another form of arthritis in childhood, systemic juvenile arthritis, presents with systemic abnormalities and not joint lesions. Its equivalent in adults is adult Still's disease. Rheumatic fever usually presents with a systemic abnormality (fever) in combination with a nonerosive form of arthritis, and has a neurological abnormality (Sydenham's chorea) as another major manifestation. It is the only inflammatory connective tissue disease (ICTD) of which the causative environmental factor has been established. The neurological and myological aspects of RA have recently been reviewed by Change and Paget (1993).

RHEUMATOID ARTHRITIS: A SHORT GENERAL DESCRIPTION

EPIDEMIOLOGY

RA is widely distributed all over the world and affects all races (see Felson, 1997). The prevalence in the adult population is assessed at approximately 0.8 to 1.0%. The annual incidence in Europe varies in different geographical areas from 27 to

8/100000 (Symmons *et al.*, 1994; Guillemin *et al.*, 1994; Bregeon *et al.*, 1985). Prevalence and incidence are about 3 times higher in women than in men and increase with age. RA is rare in young men.

AETIOLOGY

As in other ICTDs, both genetic predisposition and environmental factors are likely to play a role (see Albani and Carson, 1997). A modest genetic role has been demonstrated in a nationwide British twin study (Silman *et al.*, 1993). The concordance in monozygotic twins is approximately 15% and is proportional to the severity of the disease: more severely affected patients have a higher chance of an affected twin. RA is associated with class II major histocompatibility complex (MHC) haplotype HLA-DR4. Patients who are DR4-positive show, in comparison to others, more disease activity and continued progression of arthrogenic changes (van Zeben *et al.*, 1992).

Possible environmental factors that provoke RA in genetically predisposed individuals are infectious agents, but evidence for a role of any specific micro-organism has not been discovered yet (see Firestein, 1997).

PATHOGENESIS

Very schematically, the following might happen: an as yet unidentified, arthritogenic stimulus triggers an immuno-inflammatory cascade in an immuno-genetic susceptible individual. Inflammation is mediated by inflammatory cells, prostaglandins, and cytokines. The inflammation causes local joint damage and widespread bone loss (Emery, 1997; Bijlsma and Velthuis, 1995; Gough *et al.*, 1994).

Rheumatoid factor (RF), one of the altered immunoglobulins in RA, has a special significance. RF is an auto-antibody against IgG. It is present in approximately 80% of RA patients, and is not specific for RA despite its name. RFs are found in other auto-immune (connective tissue) diseases (such as SLE and Sjögren's syndrome) in infectious and haematologic diseases, and in about 5% of the normal population. RFs in the normal population are mainly of the IgM phenotype in contrast to the IgG phenotype present in RA. RFs are involved in immune-complex formation and induce recruitment of macrophages and other white blood cells (Soltys and Axford, 1997). RA patients with a positive test for RF in blood have a more severe clinical disease (Cats and Hazevoet, 1970). Extra-articular manifestations occur mostly in RF-positive patients with progressive joint inflammation, suggesting these manifestations are immune-mediated (Albani and Carson, 1997).

PATHOLOGY

Synovia

At onset, lymphocytes and macrophages are spread diffusely in the synovia or gathered in small aggregates. The lymphocytes are predominantly T-cells, most of them of CD4+ T-helper cell-phenotype. In more advanced stages, the infiltrates consist of a considerable portion of plasma cells; mast cells are also present. The synovia become thickened, in part due to this infiltrate and to oedema, but also because of growth of blood vessels, proliferation of synovial fibroblasts, and multiplication and enlargement of synovial lining cells. This granulation tissue is called pannus. The pannus attacks the cartilage and causes destructive changes. It also invades the bone cortex near the joints.

Rheumatic nodules

Nodules are found in 20 to 35% of patients with definite, seropositive (*i.e.* RF positive) RA (Fig. 9.1). The nodule has a yellow, necrotic centre that has at microscopy a fibrinoid aspect; it contains fibrillary proteins, immunoglobulins, cellular debris, collagen mucopolysacharides, and nucleoproteins, and is surrounded by palissading histiocytes and a mixed inflammatory infiltrate (see Hale and Haynes, 1997). At an early stage, the nodule consists of a nest of granulation tissue (Mellbye *et al.*, 1991); it grows by accumulating cells at the periphery.

Mainly, the nodules are located subcutaneously at pressure points: at the extensor side of the olecranon (Fig. 9.2), the proximal part of the ulna, and in bedridden patients at the occiput. They are found less frequently in tendons and tendon sheaths, in periarticular subcutaneous tissue, and in many other tissues and organs, including the meninges and the spine (Pearson *et al.*, 1987).

Vasculitis

Vasculitis in RA may affect arteries of all sizes as well as small vessels, but has a preference for medium and small arteries. Vasculitis may be indistinguishable from periarteritis nodosa (see Hale and Haynes, 1997) (see Fig. 5.14). Venules may be involved also. Though all layers may be infiltrated, inflammation is generally greatest in the adventitia. The infiltrates consist predominantly of lymphocytes and macrophages, but there are also neutrophils and plasma cells. The intima may show fibrinoid degeneration or proliferation, and the lumina may show thrombosis and recanalization. Vasculitis in RA is considered to be mediated by the deposition of circulating immune complexes. IgG, IgM and C3 have been demonstrated in some of the involved vessel walls (Chalk *et al.*, 1993), and RF can be demonstrated by

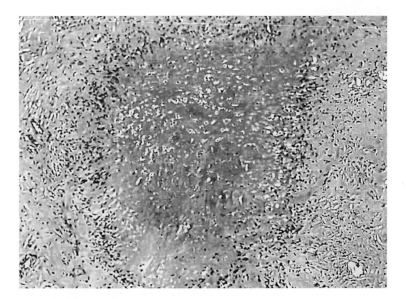

Figure 9.1 Rheumatic nodule. Transverse, H & E stained section at low magnification, showing central necrotic area, surrounded by palissading cells, and a mixed inflammatory infiltrate. (Courtesy of Prof. Piet Slootweg.)

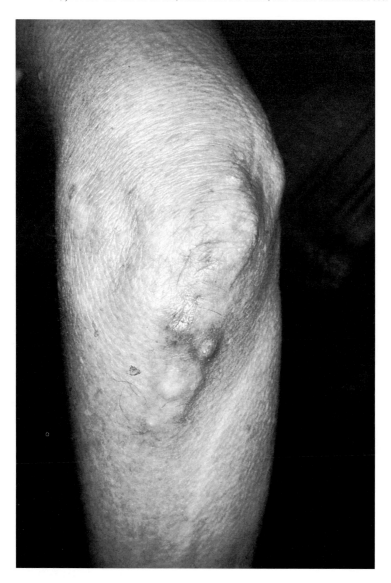

Figure 9.2   Rheumatic nodules just below the elbow, at a characteristic place.

immuno-histochemical methods at places where immunoglobulins and complement are present (van Lis and Jennekens, 1977).

CLINICAL FEATURES AND DIAGNOSIS

RA presents either with systemic manifestations (malaise, subfebrile temperature, anaemia) or with symptoms and signs of arthritis of the metacarpophalangeal joints (MCP), proximal interphalangeal joints (PIP), or wrists (Bijlsma and Velthuis, 1995).

More proximal, larger joints may become involved with time. Onset is gradual or occasionally acute. Joint inflammation causes morning stiffness, limitation of movement, pain, swelling, redness, and deformity. Not all of these changes are always detectable at examination. Active vasculitis is seen in ill patients with joint deformities and high RF titre, and is, in some cases (not always!), acute and dramatic in onset (Harris, 1997). It may cause a large number of clinical manifestations, including nailfold teleangiectasia, digital gangrene, purpura, skin ulcers, visceral infarcts, and mononeuritis multiplex. CNS involvement is rare but has been reported (Bacon and Moots, 1997; see also this Chapter, *Neurology of RA*).

Laboratory examination in patients with RA shows increase of erythrocyte sedimentation rate (ESR) and some degree of anaemia and leukocytosis. A raised RF is in favour of the diagnosis. X-rays reveal periarticular osteopenia and marginal erosions.

Diagnosis is made mainly on clinical grounds. As a rule, joints are affected in a symmetrical fashion or with some degree of asymmetry. The main exceptions to this rule are the joints in the paretic side of hemiplegic individuals, which are much less involved probably due to limitation of activity (Bland and Eddy, 1968). The classification criteria for definite RA are given in Table 9.1. Extra-articular manifestations are enumerated in Table 9.2; some of them eventually occur in most patients.

THERAPY

Therapy aims at relief of pain and stiffness and preservation or improvement of function. Scales have been developed to assess the functional status of patients and to measure disease activity (Kater and Provost, 1995). Non-pharmaceutical interventions (psychosocial assistance, physical therapy, occupational therapy, splints and orthoses, surgery) have an important place in treatment plans. Pharmaceutical interventions are either local (intra-articular injections, ulcer treatment) or systemic. Among the latter, one makes a distinction between non-steroidal inflammatory drugs (NSAIDs), corticosteroids, and a heterogeneous group of disease-modifying antirheumatic drugs (DMARDs), which are also called slow-acting antirheumatic drugs (SAARDs). Drugs belonging to this last group are hydroxychloroquine, gold-salts, sulfasalazine, D-penicillamine, azathioprine, methotrexate, cyclosporine, and cyclophosphamide. Early intensive therapy with prednisolone and methotrexate is at present advocated (Broers *et al.*, 1997).

COURSE OF THE DISEASE AND PROGNOSIS

In some patients, the course is intermittent (15–20%); occasionally, it has long clinical remissions (10%); but in most patients, it is progressive (60–70%). Life expectancy is shortened, more for males than for females (see Harris, 1997). Seropositivity and onset at a young age are associated with a poorer prognosis.

NEUROLOGY OF RHEUMATOID ARTHRITIS

MOOD AND COGNITION

Patients with RA are more often depressed and anxious than age and sex matched controls (Pincus *et al.*, 1996). Feelings of distress are increased by pain, disability,

Table 9.1 1988 revised ARA classification criteria for rheumatoid arthritis

Criterion	Definition
1. Morning stiffness	Morning stiffness in and around the joints lasting at least 1 hour before maximal improvement
2. Arthritis of three major joint areas	At least three joint areas having soft-tissue swelling or fluid (not bone overgrowth alone) observed by a physician (the possible joint areas are right or left PIP, MCP, wrist, elbow, knee, ankle, and MTP joints)
3. Arthritis of hand joints	At least one joint area swollen as above in wrist, MCP, or PIP
4. Symmetrical arthritis	Simultaneous involvement of the same joint areas (as in criterion 2) on both sides of the body (bilateral involvement of PIP, MCP, or MTP joints is acceptable without absolute symmetry)
5. Rheumatoid nodules	Subcutaneous nodules over bony prominences or extensor surfaces, or in juxta-articular regions, observed by a physician
6. Serum rheumatoid factor	Demonstration of abnormal amounts of serum 'rheumatoid factor' by any method that has been positive in less than 5% of normal control subjects
7. Radiographic changes	Changes typical of RA on postero-anterior hand and wrist radiographs which must include erosions or unequivocal bony decalcification localized to or most marked adjacent to the involved joints (osteoarthritic changes alone do not qualify)

A patient is said to have RA if he or she has satisfied at least 4 of the above 7 criteria. Criteria 1 to 4 must be present for at least 6 weeks. Patients with two clinical diagnoses are not excluded. Abbreviations: ARA, American Rheumatism Association; PIP, proximal interphalangeal; MCP, metacarpophalangeal; MTP, metatarsophalangeal; RA, rheumatoid arthritis.
From Arnett *et al.* (1988), with permission.

and fatigue (Smedstad *et al.*, 1996). Mild cognitive deficits were found in a recent well-controlled, extensive neuropsychological investigation of a group of non-neurological patients with RA. The result came as a surprise and could not be explained as an effect of psychological distress (Kozora *et al.*, 1996).

MENINGEAL NODULES, PACHYMENINGITIS, AND CNS VASCULITIS

Rheumatic nodules occur occasionally in the dura, falx cerebri, the leptomeninges, and the chorioid plexus (see Kim and Collins, 1981; Bathon *et al.*, 1989). Some of the nodules adhere to the brain or spinal cord and compress structures, but they do not intrude into the parenchyma and probably do not occur in the parenchyma of the nervous tissue. In some cases, not only nodules are present; there is also a more widespread, plaque-like inflammation of the meninges with necrosis, lymphocytes, and a variable percentage of plasma cells. This aseptic pachymeningitis may also occur on its own without any rheumatic nodules (Schachenmayr and Friede, 1978).

Table 9.2 Extra-articular features of rheumatoid arthritis

I.	Essential to systemic rheumatoid disease
	Nodules (granulomata)
	Pericarditis, pleuritis
	Vasculitis
II.	Other features and associated syndromes
	Anaemia
	Lymphadenopathy
	Osteopenia
	Sjögren's syndrome
	Interstitial lung fibrosis
	Amyloidosis
	Felty's syndrome*
III.	Side effects of drugs**

*Felty's syndrome: splenomegaly and leukopenia (neutrophils) in patients with RA.
**See Chapter 4.

Vasculitis, extending in some cases from a region of pachymeningitis into the brain, has also been reported (Ramos and Mandybur, 1975; Beck and Corbett, 1983).

Mental obtundation, organic brain syndrome, severe headache (Rodman 1984; Bathon *et al.*, 1989), seizures (Beck and Corbett, 1983), cranial neuropathy including optic neuropathy (Kim, 1980; Bathon *et al.*, 1989), paresis and agnosia (Ramos and Mandybur, 1975; Rodman, 1984), thoracic myelopathy (Fairburn, 1975; Sasaki *et al.*, 1997), and radiculopathy (Friedman, 1970; Markenson *et al.*, 1979) due to rheumatic nodules or pachymeningitis have all been reported. The number of patients with these syndromes is small and few reports are of recent date. Inflammatory CNS disease as described here occurs usually, but not exclusively, in patients with long-standing seropositive disease and considerable deformities. Not all patients with inflammatory CNS disease have subcutaneous nodules (Bathon *et al.*, 1989).

When performed, CSF examination reveals a raised protein content and a modest degree (or no) pleocytosis (Kim, 1980; Bathon *et al.*, 1989). Imaging has been helpful in a few cases by showing enhancement of meningeal structures (Allison and Mazano, 1985). In the reported cases, vasculitis has never been discovered by angiography. In fact, the introduction of new imaging techniques has somewhat simplified making the diagnosis of cerebral vasculitis. These new techniques have stimulated interest in cerebral vasculitis (see Chapter 5, *Diagnosing CNS Vasculitis*), but have not increased the publication of new cases of rheumatoid vasculitis, and this casts some doubt on the entity 'rheumatoid cerebral vasculitis'. Meningeal rheumatic nodules are sometimes discovered at autopsy in patients without any neurological manifestations (Schachenmayr and Friede, 1978; Jackson *et al.*, 1984).

NORMAL PRESSURE HYDROCEPHALUS AND RHEUMATOID ARTHRITIS

Normal pressure hydrocephalus is characterized by dementia, unstable gait, and urinary incontinence, and can be treated by ventriculo-peritoneal shunting. It was described by Rasker *et al.* (1985) in six patients with RA. The relation between the two diseases, if any, remains unclear. In 1995, Markusse *et al.* reported on two further possible cases and suggested that it might be caused by obstruction of CSF absorption by chronic meningitis. The authors observed improvement in their patients upon treatment with corticosteroids, and considered this as support for their hypothesis. In established and published cases of 'rheumatoid meningitis', normal pressure hydrocephalus has so far not been observed and reported.

RHEUMATOID ARTHRITIS OF THE CERVICAL SPINE

Epidemiology
Cervical spine lesions in patients with long-standing RA often form a point of great concern. Two years after the diagnosis of RA has been established, 10% of patients already show a mild degree of one of the different forms of cervical rheumatoid subluxations (Winfield *et al.*, 1981; Paimela *et al.*, 1997). After approximately 10 years, one third of the patients have a form of cervical subluxation (Winfield *et al.*, 1983), and after a mean disease duration of 15.7 years, the prevalence of cervical subluxations is 52%, as was shown in a population-based study in Finland (Kauppi and Hakala, 1994). The severity of the neck lesions correlates with the degree of erosion of metacarpo- and metatarsophalangeal joints (Winfield *et al.*, 1983). In contrast to cervical rheumatoid arthritis, thoracic arthritis rarely causes subluxations (see this Chapter, *The Thoracic and Lumbar Spine*).

The reason for the excessive vulnerability of the cervical spine is not definitely clarified, but two factors are likely to play a significant role: the extreme mobility of the cervical spine and the heavy load it has to carry (Agarwal *et al.*, 1993). It is of interest that the protective effect of hemiplegia on the development of rheumatoid joint lesions is explained by the decreased use of the joints on the lame side of the body (Martel, 1977; Bland and Eddy, 1968).

Destructive changes
Destructive changes occur in particular at the atlanto-occipital and atlanto-axial levels and to a lesser degree in the subaxial cervical segments (Box 9.1). At each cervical segment, from the atlanto-occipital level downward, there are two lateral synovia-lined joints. The dens has, in addition, a small synovia-lined joint with the anterior arch of the atlas and another one with the strong transverse ligament that covers the dens at the posterior side. This transverse ligament prevents posterior movement of the odontoid process towards or against the spinal cord during flexion of the cervical spine. From C2 downward there are small synovia-lined joints between the lateral edges of the cervical vertebrae (Stockwell, 1981). All these synovia-lined joints, as well as nearby ligaments, cartilage, and bone, may become affected and destroyed by the inflammatory rheumatoid process. This may result in abnormal mobility and some degree of luxation of cervical vertebrae, which potentially endangers the spinal cord (Fig. 9.3).

Bulbo-myelopathy and radiculopathy
The neurological manifestations, as summarized in Box 9.2, are in broad outline similar to other cranio-vertebral syndromes. Displacement of vertebrae may narrow the space available for the radices in foramina intervertebralia, for the spinal cord in the spinal canal, and for the medulla oblongata in the foramen magnum (Fig. 9.4).

Box 9.1. Five forms of cervical subluxation

---

1. Anterior atlanto-axial subluxation (AAS) is caused mainly by laxity and destruction of the transverse ligament. The distance between the posterior side of the atlas and the anterior side of the odontoid process (normal less than 3 mm, Martel, 1961) is increased, and the diameter of the vertical canal (normal 18–26 mm) is decreased. At flexion of the neck, AAS increases (reducible AAS). This is the most frequent form of cervical subluxation.

2. Posterior AAS is due to severe erosion or fracture of the odontoid process that allows the atlas to move backward. This form of subluxation is uncommon.

3. Atlanto-occipital impaction (AAI) or vertical subluxation happens when the cranium descends on the cervical spine and the odontoid process moves upward through the foramen magnum (normally, the odontoid process is below the foramen magnum), due to destruction of bone and cartilage at the occipito-atlanto- and atlanto-axial joints. Authors use different criteria for AAI and the figures for its prevalence vary accordingly (McGregor, 1948; Ranawat et al., 1979; Redlund-Johnell and Petterson, 1984; Kauppi et al., 1990). It is probably the second most frequent form of cervical subluxation (Halla and Hardin, 1990; Kauppi et al., 1990; Kauppi and Hakala, 1994; Chang and Paget, 1993) after AAS, and occurs after a longer period of disease than AAS (Casey et al., 1997a). AAI has a stabilizing effect on AAS due to loss of mobility in the atlanto-axial joints (Oda et al., 1995; Kauppi et al., 1996a).

4. Lateral AAS is due to unilateral or asymmetrical joint disease and destruction of the lateral mass of the atlas at that side. Patients show rotational tilting of the head towards the affected side.

5. Subaxial subluxation is due to intervertebral joint lesions and weakening of ligaments (Hughes, 1977). Subaxial subluxation is held to be present when there is displacement of adjacent vertebral bodies of more than 3.5 mm as measured from the posterior side of the bodies (White et al., 1975; Paimela et al., 1997; Eulderink and Meijers, 1976; Pellici et al., 1981). Subaxial subluxation tends to become more severe by fixation of the two upper cervical vertebrae, either by AAI or by operation (Kraus et al., 1991; Oda et al., 1995). Long-standing cervical RA may occasionally result in progressive kyphosis from C2–C7, with compensatory lordosis at the craniocervical junction (King, 1994).

Compression of nervous structures may be intermittent, as in patients with reducible AAS, (see Box 9.1) or permanent, as in most vertebral subluxations. Neurological symptoms and signs may therefore be intermittent also, though they are mostly definite.

How often and when

Neurological evaluation of handicapped, deformed patients with long-standing rheumatoid arthritis and atrophy of peri-articular muscles is not easily performed. This is reflected by the descriptions in the literature on the neurology of the cervical spine lesions, which are usually put in very general terms. Spinal cord compression develops only in a small minority of patients, after many years or even decades. Winfield et al. (1983) followed a group of 100 patients from the first year after RA had been diagnosed. At the end of a 10 year period, one patient had developed

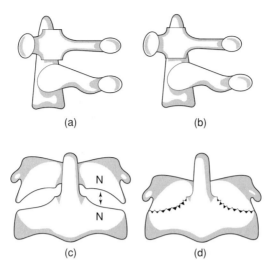

Figure 9.3 Diagrams of atlanto-axial subluxation and vertical subluxation. Top left: lateral view of neutral upright position. Top right: lateral view during flexion. The distance of the dens to the anterior part of the atlas has increased, and the distance towards the posterior part has decreased, thus leaving less space for the spinal cord. Bottom left: anterior-posterior view of atlanto-axial lateral intervertebral facets. Bottom right: anterior-posterior view. The atlanto-axial lateral facets have eroded and rest upon one another. The dens extends abnormally above the atlas. [Adapted from Kauppi *et al.* (1996a), with permission.]

Box 9.2 Neurological symptoms and signs in patients with cervical subluxations

1. In comparison to the degree of the cervical abnormalities and the evidence of bulbospinal compression, neurological signs are commonly less marked than one would expect. Symptoms and signs of the spinal cord and radiculi are much more frequent than bulbar syndromes and cranial nerve lesions.
2. Myelopathy: disturbance of gnostic sensibility is more frequent than of vital sensibility. Some patients have unilateral or bilateral astereognosis of the hands. Lhermitte's sign* may be present. Pyramidal changes include raised tendon reflexes with positive Babinski reflexes, spasticity, and muscle weakness in that order. Disorders of bladder and bowel motility are not rare.
3. Radiculopathy: severe pain in the occipital region presumably of radicular origin is relatively frequent.
4. Bulbar syndromes and cranial nerve lesions: dysphagia and dysarthria, vertigo, fainting, cerebellar signs, symptoms of nn V, IX, X, XII, VII and rarely III, IV and VI. Obstructive hydrocephalus and secondary inappropriate antidiuretic hormone secretion have been reported.

*Passive or active flexion of the neck elicits a sensation of electricity irradiating along the trunk to the limbs.
From text references.

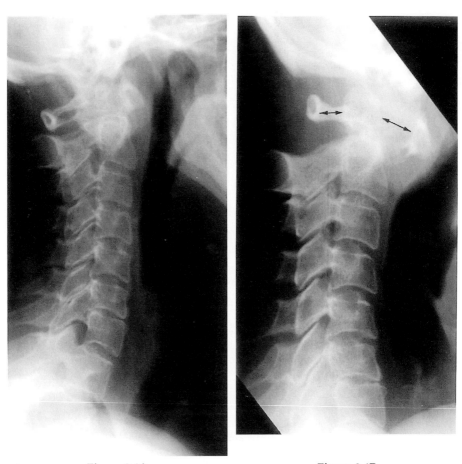

Figure 9.4A   **Figure 9.4B**

Figure 9.4 Atlanto-axial subluxation. Radiology and MRI of 62-year old female with rheumatoid arthritis. **A.** Radiology of cervico-occipital transition. Lateral view. Head and vertebral column are in neutral position. The odontoid process is not clearly discernable. **B.** Flexion of the head. The anterior arch of the atlas is moved far forward and a considerable space has arisen between the posterior side of the anterior arch of the atlas and the silhouette of the dens, which is now just visible (longest arrow). The distance between posterior side of the dens and posterior arch of the atlas has become smaller than the distance between dens and anterior arch (smallest arrow).

cervical myelopathy. Two others were operated on for severe occipital headache. Rana *et al.* (1973) and Rana (1989) followed a selected group of 41 patients who all had some degree of AAS from the onset. Eight patients had disturbance of trigeminal sensibility at onset and 19 had miscellaneous neurological symptoms and signs. During the subsequent period of 10 years, three of these 27 patients presented with progressive myelopathy. Fourteen other patients were neurologically normal at onset. One of them developed posterior column signs and severe narrowing of the canal, which had to be operated. The others did not show any signs of myelopathy.

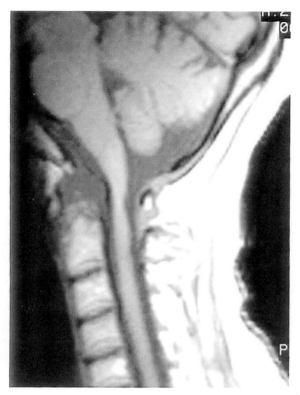

Figure 9.4C

Figure 9.4C Same patient as in Figures 9.4A and B. Sagittal MRI, T1-Wi image. Head in neutral position. The remains of the dens and pannus narrow the spinal canal and compress the spinal cord.

Pain
Patients with rheumatoid cervical spine lesions frequently complain about neck pain and occipital pain radiating toward the vertex, possibly due to compression of the second cervical root. Often, intractable occipital pain is the reason for surgical intervention (Pellici *et al.*, 1981; Casey *et al.*, 1996).

Bulbar signs
Nakano *et al.* (1978) retrospectively found, among 1100 patients admitted to a hospital that cares mainly for RA, 32 patients with neurological changes related to the cervical spine. Six patients had evidence of lower brainstem dysfunction, including vertigo, diplopia, and dysphagia. Similar symptoms were present in 24 of 45 'symptomatic' (in the neurological respect) patients with AAI (vertical subluxation) (Menezes *et al.*, 1985). Some also had transient black-out spells. One of them could provoke nystagmus and vertigo by rotating his head. The brainstem signs in the group of Menezes *et al.* (1985) were: nystagmus (in some patients downbeat), Horner's syndrome, internuclear ophthalmoplegia, and 'cerebellar' signs. The hypoglossus, glossopharyngeus and vagus nerves were the most frequently

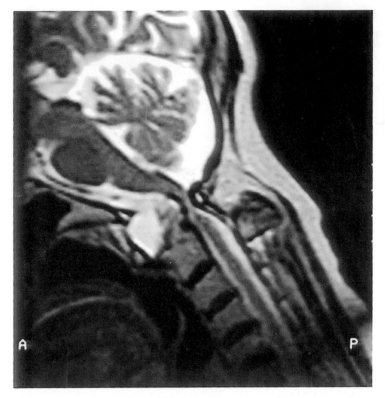

Figure 9.4D

Figure 9.4D Same patient as in Figures 9.4A, B and C. Sagittal MRI, T2-Wi image. Head in flexion. The remains of the dens are now visible. The distance between dens and anterior arch of the atlas is considerably increased and is filled with pannus. The diameter of the vertebral canal is markedly reduced and odontoid process and posterior arch of the atlas compress the spinal cord severely. (Courtesy of Dr. Lino Ramos.)

affected cranial nerves, but one of the patients of Menezes *et al.* had loss of pain and touch in the distribution of the trigeminal nerve and another even had facial diplegia. In the group of Rana *et al.* (1973) eight of 41 patients with AAS had trigeminal sensory neuropathy. Toolanen (1987) determined the cutaneous threshold for the face in patients with AAS and AAI due to RA, and discovered changes in the ophthalmic and maxillary divisions of the trigeminal nerve but not in the mandibular division, presumably due to lesions in the trigeminal spinal tract. Obstructive hydrocephalus was reported in three cases, and was associated in one with secondary inappropriate antidiuretic hormone secretion (Collee *et al.*, 1987; Rillo *et al.*, 1989; Naredo-Sanchez *et al.*, 1996). Symptoms of dysphagia and dysarthria of uncertain origin were present in 41 (respectively 35) of 186 patients operated for either AAS or AAI (Casey *et al.*, 1997a).

Myelopathy

Menezes *et al.* (1985) found hyperreflexia with positive Babinski signs in 36 of their 45 neurologically symptomatic patients with AAI. The authors had difficulty in adequately evaluating the strength of their patients. Posterior column sensory disorders were frequent, but hypalgesia was unusual. Nakano *et al.* (1977) also found weakness in patients with hyper-reflexia and Babinski signs. Astereognosis of the hands was a feature of 18 of these 32 patients. Other sensory disturbances including hypalgesia were often present. Sixteen patients had bladder and/or rectal sphincter dysfunction. Lhermitte's sign was present in 35 of 186 patients with myelopathy (Casey *et al.*, 1997a).

The Ranawat classification

The Ranawat system is used mainly by surgeons to classify patients for degree of pain and neurological deficit (Table 9.3) (Ranawat *et al.*, 1979).

Radiology of the rheumatoid cervical spine versus neurological signs

Are there any radiological parameters that reliably predict the presence or the development of severe neurological signs? The answer that is usually given to this question is in the negative. Considerable atlanto-axial subluxation, vertical subluxation, and local pannus appear to be compatible with Ranawat class I (no neurological deficit). Boden *et al.* (1993) stress that it is not the degree of subluxation that should be measured but the width of the cervical canal. On the basis of a retrospective analysis of their material (conventional radiography, tomography, and CT scans), they suggest that a postero-anterior diameter of less than 14 mm predicts neurological deficit. However, it appears from observations by others that some neurological deficit may well be present in patients with AAS and a canal width of 14 mm and that patients with canal diameters of 13 mm may be Ranawat class I. Neither is there a simple nor linear relation between the hight of the dens and the Ranawat classification. MRI may reveal serious abnormalities in patients who (still) do not have any neurological dysfunction. In one study, six of 11 patients with MRI evidence of brainstem compression and eight of 22 with MRI signs of spinal cord compression had no neurological changes (Reijnierse *et al.*, 1996). Only MRI evidence of reduction of the subaxial subarachnoid space correlated with neurological abnormalities. Decisions on the management of patients with rheumatoid cervical

Table 9.3 Ranawat classification of pain and neurological deficit in patients with rheumatoid cervical spine lesions

Class	Pain	Deficit
I	Mild, requiring aspirin intermittently	No deficit
II	Moderate, cervical collar needed	Subjective weakness with hyper-reflexia and dysaesthesia
III	Severe, pain cannot be relieved by either aspirin or collar, or both	Objective weakness and long tract signs A can still walk B not ambulatory

From Ranawat *et al.* (1979), with permission.

spine lesions should therefore be based on results of both clinical and laboratory investigations and never on radiology alone.

Neuropathology of rheumatoid cervical spinal cord lesions

There is one large neuropathological study of brainstems and cervical spinal cords in the literature that has several unexpected findings (Henderson *et al.*, 1993). This report concerned nine cases, eight of which had been operated for craniocervical compression or instability. Most patients were Ranawat III B, and none had cranial nerve lesions. All had a marked vertical subluxation with a variable degree of AAS, and all but one had subaxial changes. Changes in the brainstem, notably the cranial nerve nuclei, were mild. Spinal cords showed necrosis at severely compressed places. Where compression was less severe, pathology was restricted mainly to the dorsal white columns. The fasciculus cuneatus was more affected than the fasciculus gracilis. At several levels in eight of the nine cases, anterior horn cells showed chromatolysis but no obvious cell loss. Chronic inflammation of the pia-arachnoid was seen in several cases at sites of compression. The spinal cord changes were best explained by stretch and compression and not by ischaemia or vasculitis. The preferential involvement of the fasciculus cuneatus also has been observed by others, but has not been sufficiently clarified (Nakano *et al.*, 1978). The authors concluded that the extent of compression at the subaxial levels was underestimated. They suggested that patients be operated on before they reached neurological deficit Ranawat III B (see the following sections).

Prevention and treatment of cervical spine lesions

Medical treatment of RA aims at suppression of disease activity as a whole and is not directed to one specific joint area. Local approaches to prevent progress of lesions to the cervical spine and the spinal cord aim at reduction of mobility and instability of the cervical spine, and at increase of the width of the spinal canal. Surgical and conservative policies have each their advocates.

The surgical viewpoint. According to Casey *et al.* (1996), in general, rheumatologists favour a conservative approach until neurological signs or symptoms force them to opt for surgery. Many patients are in the neurological deficit class Ranawat III B before they come for operation. At this stage, surgery does not have much to offer anymore. Pain relief is indeed frequently obtained, but only few patients improve functionally (improvement to neurological deficit classes Ranawat I or II). Post-operative complications are frequent and post-operative mortality is high (Casey *et al.*, 1997b). Neurological deficit Ranawat III A patients do much better than Ranawat III B patients. Therefore, surgeons feel that patients should be operated on when they are in stage Ranawat II or III A.

The viewpoint of a rheumatologist. There are far too many patients with subluxations for them all to be operated on, and the risks related to surgical interventions are considerable. Conservative treatment is unavoidable and should be pursued more actively. According to Kauppi (1996) and Kauppi *et al.* (1996b) an active policy to prevent progressive cervical spine lesioning and to reduce pain involves: (1) patient education, (2) a stiff collar, (3) a number of practical aids, and (4) treatment with active disease-modifying anti-rheumatic drugs (DMARD). With this treatment regime, the number of patients that have to be operated on can be reduced considerably. Using this approach in a group of 20 patients, it appeared that 17 adapted well to the instructions. After one year, there was a favourable effect on cervical pain and there were 'promising changes in some cervical radiographs' (Kauppi *et al.*, 1998).

THE THORACIC AND LUMBAR SPINE

Widespread bone loss is one of the characteristic features of RA and is associated with disease activity (Gough *et al.*, 1994). Osteoporosis of the spine and collapse of vertebrae at the thoracic and lumbar level are common in RA (Lems *et al.*, 1995).

Bywaters discovered, according to Redlund-Johnell and Larson (1993) at autopsy of 14 patients with RA, evidence of discitis with rheumatoid erosions of the costovertebral joints in eight cases. They screened conventional X-rays of the dorsal spine in 100 consecutive cases of occipito-cervical fusion and discovered arthritis of the upper part of the thoracic spine (T1–T2, T2–T3 and T3–T4) with subluxation in four patients. MRI demonstrated spinal cord compression in one of these cases who was a paraplegic patient (Redlund-Johnell and Larson, 1993).

Sasaki *et al.* (1997) described a woman with thoracic myelopathy due to vertebral compression fractures at several levels and compression of the cord at these levels by a mass of extradural granulation tissue. Fairburn (1975) observed a patient with cord compression at T–5 by an extradural rheumatic nodule. Destruction of the body of the fourth lumbar vertebra by a nodular granulation tissue was reported by Pearson *et al.* (1987), and pachymeningitis with lumbar radiculopathy was observed by Markenson *et al.* (1979). One should be aware that spastic paraparesis, not sufficiently explained by subluxation at the cervical level, can be caused by a rheumatoid disorder at the thoracic level.

SENSORY OR SENSOMOTOR POLYNEUROPATHIES AND MONONEURITIS MULTIPLEX

Epidemiology

Sensory or sensomotor neuropathies do not often create management problems in RA, and for that reason the epidemiology of these disorders is probably not fully elucidated yet. Conn and Dyck (1975) detected, in a survey of 2162 patients with RA all seen in 1971 in the Mayo Clinics (!), 25 cases with symptomatic peripheral neuropathy. There is a possibility that these were only the more severe cases, as the authors did not explain how they traced the patients. The findings of Bekkelund *et al.* (1996) concerning nerve conduction in 52 women with seropositive and erosive RA and the lack of any evidence of neuropathy in this group support the view that peripheral neuropathies are infrequent. The disease duration of the patients was not mentioned. On the other hand, Fleming *et al.* (1976), in a large longitudinal investigation of extra-articular features during the first five or six years after onset of RA, diagnosed 'distal sensory' or 'distal motor neuropathy' in 18 of 102 patients. Distal sensory neuropathy was more frequent than sensomotor or motor neuropathy. This confirmed previous observations by Pallis and Scott (1965), Chamberlain and Bruckner (1970), and Weller *et al.* (1970) indicating that a relatively mild sensory neuropathy could be distinguished from more severe forms with motor and sensory symptoms.

Clinical features and course

Mild sensory neuropathy is stated to recover mostly spontaneously (Chang and Paget, 1993) and to occasionally become severe and sensomotor (Conn and Dyck, 1975). Some of the more severe sensomotor polyneuropathies present at onset as mononeuritis multiplex. In such cases, the patient complains suddenly about pain and dysaesthesia in the course of a peripheral nerve at one of the lower limbs and feet or, more rarely, at one of the hands and underarms. Weakness develops, thereafter, within hours or days. Gradually more nerves become involved and the clinical picture becomes symmetrical. This type of rheumatoid peripheral neuropathy is caused by vasculitis of small or medium-sized epineurial vessels (between 70–250 µm; Chalk *et al.*, 1993; Puéchal *et al.*, 1995). The vascular changes resemble those of periarteritis nodosa (see this Chapter, *Vasculitis*).

In a retrospective investigation, Puéchal *et al.* (1995) studied the clinical features of 32 patients with RA, peripheral neuropathy, and vasculitis established by nerve or muscle biopsy. Nearly 50% of the patients had a predominantly sensory neuropathy. Others had a sensomotor polyneuropathy, a predominantly motor neuropathy, or mononeuritis multiplex, which demonstrated that all these types of neuropathies could potentially be caused by vasculitis. It is of interest that in a retrospective investigation of 61 patients with RA and histologically-proven vasculitis done by Voskuyl *et al.* (1996a), 12% had mononeuritis multiplex and 15% had distal sensory neuropathy. These observations indicate, but do not prove, that all forms of neuropathy, including mild sensory neuropathy, may be caused by vasculitis. No less than 25% of the patients of Puéchall *et al.* (1995) had a relapse after recovery of their neuropathy. Vasculitic neuropathy, in this study, was a feature of long-standing, seropositive RA with rheumatic nodules; the range of RA disease duration was, however, wide (mean 16 years, range 2–47!). The five-year survival rate of patients with rheumatoid vasculitis varies in different studies: in Puéchall *et al.* it was 57% and in Voskuyl *et al.* (1996a) it was 67%.

Diagnosis and management

Patients with mild sensory neuropathy should be examined for evidence of vasculitis. There is a reasonable chance that vasculitis can be discovered by the presence of skin lesions (in up to 40% of cases with vasculitis) (Puéchall *et al.*, 1995) (see this Chapter, *Vasculitis*). Less frequent are kidney or gastrointestinal lesions. Nailfold infarcts and splinter haemorrhages are also due to vasculitis, but only of small arteries. These are often present, but need no therapy as they tend to recover spontaneously. They should not be considered as signs in support of a vasculitic origin of neuropathy. On its own, mild sensory neuropathy requires regular careful control. The available data suggest that one should wait and see what happens, as spontaneous recovery seems to occur in at least some cases. When there is progress towards a sensomotor neuropathy or in cases of mononeuritis multiplex, invasive diagnostic methods may be used and aggressive therapy should be started without delay. Muscle biopsies, preferably of a distal limb muscle, are at least as often diagnostic as sural nerve biopsies (Puéchall *et al.*, 1995), and are to be preferred as they cause disagreeable sequelae less often than sural nerve biopsies. Patients with rheumatoid vasculitis and severe organ involvement are likely to benefit from prompt initiation of therapy with high-dose corticosteroids and cytostatic agents (Voskuyl *et al.*, 1996a; Voskuyl *et al.*, 1996b; see also Chapter 5). Luqmani *et al.* (1994) prefer, however, intermittent high-dose pulses of cyclophosphamide, initially at two week intervals (see Chapter 4 for doses), with low dose oral corticosteroids as supportive therapy. With this strategy, remission is, according to the experience of the authors, obtained usually within a few months, following which maintenance therapy is required. However, the ideal medication for maintenance therapy is not available yet. Azathioprine does not sufficiently prevent relapses and low-dose corticosteroids have too many side effects.

COMPRESSION NEUROPATHIES

Carpal tunnel syndrome

Compression of the median nerve in the carpal tunnel is frequently in RA. In their prospective longitudinal investigation of 102 frequently controlled patients with RA of recent onset, Fleming *et al.* (1976) registered, in a mean period per patient of 44 months, clinical evidence of median nerve compression in 52% of the patients overall. Other authors reported slightly lower percentages (see Chang and Paget, 1993). Patients complain about numbness and tingling in digits 1 (the thumb) to 4. Pain in the median nerve-innervated part of the hand may irradiate up to the elbow and even higher. Neurological investigation may reveal disturbance of skin sensibility in the area innervated by the median nerve. Weakness of thumb opposition and abduction and atrophy of the abductor pollicis brevis muscle may develop later on, but may not be so easy to assess in RA patients. The laboratory technique that is used mostly for confirmation of the clinical diagnosis is comparison of sensory conduction from the fourth finger along the median nerve with sensory conduction from the same finger along the ulnar nerve (de Krom *et al.*, 1990; Stevens, 1997). Therapy is conservative when the complaints are slight and includes local injection of corticosteroids in case of active carpal synovitis. When the complaints are more severe or when there is evidence of neurogenic thumb weakness surgery is required.

Tarsal tunnel syndrome

The tibial nerve may become compressed behind and below the medial side of the ankle where it passes under the flexor retinaculum. Clinical manifestations are infrequent and comprise pain, tingling, and numbness of the toes and the soles (Grabois *et al.*, 1981; McGuigan *et al.*, 1983). The diagnosis requires electrophysiological confirmation. The tibial nerve divides in the tunnel in two or three branches. Not all these branches need to be compressed to the same degree. When only one of the branches is involved, differentiation is necessary of tarsal tunnel syndrome from plantar nerve compression distal to the tarsal tunnel, and additional nerve conduction studies, which are not easy to perform, are required (Spaans, 1987).

Finger drop by posterior interosseus nerve entrapment

The motor branch of the radial nerve separates from the sensory branch at the level of the elbow and passes below the elbow between the superficial and the deep part of the supinator muscle. At the site of entrance in the supinator muscle, the nerve may be compressed by the fibrous arch of the superficial part of the m. supinator or by the extensor carpi radialis brevis muscle. It may also be compressed, at a slightly higher level, by fibrous bands, which may form the radialis tunnel. In all these cases, the main symptom is very characteristic, and comprises inability to extend the fingers due to weakness of the extensor digitorum communis muscle and the extensor pollicis (Spaans, 1987). Wrist extension is usually preserved and sensibility remains intact. Rupture of the tendon of the extensor digitorum muscle is the main differential diagnosis. However, tendon rupture usually occurs suddenly, which is in contrast to posterior interosseus nerve compression which progresses gradually. Tendon rupture concerns the fourth and fifth fingers mostly and not the thumb. Prevention of initiation of finger extension also may be due to metacarpophalangeal dislocation, but in this case, extension of the fingers can be maintained after passive stretching. Posterior interosseus nerve lesion can be confirmed by electromyography. In patients with RA, the nerve is compressed or stretched by bulging, proliferating elbow synovium, which is often palpable and best visualized by MRI. Up until now, at least 13 cases have been reported (Marshall and Murray, 1974; Fernandez and Tiku, 1994; McDonald and Smith, 1996). Treatment with local intra-articular steroids, systemic anti-inflammatory drugs, or both has been successful in several cases. Surgical decompression is advised when medical treatment is unsuccessful (McDonald and Smith, 1996).

Compression of other nerves
Compression of nerves at other sites is possible but exceptional. All cases of mononeuropathy in patients with RA deserve accurate diagnosis, as they may in fact be the onset of mononeuritis multiplex.

MYASTHENIA GRAVIS AND RA

Myasthenia gravis (MG) is often associated with other auto-immune diseases. The RA prevalence in patients with MG varies in different studies. It is, according to Oosterhuis (1993), from 0–10%. In a 37 year period, this author followed 813 patients with MG: 34 of them developed RA (eight males and 26 females) (Oosterhuis, 1997). MG may be induced by treatment with D-penicillamine (see Chapter 4 for side-effects of D-penicillamine).

MUSCLE ATROPHY, MYOPATHY, AND MYOSITIS

Muscular strength and endurance in RA are, in general, less than in a control population, and patients have less muscle volume (Ekdahl *et al.*, 1989). These changes are conceived to be due to factors related to the inflammatory process and to inactivity. Muscles around arthritic joints may become obviously atrophic; this is one of the most common features of RA. Fleming *et al.* (1976), in their prospective longitudinal study of 102 patients, registered evidence of hand-muscle wasting in 58% of patients. The pathological substrate of the general loss of muscle strength is atrophy of muscle fibres, predominantly type II fibres (Brook and Kaplan, 1972). In some cases, there are also occasional focal mononuclear cell infiltrates around vessels or in between muscle fibres (Mastaglia and Walton, 1992). For unexplained reasons, mean values for CK activity are lower in RA than in controls. Unexplained low serum CK values also have been observed in SLE and other connective tissue diseases, in patients on corticosteroid medication, and in patients with liver diseases (Wei *et al.*, 1981; Sanmarti *et al.*, 1994; Sanmarti *et al.*, 1996).

Preferential weakness and atrophy of proximal limb muscles are infrequent in RA. In a retrospective study of all patients with RA (350) seen in their hospital over an eight year period, Miro *et al.* (1996) selected patients with limb muscle weakness and atrophy, myalgia, or cramps. Twenty one patients complied to the inclusion criteria (incidence of 6% in an eight year period). Sixteen had limb muscle weakness, which was predominantly proximal, and eight had limb muscle atrophy. They were diagnosed as: true dermatomyositis (2), dermatomyositis following initiation of D-penicillamine treatment (2), true polymyositis (4), polyarteritis nodosa (1), corticosteroid myopathy (5), and chloroquine myopathy (1). Interestingly, ragged red fibres were seen in six biopsies; ragged red fibres can occur in inflammatory muscle disorders, but the authors provide no information on this association in their material. The study of Miro *et al.* (1996) shows that predominantly proximal weakness in RA is due mostly to either myositis (DM or PM) or to an unwanted effect of medication (corticosteroids, D-penicillamine, chloroquine). The association of RA and inclusion body myositis (IBM) has been reported (Soden *et al.*, 1994) (see Chapter 6).

SUMMARY

Inflammatory processes of the synovia of intervertebral articulations, particularly at the atlanto-occipital and atlanto-axial levels, may result in subluxations of cervical vertebrae and compression of the spinal cord, bulbar structures, and radiculi. These are the most frequent causes of CNS manifestations in RA and occur predominantly in the advanced stages of the disease. There are case reports on rheumatic nodules in the meninges and on pachymeningitis with local vasculitis extending in superficial brain structures, but these changes are seldom. Polyneuropathies or multiple neuropathies are more frequent than CNS manifestations, and are due mostly to peripheral nerve vasculitis. Skeletal deformities and inflammatory changes may cause carpal tunnel syndrome and other peripheral nerve compression syndromes. In relatively few patients, RA is associated with myositis or MG.

JUVENILE CHRONIC ARTHRITIS (JCA) AND ADULT STILL'S DISEASE

According to the classification by a task force of the International League against Rheumatism, seven idiopathic arthritides, all with onset before the age of 16 years, have to be distinguished (Box 9.3). The overall incidence rate of the diseases in this group is estimated to be approximately 10/100 000 per year. Different genetic and environmental factors are likely to be involved in each of these diseases (see Woo and Wedderburn, 1998). The following descriptions are limited to arthritides with neurological manifestations.

SYSTEMIC JUVENILE ARTHRITIS (SJA)

Of all patients with JCA, 12 to 14% have systemic arthritis. It is a disease of preschool-age children without any gender preference. Onset can be at any age during childhood with a peak age of 2 years (Woo and Wedderburn, 1998; Laxer and Schneider, 1998). The disease presents with systemic features, primarily a high intermittent fever of up to 40°C, transient maculopapular skin rash, polyserositis, hepatosplenomegaly, lymphadenopathy, high erythrocyte sedimentation rate (ESR), high C-reactive protein concentration, anaemia, and increase of granulocytes

Box 9.3 Classification of different forms of juvenile idiopathic arthritides, according to The International League against Rheumatism Task Force

---

1. Systemic arthritis
2. Oligoarthritis (persistent)
3. Oligoarthritis (extended)
4. Polyarticular arthritis, rheumatoid factor positive
5. Polyarticular arthritis, rheumatoid factor negative
6. Enthesitis arthritis
7. Psoriatic arthritis
8. Unclassified

From Woo and Wedderburn (1998), with permission.

and thrombocytes. Serum auto-antibodies, such as antinuclear antibodies (ANAs) and RF, are absent. Most patients develop chronic polyarthritis within the first three months after onset, but in some cases it takes up to three years; a small minority remains free from arthritis. Knees, ankles, and wrists are the most affected, but the cervical spine, hips, and temperomandibular joints may be involved also. One third of the patients have destructive joint lesions. Rarely, the affected children acquire pulmonary disease and myocarditis.

After the initial stage, the polyarthritis becomes gradually more prominent, while the systemic features decrease. During infections, however, the systemic features may transiently recur. Patients experience malaise, joint pain and destruction, growth retardation, and in the chronic cases, there is a risk of amyloidosis. The course is variable: either monophasic with complete remission in two years, polyphasic with exacerbations of systemic disease activity, or chronic and persistent. The mean duration of the disease is approximately 5–6 years, but approximately 25% of patients have persistent symptoms 10–15 years after onset (Woo and Wedderburn, 1998). Mortality in systemic onset juvenile arthritis is related to amyloidosis, infections, and hepatic failure and amounts to approximately 14% of patients.

Management. Treatment consists initially of NSAIDs, such as acetylsalicylic acid (80–100 mg/kg), indomethacin (1–2 mg/kg), or naprosyne (approximately 10 mg/kg). Usually a second agent must be added. Prednisone is used both orally in low doses (0.3–0.5 mg/kg) or in pulses (methylprednisolone 15–30 mg/kg/day for several days). Other drugs (methotrexate orally 0.3 mg/kg once weekly or high-dose intramuscular or subcutaneous 1 mg/kg/week; cyclosporine 2–5 mg/kg/day; salazopyrin 50 mg/kg) are added in case of ongoing disease activity in an effort to prevent the chronic use of corticosteroids.

However, randomized placebo-controlled intervention studies into the efficacy of these drugs are lacking. Intravenous immunoglobulin (IVIG) infusions are helpful in severe cases, as they induce clinical improvement in most patients, but the duration of the beneficial effect is short and the course of the diseases is not altered (Pediatric Rheumatology Collaborative Study Group, 1997; Uziel *et al.*, 1996). For the most severe and drug resistant cases, autologous bone marrow transplantation may be an option (Wulffraat *et al.*, 1997). Without treatment, systemic arthritis can progress to the macrophage activation syndrome.

Neurological manifestations in systemic arthritis

It is only in few patients that CNS or PNS manifestations create management problems. Most attention is needed for cervical spine lesions.

1. *Macrophage activation syndrome* (MAS) (Stephan *et al.*, 1993), also known as *haemophagocytic syndrome* (Woo and Wedderburn, 1998) or *haematophagic histiocytosis* (Reiner and Spivak, 1988), may develop in children with untreated or insufficiently treated systemic juvenile arthritis. It is notorious for its high mortality rate. The syndrome is characterized by fever, depressed blood cell counts, hepatic dysfunction, decreased fibrinogen levels, and hepatosplenomegaly. Macrophage activation, which is revealed at bone marrow examination by the presence of histiocytes containing haematopoietic elements and by the overproduction of cytokines [in particular tumour necrosis factor alpha (TNF-α)] is considered an essential feature of the syndrome. Meningeal and cerebral complications (infiltration of the meninges by non-malignant histiocytes, seizures, 'encephalopathy', coma) are frequent. MAS may be provoked by a viral infection or a change in therapy, or it may occur spontaneously. Reiner and Spivak (1988), who described MAS under the name of haematophagic histiocytosis, state that the syndrome occurs generally in the setting of a pre-existing immunological abnormality. Early diagnosis and treatment with methylprednisolone pulse-doses or cyclosporine are required to prevent serious complications.

2. Lang *et al.* (1995) retrospectively reviewed radiological findings in 42 patients with systemic onset of juvenile arthritis and established spine abnormalities in 17%. Five of 42 patients had joint ankylosis of apophysial joints of the cervical spine: in each case at the C2–C3 level, in two cases at the C3–C4 level, and in another two at C4–C5. It may present clinically with pain, limitation of neck movements, and torticollis. Atlanto-axial subluxation is much less frequent than ankylosis of apophysial joints and it causes generally no neurological abnormalities. Neurosurgical intervention is required in some cases for correction of atlanto-axial rotatory fixation and subluxation (Uziel *et al.*, 1998).

3. Acquired neuromyotonia or *Isaacs' syndrome* has recently been described in association with juvenile systemic arthritis. It is due to antibodies against voltage-gated potassium channels in the membrane of the terminal motor axon near the neuromuscular synapse, and it is clinically characterized by muscle twitching, aching or cramps, and myotonia-like features during muscle activity. It has been observed in association with other auto-immune disorders and is treated in the first instance with the anti-convulsants, carbamazepine or phenytoin (see Chapter 2) (Le Gars *et al.*, 1997).

4. Brown's syndrome gives rise to vertical diplopia on upward and inward gaze, and is due to an inflammatory disorder of the posterior part of the tendon of the m.obliquus superior. It disappears spontaneously or by treatment with a NSAID or a low dose of prednisone (see Chapter 6) (Wang *et al.*, 1984; Moore and Morin, 1985).

5. Though anticardiolipin antibodies (ACAs) in JCA are generally not associated with vessel occlusions, an exception to this has been reported (Andrews and Hickling, 1997).

POLYARTICULAR AND OLIGOARTICULAR JUVENILE CHRONIC ARTHRITIS

The rheumatoid factor positive (seropositive) variety of polyarticular JCA usually occurs in children over the age of eight years. In most respects, it is indistinguishable from RA in adults and may be associated with all the neurological manifestations of the adult form (Ansell, 1998). The seronegative variant of polyarticular JCA may occur at younger ages than the seropositive form and is more frequent. There is a female preponderance among patients with polyarticular JCA. ANAs occur in both forms. The seropositive variant has a worse prognosis than the seronegative form. Atlanto-axial subluxation occurs both in the seropositive and the seronegative form, and causes in general no neurological abnormalities (Espada *et al.*, 1987). Apophysial joint fusion is more frequent than atlanto-axial subluxation in both forms of polyarticular JCA, and is one of the few manifestations in which adult and juvenile seropositive RA differ. Joint ankylosis is rare in the adult form of RA. In particular, joint fusion occurs at the level of C2–C3 (Fig. 9.5). Cervical spine disorders most often present clinically with limitation of neck movements and torticollis. Synovitis of apophysial joints may occur also at the thoracic and lumbar level (Prieur, 1998).

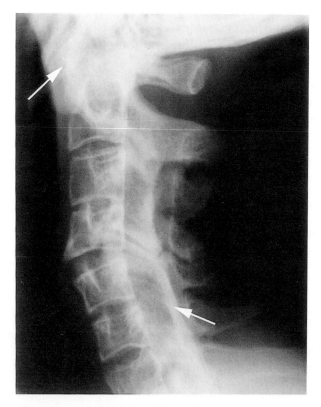

Figure 9.5 Juvenile chronic polyarthritis. Cervical spine of a young adult known for juvenile chronic arthritis showing apophysial joint ankylosis and atlanto-axial subluxation (arrows). (Courtesy of Dr Lino Ramos.)

Oligoarticular JCA affects fewer joints than polyarticular JCA and does not give rise to neurological abnormalities. Muscular atrophy secondary to the joint lesions can be prominent, however, both in oligoarticular and in polyarticular juvenile arthritis.

ADULT STILL'S DISEASE

Adult Still's disease is a rare disorder that has been described in very different parts of the world (Laxer and Schneider, 1998). It is the equivalent of systemic arthritis in juveniles, and occurs predominantly in young adults (16–35 years) and more often in females than males. The incidence decreases with age, but the disease has been reported in individuals as old as 82 years (Sanada *et al.*, 1997). RF and ANAs are usually not present. Serum IgG may be raised, however. The ESR and white blood cell counts are raised during active stages of the disease. Neurological manifestations are very exceptional and have been described only in case reports. They include, according to a review by Denault and others (1990), brainstem haemorrhage, seizures, sensorineural deafness, aseptic meningitis, inflammatory orbital pseudotumour, and peripheral neuropathy. Brown's syndrome has been reported also (see this Chapter, *Systemic Juvenile Arthritis* and Chapter 6, *Brown's Syndrome* (Kaufman *et al.*, 1987).

ACUTE RHEUMATIC FEVER

As in nearly all other ICTDs, rheumatic fever is conceived to be due to a combination of an environmental factor and genetic predisposition. What makes rheumatic fever exceptional is that the environmental factor has been identified and this knowledge has been used to devise an effective prevention programme. Two to four weeks after a pharyngeal infection by group-A β haemolytic streptococcus, symptoms of rheumatic fever may become manifest (see Gibofsky and Zabriskie, 1998). This occurs mostly in children between five and 15 years, though it has been described in adults also. Up to 3% of the infected individuals, but usually much less, respond in this fashion. Possible explanations for this low percentage are restriction of rheumagenicity to a limited number of strains of group-A streptococci and genetic predisposition of some individuals (Carapetis *et al.*, 1996; Stollerman, 1997). The prevalence of rheumatic fever varies greatly between countries. The marked decline in the more developed countries in the last few decades differs strikingly with the still high incidence in the underdeveloped world. Prevalence rates of rheumatic heart disease (one of the main sequelae of rheumatic fever) among children of 12–14 years in Soweto are as high as 20/1000, whereas in developed countries it is approximately 0.2–0.5/100 000 (Stollerman, 1997).

Initially, it was believed that antibodies directed against antigenic epitopes of the streptococcus might cross-react with similar epitopes in tissue components of the affected organs, and would thus cause tissue damage. Though the humoral component in the immune response is at present not contested, a cell-mediated immune response to antigens eliciting a cross–reaction may be partly responsible for the complications, as patients with acute rheumatic fever show exaggerated cellular immunity to streptococcal antigens and non-specific changes in circulating CD4 and CD8 cells. A role for cellular immunity is suggested also by the fact that the cellular infiltrate in the affected heart valves consists predominantly of T-lymphocytes.

CLINICAL FEATURES AND DIAGNOSIS

The clinical manifestations of rheumatic fever follow upon the pharyngeal infection with an interval of 2–3 weeks (Gibofsky and Zabriskie, 1998). The most common presentation of the disease consists of acute fever and polyarthritis. Concomittantly, carditis may develop and also chorea, though the latter usually becomes manifest after a delay of one or several months. Other features of the disease are a characteristic evanescent erythema, which has clear centres and round or serpiginous margins, on the trunk and proximal parts of the limbs (erythema marginatum) and subcutaneous nodules, which are somewhat smaller than the rheumatic nodules in RA and more short-lived. The arthritis affects joints for short periods, not all of them simultaneously, and thus creates the suggestion that arthritis migrates from one joint to another. It causes exudation in joints, not proliferation or destructive lesions, and can be extremely painful. The duration of polyarthritis commonly varies from 1–4 weeks. Carditis may cause valvular and cardiac muscle damage, and may give rise to new cardiac murmurs, cardiomegaly, congestive heart failure, and pericarditis. Symptoms of heart involvement are often lacking in the acute stage, but 10–20 years after the attack, valvular heart disease, primarily of the mitral and aortal valves, with stenosis or regurgitation may become apparent, necessitating surgical intervention.

The guidelines for the diagnosis of acute rheumatic fever are listed in Table 9.4.

Laboratory investigations in patients with clinical signs compatible with rheumatic fever may give answers to the query about whether an antecedent group-A streptococcal infection has taken place. The best method for obtaining an answer to this question is to measure the titre of antistreptolysin O, an antibody against an extra-cellular product of the streptococcus. The antibody response peaks at about

Table 9.4 Guidelines for the diagnosis of acute rheumatic fever: the revised Jones criteria.

Major manifestations	Minor manifestations
Clinical findings	
Carditis	Fever
Polyarthritis	Arthralgia
Chorea	Previous rheumatic fever
Erythema marginatum	Rheumatic heart disease
Subcutaneous nodules	

Laboratory findings
1. elevated acute phase reactants
   a. c-reactive protein
   b. erythrocyte sedimentation rate
2. prolonged P-R interval rate

Supportive evidence of preceding streptococcal infection
   a. increased ASO or other streptococcal antibodies
   b. positive throat culture for group A-haemolytic streptococci
   c. recent scarlet fever

Abbreviation: ASO, antistreptolysin O
With permission from Jones Criteria Update (1992) Guidelines for diagnosis of rheumatic fever. *JAMA* **268**, 2069–2073.

4–5 weeks after the streptococcal pharyngitis, and is usually demonstrable in the first few weeks of the attack of rheumatic fever. ESR and C-reactive protein levels are raised during attacks.

Management. Treatment is directed against the streptococcus infection (penicillin for at least 10 days in doses required for treatment of pharyngitis) and against the inflammatory changes by the rheumatic fever attack (aspirin 80–100 mg/kg in children) (Gibofsky and Zabriskie, 1998). Arthritis generally reacts very favourably to aspirin medication. Prednisone is given to patients with carditis (1–2 mg/kg/day for 2–3 weeks, then tapering). Recurrences of attacks occur most often, but not exclusively, in the first two years after the first attack, and they considerably increase the chance on valvular heart disease (Stollerman, 1997). Prevention of recurrent streptococcal infections is possible by oral administration of penicillin VK (250 000 units, twice daily) or depot intramuscular injection of 1.2 million penicillin G, every 3–4 weeks (Singh *et al.*, 1997). There is no consensus on the duration that preventive medication is required. Some authors suggest until the 18th year and others suggest indefinitely.

THE NEUROLOGY OF RHEUMATIC FEVER: SYDENHAM'S CHOREA

Antibodies have been discovered in patients with Sydenham's chorea that react with a component in the cytoplasm of neurones in the nucleus caudatus and nucleus subthalamicum (Husby *et al.*, 1976). They may have a role in the genesis of the choreic movements. Studies of the pathology of the brain are very few, as patients with this disorder nearly always survive. A mild vasculitis of small vessels has been found in the brain tissue, not, however, in the striatum and corpus subthalamicum (see Nausieda, 1986). Positron emission tomography (PET) in two children with choreic movements has demonstrated increase of glucose metabolism in the nucleus caudatus and putamen. Three months after full clinical recovery, the glucose metabolism in the caudate nucleus was, in both children, back to normal, but in the putamen of one of them it was still higher than in controls (*i.e.* young adults) (Goldman *et al.*, 1993; Weindl *et al.*, 1993). In one other child, repeat MRIs revealed persistent abnormal signal in the nucleus caudatus and putamen 40 months after the initial illness (Emery and Visco, 1998). MRIs of the brain of 24 children (8 boys and 16 girls) with recent onset Sydenham's chorea showed a significantly larger mean volume of the caudate nucleus, putamen, and globus pallidus than in 48 controls matched for age, gender, height, and handedness. The overlap between the groups was considerable, and in many patients the volume of the basal ganglia nuclei was in the normal range. There were no differences in the volumes of the total hemispheres, pre-frontal and mid-frontal regions and thalamus (Giedd *et al.*, 1995). These findings all support a special role of the striatum in the origin of Sydenham's chorea. It is of interest that, at least in some patients, abnormalities of the striatum persist following clinical recovery.

Sydenham's chorea is mostly a disease of children in the age range of 5–15 years, and it affects girls more often than boys (Swedo *et al.*, 1993; Fahn, 1995). It may take up to 6 months after the rheumatic fever attack before chorea becomes apparent. Some patients first have a period with arthritis and thereafter chorea. In others, the history is not very helpful and the streptococcal pharyngitis and symptoms of rheumatic fever cannot definitely be ascertained. Antistreptolysin O titres are not always raised, presumably because the delay between the infection and the appearance of abnormal movements has been too long. There is always a chance that patients have heart murmurs due to valvular lesions.

Sydenham's chorea is mostly bilateral and generalized, but in a minority of approximately 20% it is restricted to one side of the body. Abnormal movements are most frequent during activity and may almost disappear completely when lying quietly in bed. Dysarthria, inability to maintain a firm grip, and gait disturbances are due to the abnormal innervation of muscles (Cardoso *et al.*, 1997; Swedo *et al.*, 1993). Though paresis is not a feature of chorea, muscle force is limited. Patients are often emotionally labile or irritable but this need not to be of organic origin. Sydenham's chorea goes into remission after a mean period of approximately nine months. A mild degree of involuntary movements may, however, persist. Recurrences after months or years have been reported (Fahn, 1995).

Management. Therapy is entirely symptomatic. Patients may benefit from sedatives, and they should remain as quiet and inactive as possible because activity furthers choreic movements. Valproate may be helpful when sedatives are insufficient. Haloperidol is more effective than valproate in suppressing choreic movements, but is best not given because it has, similar to other neuroleptics, tardive dyskinesia as a side effect (oro-bucco-linguo-facial dyskinesia). Tardive dyskinesia is irreversible in a high percentage of patients (see Chapter 2, *Chorea* for a more extensive discussion of tardive dyskinesia as side effect of haloperidol and other neuroleptics).

REFERENCES

Agarwal AK, Peppelman WC, Kraus DR *et al.* (1993) The cervical spine in rheumatoid arthritis. *Brit Med J* **306**, 79–80.

Albani S and Carson DA (1997). Etiology and pathogenesis of rheumatoid arthritis. In: Koopman WJ (ed) *Arthritis and Allied Conditions. A Textbook of Rheumatology*, 13th ed, pp 979–992. Baltimore: Williams and Wilkins.

Allison DJ and Mazano GD (1985) Computed tomography of rheumatoid pachymeningitis. *Am J Neuroradiol* **6**, 976–977.

Andrews A and Hickling P (1997) Thrombosis associated with antiphospholipid antibody in juvenile chronic arthritis. *Lupus* **6**, 556–557.

Ansell BM (1998) Juvenile rheumatoid arthritis (rheumatoid factor positive polyarthritis). In: Maddison PJ, Isenberg DA, Woo P *et al.* (eds) *Oxford Textbook of Rheumatology*, 2nd ed, pp 1031–1036. Oxford: Oxford University Press.

Arnett FC, Edworthy SM, Bloch DA *et al.* (1988) The American Rheumatism Association 1987 revised criteria for the classification of rheumatoid arthritis. *Arthritis Rheum* **31**, 315–324.

Bacon PA and Moots RJ (1997) Extra-articular rheumatoid arthritis. In: Koopman WJ (ed) *Arthritis and Allied Conditions. A Textbook of Rheumatology*, 13th ed, pp 1071–1088. Baltimore: Williams and Wilkins.

Bathon JM, Moreland LW and DiBartolomeo AG (1989) Inflammatory central nervous system involvement in rheumatoid arthritis. *Sem Arthritis Rheum* **18**, 258–266.

Beck DO and Corbett JJ (1983) Seizures due to central nervous system rheumatoid meningovasculitis. *Neurology* **33**, 1058–1061.

Bekkelund SI, Torbergsen T, Omdal R *et al.* (1996) Nerve conduction studies in rheumatoid arthritis. *Scand J Rheumatol* **25**, 287–292.

Bijlsma JWJ and Velthuis PJ (1995) Rheumatoid arthritis. In: Kater L and Baart de la Faille H (eds) *Multi-Systemic Auto-Immune Diseases: An Integrated Approach*, pp 141–172. Amsterdam: Elsevier.

Bland JH and Eddy WM (1968) Hemiplegia and rheumatoid hemiarthritis. *Arthritis Rheum* **11**, 72–79.

Boden SD, Dodge LD, Bohlman HH *et al.* (1993) Rheumatoid arthritis of the cervical spine. *J Bone Joint Surg* **75**(A), 1282–1297.

Bregeon C, Rolland D, Masson C *et al.* (1985) Incidence of rheumatoid arthritis in Anjou, France (abstract). *Rev Rhum* **56**, 242.

Broers M, Verhoeven AC, Markusse HM *et al.* (1997) Randomized comparison of combined step-down prednisolone, methotrexate and sulphasalazine with sulphasalazine alone in early rheumatoid arthritis. *Lancet* **350**, 309–318.

Brook MH and Kaplan H (1972) Muscle pathology in rheumatoid arthritis, polymyalgia rheumatica, and polymyositis. *Arch Pathol* **94**, 101–118.

Carapetis JR, Currie BJ and Good MF (1996) Towards understanding the pathogenesis of rheumatic fever. *Scand J Rheumatol* **25**, 127–131.

Cardoso F, Eduardo C, Silva AP *et al.* (1997) Chorea in fifty consecutive patients with rheumatic fever. *Mov Disord* **12**, 701–703.

Casey ATH, Crockard HA, Bland JM *et al.* (1996) Surgery on the rheumatoid cervical spine for the non-ambulant myelopathic patient – too much, too late? *Lancet* **347**, 1004–1007.

Casey ATH, Crockard HA, Geddes JF *et al.* (1997a) Vertical translocation: The enigma of the disappearing atlantodens interval in patients with myelopathy and rheumatoid arthritis. Part I. Clinical, radiological and neuropathological features. *J Neurosurg* **87**, 856–862.

Casey ATH, Crockard HA and Stevens J (1997b) Vertical translocation. Part II. Outcomes after surgical treatment of rheumatoid cervical myelopathy. *J Neurosurg* **87**, 863–869.

Cats A and Hazevoet HM (1970) The significance of positive tests for rheumatoid factor in the prognosis of rheumatoid arthritis. *Ann Rheum Dis* **29**, 254–260.

Chalk CH, Dyck PJ and Conn DL (1993) Vasculitic neuropathy. In: Dyck PJ, Thomas PK, Griffin JW *et al.* (eds), *Peripheral Neuropathy*, 3rd ed, pp 1424–1436. Philadelphia: WB Saunders.

Chamberlain MA and Bruckner FE (1970) Clinical and electrophysiological features of rheumatoid neuropathy. *Ann Rheum Dis* **29**, 609–616.

Chang DJ and Paget SA (1993) Neurologic complications of rheumatoid arthritis. *Rheumatic Disease Clinics of North America* **19**, 955–973.

Collee G, Breedveld FC, Algra PR *et al.* (1987) Rheumatoid arthritis with vertical atlanto-axial subluxation complicated by hydrocephalus. *Brit J Rheumatol* **26**, 56–58.

Conn DL and Dyck PJ (1975) Angiopathic neuropathy in connective tissue disease.. In: Dyck PJ, Thomas PK and Lambert EH (eds) *Peripheral Neuropathy*, vol 2, pp 1149–1165. Philadelphia: WB Saunders Co.

de Krom MCTFM, Knipschild PG, Kester ADM *et al.* (1990) Efficacy of provocative tests for diagnosis of carpal tunnel syndrome. *Lancet* **335**, 393–395.

Denault A, Dimopoulos MA and Fitzcharles MA (1990) Meningoencephalitis and peripheral neuropathy complicating adult Still's disease. *J Rheumatol* **17**, 698–700.

Ekdahl C, Andersson SI and Svenson B (1989) Muscle function of the lower extremities in rheumatoid arthritis and osteoarthrosis: A descriptive study of patients in a primary health care district. *J Clin Epidemiol* **42**, 947–954.

Emery P (1997) Rheumatoid arthritis: Not yet curable with early intensive therapy. *Lancet* **350**, 304–305.

Emery ES and Visco PT (1997) Sydenham chorea: Magnetic resonance imaging reveals permanent basal ganglia injury. *Neurology* **48**, 531–533.

Espada G, Babini JC, Maldonado-Cocco JA *et al.* (1987) Radiological review: the cervical spine in juvenile rheumatoid arthritis. *Sem Arthritis Rheum* **17**, 185–195.

Eulderink F and Meijers KAE (1976) Pathology of the cervical spine in rheumatoid arthritis: A controlled study of 44 spines. *J Pathol* **120**, 91–108.

Fahn S (1995) Sydenham and other forms of chorea. In: Rowland LP (ed) *Merritt's Textbook of Neurology*, 9th ed, pp 699–705. Baltimore: Williams and Wilkins.

Fairburn B (1975) Spinal cord compression by a rheumatoid nodule: A case report. *J Neurol Neurosurg Psychiat* **38**, 1056–1058.

Felson DT (1997) Epidemiology of the rheumatic diseases. In: Koopman WJ (ed) *Arthritis and Allied Conditions. A Textbook of Rheumatology*, 13th ed, pp 3–34. Baltimore: William and Wilkins.

Fernandez AM and Tiku ML (1994) Posterior interosseus nerve entrapment in rheumatoid arthritis. *Sem Arthritis Rheum* **24**, 57–60.

Firestein GS (1997) Etiology and pathogenesis of rheumatoid arthritis. In: Kelley WN, Ruddy S and Harris ED *et al.* (eds) *Textbook of Rheumatology*, 5th ed, pp 851–897. Philadelphia: WB Saunders.

Fleming A, Dodman S, Crown JM *et al.* (1976) Extra-articular features in early rheumatoid disease. *Brit Med J* **1**, 1241–1243.

Friedman H (1970) Intraspinal rheumatoid nodule causing nerve root compression. *J Neurosurg* **32**, 689–691.

Gibofsky H and Zabriskie JB (1998) Rheumatic fever. In: Maddison PJ, Isenberg DA, Woo P *et al.* (1998) *Oxford Textbook of Rheumatology*, 2nd ed, pp 972–982. Oxford: Oxford University Press.

Giedd JN, Rapoport JL, Kruesi MJP *et al.* (1995) Sydenham's chorea: Magnetic resonance imaging of the basal ganglia. *Neurology* **45**, 2199–2202.

Goldman S, Amron D, Szliwowski HB *et al.* (1993) Reversible striatal hypermetabolism in a case of Sydenham's chorea. *Mov Disord* **8**, 355–388.

Gough AK, Lilley J, Eyre S *et al.* (1994) Generalised bone loss in patients with early rheumatoid arthritis: Time to aim for remission. *Lancet* **344**, 23–27.

Grabois M, Puentes J and Lidsky M (1981) Tarsal tunnel syndrome in rheumatoid arthritis. *Arch Phys Med Rehabil* **62**, 401–403.

Guillemin F, Briancon S and Klein JM *et al.* (1994) Low incidence of rheumatoid arthritis in France. *Scand J Rheumatol* **23**, 264–268.

Hale LP and Haynes BF (1997) Pathology of rheumatoid arthritis and associated disorders. In: Koopmans WJ (ed) *Arthritis and Allied Conditions. A Textbook of Rheumatology*, 13th ed, pp 993–1016. Baltimore: Williams and Wilkins.

Halla JT and Hardin Jr JG (1990) The spectrum of atlantoaxial facet joint involvement in rheumatoid arthritis. *Arthritis Rheum* **33**, 325–329.

Harris ED Jr (1997) Clinical features of rheumatoid arthritis. In: Kelley WN, Ruddy S, Harris ED *et al.* (eds) *Textbook of Rheumatology*, 5th ed, pp 898–932. Philadelphia: WB Saunders.

Henderson FC, Geddes JF and Crockard HA (1993) Neuropathology of the brainstem and spinal cord in end stage rheumatoid arthritis: Implications for treatment. *Ann Rheum Dis* **52**, 629–637.

Hughes JT (1977) Spinal cord involvement by C4–C5 vertebral subluxation in rheumatoid arthritis: A description of 2 cases examined at necropsy. *Ann Neurol* **1**, 575–582.

Husby G, van de Rijn I, Zabriskie JB *et al.* (1976) Antibodies reacting with cytoplasm of subthalamic and caudate nuclei neurons in chorea and acute rheumatic fever. *J Exp Med* **144**, 1094–1110.

Jackson CG, Chess RL and Ward JR (1984) A case of rheumatoid nodule formation within the central nervous system and review of the literature. *J Rheumatol* **11**, 237–240.

Jones Criteria Update (1992) Guidelines for diagnosis of rheumatic fever. *JAMA* **268**, 2069–2073.

Kater L and Provost TT (1995) Classification criteria, disease activity and chronicity criteria. In: Kater L and Baart de la Faille H (eds) *Multi-Systemic Autoimmune Diseases*, pp 43–59. Amsterdam: Elsevier.

Kaufman LD, Sibany PA, Anand AK *et al.* (1987) Superior oblique tenosynovitis (Brown's syndrome) as a manifestation of adult Still's disease. *J Rheumatol* **14**, 625–627.

Kauppi M (1996) Conservative treatment for rheumatoid cervical spine. *Lancet* **347**, 1695.

Kauppi M. Sakaguchi M, Konttinen YT *et al.* (1990) A new method of screening for vertical atlanto-axial dislocation. *J Rheumatol* **17**, 167–172.

Kauppi M and Hakala M (1994) Prevalence of cervical spine subluxations and dislocations in a community-based rheumatoid arthritis population. *Scand J Rheumatol* **23**, 133–136.

Kauppi M, Sakaguchi M, Konttinen YT *et al.* (1996a) Pathogenetic mechanism and prevalence of the stable atlantoaxial subluxation in rheumatoid arthritis. *J Rheumatol* **23**, 831–834.

Kauppi M, Antilla P (1996b) A stiff collar for the treatment of rheumatoid atlantoaxial subluxation. *Brit J Rheumatol* **35**, 771–774.

Kauppi M, Leppanen L, Heikkila S *et al.* (1998) Active conservative treatment of atlanto-axial subluxation in rheumatoid arthritis. *Br J Rheumatol* **37**, 417–420.

Kim RC (1980) Rheumatoid disease with encephalopathy. *Ann Neurol* **7**, 86–91.

Kim RC and Collins GH (1981) The neuropathology of rheumatoid disease. *Hum Pathol* **12**, 5–15.

King TT (1994) Progressive kyphosis with cord compression in the rheumatoid cervical spine. (abstract) *J Neurol Neurosurg Psychiat* **57**, 1148.

Kozora E, Thompson LL, West SG *et al.* (1996) Analysis of cognitive and psychological deficits in systemic lupus erythematosus patients without overt central nervous system disease. *Arthritis Rheum* **39**, 2035–2045.

Kraus DR, Peppelman WC, Agarwal AK *et al.* (1991) Incidence of subaxial subluxation in patients with generalized rheumatoid arthritis who have had previous occipital cervical fusions. *Spine* **16**, S486–S489.

Lang BA, Schneider R, Reilly BJ *et al.* (1995) Radiologic features of systemic onset juvenile rheumatoid arthritis. *J Rheumatol* **22**, 168–173.

Laxer RM and Schneider R (1998) Systemic onset juvenile chronic arthritis. In: Gibosky H, Maddison PJ, Isenberg DA *et al.* (eds) *Oxford Textbook of Rheumatology*, 2nd ed, pp 1114–1131. Oxford: Oxford University Press.

Le Gars L, Clerc D, Cariou D *et al.* (1997) Systemic juvenile rheumatoid arthritis and associated Isaacs' syndrome. *J Rheumatol* **24**, 178–180.

Lems WF, Jahanger ZN, Jacobs *et al.* (1995) Vertebral fractures in patients with rheumatoid arthritis treated with corticosteroids. *Clin Exp Rheum* **13**, 293–297.

Luqmani RA, Watts RA, Scott DG *et al.* (1994) Treatment of vasculitis in rheumatoid arthritis. *Ann Med Intern* (Paris) **145**, 566–576.

Markenson JA, McDougal JS, Tsairis P *et al.* (1979) Rheumatoid meningitis: A localized immune process. *Ann Int Med* **90**, 786–789.

Markusse HM, Hilkens PHE, van den Bent MJ *et al.* (1995) Normal pressure hydrocephalus associated with rheumatoid arthritis responding to prednisone. *J Rheumatol* **22**, 342–343.

Marshall SC and Murray WR (1974) Deep radial nerve palsy associated with rheumatoid arthritis. *Clin Orthop Relat Res* **103**, 157–162.

Martel W (1961) The occipito-atlanto-axial joints in rheumatoid arthritis and ankylosing spondylitis. *Am J Roentgenol* **86**, 223–240.

Martel W (1977) Pathogenesis of cervical discovertebral destruction in rheumatoid arthritis. *Arthritis Rheum* **20**, 1217–1225.

Mastaglia FL and Walton JN (1992) Inflammatory myopathies. In: Mastaglia FL and Lord Walton of Detchant (eds) *Skeletal Muscle Pathology*, 2nd edn, pp 453–491. Edinburgh: Churchill Livingstone.

McDonald SP and Smith MD (1996) An uncommon cause of fingerdrop in a patient with rheumatoid arthritis. *Ann Rheum Dis* **55**, 728–730.

McGregor M (1948) The significance of certain measurements of the skull in the diagnosis of basillar impression. *Brit J Radiol* **21**, 171–181.

McGuigan L, Burke D and Fleming A (1983) Tarsal tunnel syndrome and peripheral neuropathy in rheumatoid disease. *Ann Rheum Dis* **42**, 128–131.

Mellbye OJ, Forre O, Mollness TE *et al.* (1991) Immunopathology of subcutaneous rheumatic nodules. *Ann Rheum Dis* **50**, 909–912.

Menezes AH, VanGilder JC, Clark CR *et al.* (1985) Odontoid upward migration in rheumatoid arthritis. An analysis of 45 patients with 'cranial settling'. *J Neurosurg* **63**, 500–509.

Miro O, Pedrol E, Casademont J *et al.* (1996) Muscle involvement in rheumatoid arthritis: Clinicopathological study of 21 symptomatic cases. *Sem Arthritis Rheum* **25**, 421–428.

Moore AT and Morin JD (1985) Bilateral acquired inflammatory Brown's syndrome. *J Pediatric Ophthalmol Strabism* **22**, 26–30.

Nakano KK, Schoene WC, Baker RA *et al.* (1978) The cervical myelopathy associated with rheumatoid arthritis: Analysis of 32 patients, with 2 postmortem cases. *Ann Neurol* **3**, 144–151.

Naredo-Sanchez E, Carceller F, Campos Fernandez C *et al.* (1996) Hydrocephalus and secondary syndrome of inappropriate antidiuretic hormone due to rheumatoid vertical atlantoaxial subluxation. *J Rheumatol* **23**, 1098–1102.

Nausieda PA (1986) Sydenham's chorea, chorea gravidarum and contraceptive-induced chorea. In: Vinken PJ, Bruyn GW and Klawans HL (eds) *Handbook of Clinical Neurology. Extrapyramidal Disorders*, vol 5, pp 359–367. Amsterdam: Elsevier.

Oda T, Fujiwara K, Yonenobu K *et al.* (1995) Natural course of cervical spine lesions in rheumatoid arthritis. *Spine* **10**, 1128–1135.

Oosterhuis HJGH (1993) Clinical aspects. In: De Baets MH and Oosterhuis HJGH (eds) *Myasthenia Gravis*, pp 13–42. Boca Raton: CRC Press.

Oosterhuis HJGH (1997) *Myasthenia Gravis*. Groningen: Groningen Neurology Press.

Pearson ME, Kosco M, Huffer W *et al.* (1987) Rheumatoid nodules of the spine: case report and review of the literature. *Arthritis Rheum* **30**, 709–713.

Paimela L, Laasonen L, Kankaanpaa E *et al.* (1997) Progression of cervical spine changes in patients with early rheumatoid arthritis. *J Rheumatol* **24**, 1280–1284.

Pallis CA and Scott JT (1965) Peripheral neuropathy in rheumatoid arthritis. *Brit Med J* **1**, 1141–1147.

Pearson ME, Kosco M, Huffer W *et al.* (1987) Rheumatoid nodules of the spine: A case report and review of the literature. *Arthritis Rheum* **30**, 709–713.

Pediatric Rheumatology Collaborative Study Group (1997) Intravenous immunoglobulin in the treatment of polyarticular juvenile rheumatoid arthritis: A phase I/II study. *J Rheumatol* **23**, 919–924.

Pellici PM, Ranawat CS, Tsairis P *et al.* (1981) A prospective study of the progression of rheumatoid arthritis of the cervical spine. *J Bone Joint Surg* **63** (A), 342–350.

Pincus T, Griffith J, Pearce S *et al.* (1996) Prevalence of self-reported depression in patients with rheumatoid arthritis. *Brit J Rheumatol* **35**, 879–883.

Prieur AM (1998) Rheumatoid factor negative polyarthritis in children (seronegative polyarthritis). In: Maddison PJ, Isenberg DA, Woo P *et al.* (eds) *Oxford Textbook of Rheumatology*, 2nd ed, pp 1131–1143. Oxford: Oxford University Press.

Puéchall X, Said G, Hilliquin P *et al.* (1995) Peripheral neuropathy with necrotising vasculitis in rheumatoid arthritis. A clinicopathologic and prognostic study of 32 patients. *Arthritis Rheum* **38**, 1618–1629.

Ramos M and Mandybur TI (1975) Cerebral vasculitis in rheumatoid arthritis. *Arch Neurol* **32**, 271–275.

Rana NA (1989) Natural history of atlanto-axial subluxation in rheumatoid arthritis. *Spine* **14**, 1054–1056.

Rana NA, Hancock DO, Taylor *et al.* (1973) Atlanto-axial subluxation in rheumatoid arthritis. *J Bone Joint Surg* **55**(B), 458–475.

Ranawat CS, O'Leary P, Pellici P *et al.* (1979) Cervical spine fusion in rheumatoid arthritis. *J Bone Joint Surg* **61**(A), 1003–1010.

Rasker JJ, Jansen ENH, Haan J *et al.* (1985) Normal pressure hydrocephalus in rheumatic patients. A diagnostic pitfall. *N Engl J Med* **312**, 1239–1241.

Redlund-Johnell IR and Petterson H (1984) Vertical dislocation of the C1 and C2 vertebrae in rheumatoid arthritis. *Acta Radiol (Diagn)* **25**, 133–141.

Redlund-Johnell IR and Larson EM (1993) Subluxation of upper thoracic spine in rheumatoid arthritis. *Skeletal Radiol* **22**, 105–108.

Reiner AP and Spivak JL (1988) Hematophagic histiocytosis. *Medicine* **67**, 369–388.

Reijnierse M, Bloem JL, Dijkmans BAC *et al.* (1996) The cervical spine in rheumatoid arthritis: Relationship between neurologic signs and morphology on MRI imaging and radiographs. *Skeletal Radiol* **25**, 113–118.

Rillo OL, Rabadan A, Houssay R *et al.* (1989) Atlantoaxial subluxation and hydrocephalus in rheumatoid arthritis. *J Rheumatol* **16**, 121–125.

Rodman GP (1984) Clinical pathological conference. *J Rheumatol* **11**, 855–861.

Sanada I, Kawano F, Tsukamoto A *et al.* (1997) Disseminated intravascular coagulation in a case of adult onset Still's disease. *Rinsho-Ketsueki* **38**, 1194–1198.

Sanmarti R, Collado A, Gratacos J *et al.* (1996) Reduced serum creatine kinase activity in inflammatory rheumatic diseases. *J Rheumatol* **23**, 310–312.

Sanmarti R, Collado A, Gratacos J *et al.* (1994) Reduced activity of serum creatine kinase in rheumatoid arthritis: A phenomenon linked to the inflammatory response. *Brit J Rheumatol* **33**, 231–234.

Sasaki S, Nakamura H, Oda K *et al.* (1997) Thoracic myelopathy due to intraspinal rheumatoid nodules. *Scand J Rheumatol* **26**, 227–228.

Schachenmayr W and Friede RL (1978) Dural involvement in rheumatoid arthritis. *Acta Neuropath* **42**, 65–66.

Silman AJ, MacGregor AJ, Thomson W *et al.* (1993) Twin concordance for rheumatoid arthritis: Results from a nationwide study. *Brit J Rheumatol* **32**, 903–907.

Singh M, Malhotra P and Thakur JS (1997) Rheumatic heart disease in developing countries. *Lancet* **349**, 1700.

Smedstad LM, Moum T, Vaglum P *et al.* (1996) The impact of early rheumatoid arthritis on psychological distress. A comparison between 238 patients with rheumatoid arthritis and 116 matched controls. *Scand J Rheumatol* **25**, 377–382.

Soden M, Boundy K, Burrow D *et al.* (1994) Inclusion body myositis in association with rheumatoid arthritis. *J Rheumatol* **21**, 344–346.

Soltys AJ and Axford JS (1997) Rheumatoid factors: Where are we now. *Ann Rheum Dis* **56**, 281–286.

Spaans F (1987) Compression and entrapment neuropathies. In: Vinken PJ, Bruyn GW, and Klawans HL *et al.* (eds) *Neuropathies. Handbook of Clinical Neurology* 51, pp 85–118. Amsterdam: Elsevier.

Stephan JL, Zeller J, Hubert Ph *et al.* (1993) Macrophage activation syndrome and rheumatic disease in childhood: A report of four new cases. *Clin Exp Rheumatol* **11**, 451–456.

Stevens JC (1997) Electrodiagnosis of carpal tunnel syndrome. *Muscle Nerve* **12**, 1477–1486.

Stockwell RA (1981) Joints. In: Romanes GJ (ed) *Cunningham's Textbook of Anatomy*, 12th edn, pp 211–264. Oxford: Oxford University Press.

Stollerman GH (1997) Rheumatic fever. *Lancet* **349**, 935–942.

Symmons D, Barrett EM, Bankhead CR *et al.* (1994) The incidence of rheumatoid arthritis in the United Kingdom; Results from the Norfolk arthritis register. *Brit J Rheumatol* **33**, 735–739.

Swedo SE, Leonard HL, Schapiro MB *et al.* (1993) Sydenham's chorea: Physical and psychologic symptoms of St Vitus dance. *Pediatrics* **91**, 706–713.

Toolanen G (1987) Cutaneous sensory impairment in rheumatoid atlanto-axial subluxation assessed quantitatively by electrical stimulation. *Scand J Rheumatol* **16**, 27–32.

Uziel Y, Laxer RM, Schneider R *et al.* (1996) Intravenous immunoglobulin therapy in systemic onset juvenile rheumatoid arthritis: A follow-up study. *J Rheumatol* **23**, 910–918.

Uziel Y, Rathaus V, Pomeranz A *et al.* (1998) Torticollis as the sole initial presenting sign of systemic onset juvenile rheumatoid arthritis. *J Rheumatol* **25**, 166–168.

van Lis JMJ and Jennekens FGI (1977) Immunofluorescence studies in a case of rheumatoid neuropathy. *J Neurol Sci* **33**, 313–321.

van Zeben D, Hazes JMW, Zwindeman AH *et al.* (1992) Association of HLA-DR4 with a more progressive disease course in patients with rheumatoid arthritis. *Arthritis Rheum* **34**, 822–830.

Voskuyl AE, Zwinderman AH, Westedt ML *et al.* (1996a) The mortality of rheumatoid vasculitis compared with rheumatoid arthritis. *Arthritis Rheum* **39**, 266–271.

Voskuyl AE, Zwinderman AH, Breedveld FC *et al.* (1996b) Prognosis in rheumatoid arthritis: Reply. *Arthritis Rheum* **39**, 1937–1938.

Wang FM, Wertenbaker C, Behrens MM *et al.* (1984) Acquired Brown's syndrome in children with juvenile rheumatoid arthritis. *Ophthalmology* **91**, 23–26.

Wei N, Pavlidis N, Tsokos G *et al.* (1981) Clinical significance of low creatine phosphokinase values in patients with connective tissue diseases. *JAMA* **246**, 1921–1923.

Weindl A, Kuwert T, Leenders KL *et al.* (1993) Increased striatal glucose consumption in Sydenham's chorea. *Mov Disord* **8**, 437–444.

Weller RO, Bruckner FE and Chamberlain MA (1970) Rheumatoid neuropathy: A histological and electrophysiological study. *J Neurol Neurosurg Psychiat* **33**, 592–604.

White AA, Johnson R, Panjabi MM *et al.* (1975) Biomechanical analysis in clinical stability of the cervical spine. *Clin Orthop* **109**, 85–96.

Winfield J, Cooke D, Brooke AS *et al.* (1981) A prospective study of the radiological changes in the cervical spine in early rheumatoid disease. *Ann Rheum Dis* **40**, 109–114.

Winfield J, Young A, Williams P *et al.* (1983) Prospective study of the radiological changes in hands, feet, and cervical spine in adult rheumatoid disease. *Ann Rheum Dis* **42**, 613–618.

Wulffraat NW, van Royen A, Slaper I *et al.* (1997) Autologous bone marrow transplantation in a case of refractory systemic juvenile chronic arthritis. (Abstract). *Arthritis Rheum* **40**, S46.

Woo P and Wedderburn LR (1998) Juvenile chronic arthritis. *Lancet* **351**, 969–973.

10

Scleroderma

INTRODUCTION

Scleroderma is a chronic disorder of connective tissue of unknown origin, and is characterized by proliferation and accumulation of collagen and accumulation of other extracellular matrix proteins. The systemic form of scleroderma, with cutaneous sclerosis and collagen proliferation in other organs, has to be distinguished from localized forms, which affect only the skin and the local underlying tissues. Systemic scleroderma, or more aptly *systemic sclerosis*, has two variants: a diffuse one and a limited one. The difference between the two primarily concerns the extent to which the skin is involved. Diffuse sclerosis affects the skin of the limbs not only distally but also more proximally and spreads to the face, neck, and trunk. Limited sclerosis, previously called CREST syndrome (*Calcinosis, Raynaud's phenomenon, Esophageal dysmotility, Sclerodactyly, and Telangiectasia*), is confined to the distal parts of the limbs and face (Table 10.1). Vascular changes are ubiquitous in both variants. Internal organs (muscles, lungs, heart, oesophagus and gastrointestinal tract, liver, pancreas, and kidneys) are affected earlier in the course of the diffuse variant than with limited sclerosis, with the exception of the kidneys which are spared in limited

Table 10.1 Classification of scleroderma

Localized scleroderma	Limited form of systemic sclerosis, formerly CREST syndrome	Diffuse form of systemic sclerosis
Either:	With:	Main features:
Linear	calcinosis	progressive
En plaque	Raynaud's phenomenon	diffuse cutaneous sclerosis
Guttata	(o)esophageal dysmotility	(extensive) visceral
Generalized	sclerodactyly	involvement (pulmonal,
Subcutaneous only	telangiectasia	renal, gastrointestinal,
		heart)

sclerosis. Neurological changes are reputed to occur more often in the diffuse than in the limited variant. Muscles may become involved in all forms.

This chapter has three parts. The first part contains a short general description of systemic sclerosis, and the second is an extensive review of the neurological and myological aspects of systemic sclerosis. The localized forms of scleroderma are the subject of the third part. A review of the neurological and myological changes in systemic sclerosis has recently been published (Mattuci Cerinic *et al.*, 1996).

SHORT GENERAL DESCRIPTION OF SYSTEMIC SCLEROSIS

EPIDEMIOLOGY

In the USA, the annual incidence figures are about 18–19 per 10^6 (Mayes *et al.*, 1996; Steen *et al.*, 1997). The incidence increases with age and is highest between 44 and 65 years. Overall, the incidence is much higher in females than males (ratio 3:1), and is (in the USA) more frequent in young black than in young white women (Steen *et al.*, 1997). Systemic sclerosis is very rare in children; new cases in the 7th and 8th decade are not very exceptional.

AETIOLOGY

As in other inflammatory connective tissue diseases (ICTDs), the aetiology is unknown. The evidence for a genetic predisposition has been fairly weak up until now (see Mayes, 1997; Medsger Jr, 1997). Familial cases of systemic sclerosis have been described but are exceptional, and findings in identical twins do not support a predominant genetic predisposition (Tuffanelli, 1969; Rendall and McKenzie, 1974; Stephens *et al.*, 1995; Mayes, 1997). Investigations on the association of systemic sclerosis with HLA factors have not led to a definite conclusion yet (see Silman and Newman, 1996). The percentage of family members and spouses with non-specific antinuclear antibodies (ANAs) is increased in comparison to controls, which is compatible with the effect of an environmental factor (Maddison *et al.*, 1986; see also Mayes, 1997). Scleroderma-like skin changes may occur in subjects exposed to vinylchloride, silica, or trichloroethylene (Carwile Roy, 1997).

PATHOLOGY AND PATHOGENESIS

Tightening and hardening of the skin are hallmarks of systemic sclerosis and are due to the accumulation of collagen and the increase of other extracellular matrix components in the dermis. The collagen proteins are not abnormal, and the proportion of the two main collagen types of the skin, type I and type III, is also normal. No disorder of the breakdown processes of the matrix proteins have been demonstrated. Therefore, increased synthesis is a more likely explanation for the accumulation of collagen than insufficient breakdown (see Carwile Roy, 1997). The question is then, what is the signal for the increased synthesis. Biopsy specimens of the dermis in early stages of systemic sclerosis reveal infiltration by lymphocytes, predominantly CD4+ T-helper cells and macrophages, both diffusely and perivascularly. The increased expression of DR by dermal T-cells and the increased circulation of interleukine 2 receptors (IL-2R) and IL-1, IL-2, IL-4, and IL-6 indicate that the lymphocytes are activated (Report of a meeting of physicians and scientists, 1996). Apparently, the disease has, in addition to biochemical aspects, immunological ones, which has lead to the suggestion that the two are linked by the effects of cytokines. It is of interest that IL-1 and IL-4 stimulate fibroblast proliferation and collagen synthesis. The favourable effects of immunomodulation on the course of the disease are also in support of an immune-mediated mechanism in the pathogenesis of systemic sclerosis (see this Chapter, *Therapy*).

Recent findings indicate that fetal microchimerism may be involved in scleroderma. This hypothesis relies on the similarity of some features of auto-immune diseases with chronic graft-versus-host disease (Shulman and Sullivan, 1988). Fetal cells may cross the placenta during pregnancy and either remain in the circulation or migrate to various tissue sites. A subsequent event, *e.g.* environmental exposure to a viral or chemical agent, may activate the fetal cells and initiate a cascade of events resulting in disease. Fetal DNA and cells have been identified in skin lesions of women with systemic sclerosis (Artlett *et al.*, 1998; Nelson, 1998).

Vascular changes are ubiquitous in systemic sclerosis. From an early stage, digital arteries often show marked intima thickening, with an increase of collagen and ground substance, and fibrosis of the adventitia. As a consequence, the arteries are severely narrowed. A normal vasoconstrictor response to cold may then be sufficient to cause Raynaud's phenomenon. One should bear in mind that there are several pathophysiological mechanisms for cold-induced vasospasms.

Increase in connective tissue and changes in small vessels occur not only in skin but also in other internal organs, *e.g.* muscle, lung, heart, kidney, oesophagus and gastrointestinal tract, liver and biliary tract, and pancreas.

CIRCULATING AUTO-ANTIBODIES

ANAs are present in virtually all patients with systemic sclerosis, which is similar to SLE. Two of the various ANAs are characteristic for systemic sclerosis and may be helpful in diagnostic investigations. Anti-topoisomerase I, also designated anti-Scl70, is considered as a specific marker of systemic sclerosis and is present in at least 20–40% of cases. Anticentromere antibody (ACeA) is found in 50–96% (Seibold, 1997) of patients with the limited form of systemic sclerosis and in less than 10% of patients with diffuse sclerosis. The combination of Raynaud's phenomenon and ACeA in serum is indicative for the first stage of limited sclerosis. The role of anti-Scl70 and ACeA in the pathogenesis of the disease is not known. There is no relation of the antibody titres to the severity, progression, or stage of the disease. Antinuclear ribonucleoprotein (anti-nRNP) is present in about 20% of cases, and rheumatoid factor (RF) is in 30%. Anticardiolipin antibodies (ACAs) are not present or are only in low titre.

CLINICAL FEATURES

Diffuse and limited sclerosis are different expressions of one and the same disease (Box 10.1). The diffuse variant presents with skin changes, arthralgia, and Raynaud's phenomenon, but rarely with symptoms of visceral organs (systemic sclerosis sine scleroderma) (Medsger, 1997). The changes of the skin are symmetrical and become, in nearly all cases, manifest at the fingers and the hands first (Fig. 10.1). Face and neck are involved next (Fig. 10.2). The abnormalities of the hands progress to the lower arms and spread subsequently over the whole body. Initially, there is some swelling of the skin. The skin becomes shiny, taut, thickened and adherent to the underlying tissue. Pliability decreases, hair growth is sparse, and hyperpigmented and hypopigmented areas appear. Many patients develop widely dilated nailfold capillary loops or distended venules. Ulcerations may appear where skin is tightly stretched over bony prominences. Small areas of fingertip ischaemic necrosis or ulceration are frequent and leave pitted scars after recovery. In late stages, intracutaneous or subcutaneous depositions of calcium salts are often present in the digital pads, periarticular tissue, extensor side of the forearm, prepatellar areas and buttocks. The thickening of the skin decreases in the late stages.

Limited sclerosis presents, nearly always, with Raynaud's phenomenon; it may be the only clinical symptom for months or years. The association of Raynaud's phenomenon with ACeA indicates that the patient is likely to develop limited sclerosis. Limited sclerosis is distinguished from diffuse sclerosis by limitation of the changes of the skin to the acra, face and neck; slower involvement of most internal organs; a slower course of the disease and a better prognosis (Table 10.2). The kidneys are nearly always spared. The limited and diffuse forms may be associated with features of other ICTDs. These so-called overlap syndromes will be discussed in Chapter 12.

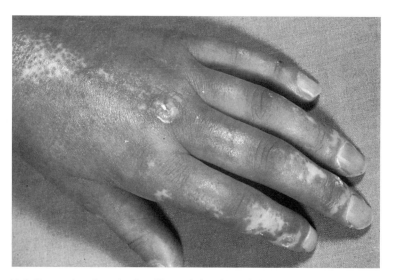

Figure 10.1 Systemic sclerosis. Swelling of the skin of the hand and puffy fingers. The skin is taut and shiny and shows hyperpigmentation and areas of hypopigmentation. There are skin defects at the level of the third metacarpophalangeal joint, the proximal interphalangeal joint of digit V, and the terminal phalanxes of digits II and III. (Courtesy of Dr. Harold Baart de la Faille.)

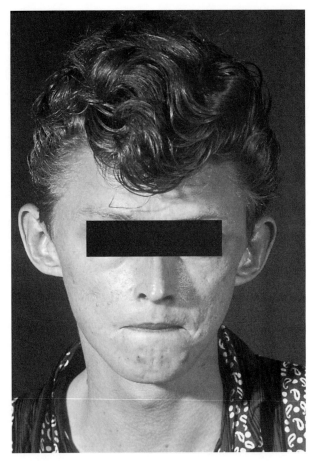

Figure 10.2 Systemic sclerosis. Sclerosis and atrophy of the skin of the face with thinning of the lips. (Courtesy of Dr. H Baart de la Faille.)

Box 10.1 Forms of systemic sclerosis

1. Systemic sclerosis sine scleroderma: Rare, initial stage of diffuse systemic sclerosis. There are symptoms of internal organ dysfunction (gastrointestinal, pulmonal, renal, cardiac) and/or arthralgia, and serum Scl70 antibodies are present.
2. Diffuse systemic sclerosis with widespread skin changes and early involvement of internal organs. Raynaud's phenomenon may be present.
3. Raynaud's phenomenon as initial manifestation of limited sclerosis with anti-centromere antibodies (ACeA) in serum.
4. Limited systemic sclerosis: Skin changes are confined to acra, face and neck. Raynaud's phenomenon is nearly always present. Early oesophageal disturbance. Most internal organs are involved at a late stage. Kidneys are nearly always spared..5
5. Systemic sclerosis associated with features of other ICTDs: Overlap syndrome.

Table 10.2 Involvement of internal organs in systemic sclerosis

Type of organ	Frequency	Presenting symptom
Oral cavity	Most pts in the course of the disease	Thinning of lips, reduced mouth opening
Oesophagus	80% of pts	Dysphagia, heart burning
Small intestine	Small proportion of pts	Bloating, abdominal cramps, episodic diarrhoea
Colon and rectum	Small proportion of pts	Constipation alternating with diarrhoea; rectal incontinence
Lungs	70% of pts	(Exertional) dyspnoea, chronic cough, rarely pleuritic chest pain
Heart	Less than 5% of pts	Congestive heart failure, arrythmias, conduction disturbances
Kidney	15 to 20% of pts with diffuse form	Malignant hypertension and renal insufficiency with headache, visual disturbances, seizures, dyspnoea, etc
Genito-urinary		Vaginal dryness, dyspareunia, impotence, etc
Thyroid gland	25% of pts	Remains often undetected
Skeletal muscle	Majority of pts	Mild weakness

Abbreviation: pts, patients.
See reviews by Jablonska *et al.* (1995), Medsger Jr (1997), Seibold (1997).

DIAGNOSIS

The proposed American Rheumatism Association (ARA) criteria for systemic sclerosis (Box 10.2) are criticized because of insufficient sensitivity for limited systemic sclerosis (Seibold, 1997). In a recent epidemiological investigation, 91% of the patients included in the study fulfilled the ARA criteria (Steen *et al.*, 1997). The patients who did not comply all had limited systemic sclerosis.

THERAPY

Therapy is either topical for minor injuries, ischaemic ulcers, and pruritis or is systemic. A majority of the patients respond favourably to some degree to methotrexate in doses of 15 to 25 mg/week (Van den Hoogen *et al.*, 1996). Up till now, this is the only formally evaluated beneficial form of treatment. Progressive systemic sclerosis is, therefore, advised to be treated with 15 mg methotrexate per week; if required, this dose can be increased after 4 months to 25 mg per week (Van den Hoogen, 1997). The effect of haematopoietic stem cell transplants is presently being investigated in patients with a progressive course who are otherwise therapy resistant. According to the American Academy of Dermatology Guidelines (1996) the calcium blocker nifedipine (thrice daily orally 10–20 mg) is the most consistently effective drug for symptoms of Raynaud's phenomenon. Patients are advised to

Box 10.2 Proposed American Rheumatism Association (ARA) criteria for scleroderma (systemic sclerosis)

Major criterion
Primary scleroderma; symmetric thickening, tightening, and induration of the skin of the fingers/digits and the skin proximal to the metacarpophalangeal or metatarsophalangeal joints. The changes may affect the entire extremity, face, neck, and trunk (thorax and abdomen).

Minor criteria
1. Sclerodactyly: above-indicated skin changes limited to the fingers.
2. Digital pitting scars or loss of substance from the finger pad: depressed area at tips of fingers or loss of digital pad tissue as a result of ischaemia.
3. Bibasilar pulmonary fibrosis; bilateral reticular pattern of linear or lineonodular densities, most pronounced in basilar portions of the lungs on standard chest roentgenogram; may assume appearance of diffuse mottling or 'honeycomb lung'. These changes should not be attributable to primary lung disease.

For the purpose of classifying patients in clinical trials, population surveys, and other studies, a person shall be said to have (progressive) systemic sclerosis (scleroderma) if 1 major or 2 or more minor criteria listed above are present. Localized forms of scleroderma, eosinophilic fasciitis and the various forms of pseudoscleroderma are excluded from these criteria. From Masi *et al.* (1980), with permission.

avoid stimuli that evoke Raynaud's phenomenon. Anti-inflammatory drugs, such as corticosteroids and cytostatic agents, are prescribed when vasculitis or other inflammatory complications are present. Symptomatic therapy is applied for various visceral manifestations as required (Farmer *et al.*, 1996).

COURSE AND SURVIVAL

Though spontaneous remission occurs in some cases, a progressive course is the rule. The overall survival rate of patients with systemic sclerosis is approximately 80% after 5 years and 60% after 10 years (Medsger, 1997). From a large cohort of patients with ICTDs, Bulpitt *et al.* (1993) selected 48 cases of scleroderma of less than 1 year duration and studied the course of the disease longitudinally. Fifteen of these 48 patients died in the first five years (survival rate 68%). Predictors of poor outcome at an early stage were cardiopulmonary and kidney involvement. The presence of circulating ACeAs makes limited systemic sclerosis the most likely diagnosis and points to a more benign course in most cases.

THE NEUROLOGY AND MYOLOGY OF SYSTEMIC SCLEROSIS

The neurological manifestations in systemic sclerosis are due either directly to the disease, or are secondary and involve other organs or systems (Table 10.3). In addition, there are some diseases that are possibly associated with systemic sclerosis (Table 10.4).

Table 10.3 Overview of the neurological disorders in systemic sclerosis

Syndromes	Pathogenesis
Focal CNS syndromes, including seizures	Secondary to disorders of internal organs Vasculitis
Transverse myelitis?	Vasculopathy or vasculitis
Spinal cord compression and radiculopathy	Intraspinal and paraspinal calcifications
Trigeminal neuropathy	Inflammatory of ganglion Gasseri
Distal subclinical axonal neuropathy	Unknown
Autonomic neuropathy	Unknown
Multiple mononeuropathy, mononeuropathy and polyneuropathy	Vasculitis
Carpal tunnel syndrome?	Speculative

See text for discussion and references.

Table 10.4 Diseases reported to be associated with systemic sclerosis

Multiple sclerosis
Myasthenia gravis
Poly-/dermatomyositis
Inclusion body myositis

See text for discussion and references.

ARE THERE ANY PRIMARY CNS DISORDERS IN SYSTEMIC SCLEROSIS?

Does systemic sclerosis cause disorders of the brain or the spinal cord? The negative response of most authors to this question is based on the results of five out of six main cohort studies. Tuffanelli and Winkelman (1961) examined the charts of 727 patients (!) with 'systemic scleroderma', and found six cases with nervous system manifestations: grand mal in two and minimal convulsive disorders in four. The authors did not explicitly mention a cause, but their description indicated that the patients may have had late stage scleroderma-related renal disease with hypertension and uraemia. Gordon and Silverstein (1970) analysed data from 130 patients and found evidence of a nervous system disorder (including the CNS) in 18.5% of cases. All CNS manifestations were considered coincidental, iatrogenic, or secondary to renal, cardiac, or gastrointestinal changes. One patient with facial hypaesthesia may have had trigeminal neuropathy. Lee *et al.* (1984) performed a prospective investigation of 125 patients, 103 of whom were females and 22 of whom were males. The patients were followed for a mean period of 31 months (S.D. 44) Nervous system manifestations were observed in seven patients (5.6%) but did not originate in the brain or spinal cord. There was one case of trigeminal neuropathy, and six patients had peripheral nerve disorders. Hietaharju *et al.* (1993a), in a small but careful retrospective study of 32 patients, found evidence of a CNS disorder in five and concluded that these were probably not primary. The only deviant view was expressed by Averbuch-Heller *et al.* (1992). These authors described findings in charts of 50 patients who were diagnosed in their hospital during a 10-year period. Sjögren's syndrome was concomitant in five patients. It appeared that four patients had symptoms or signs of what was interpreted as myelopathy, and three women in their fifties had cerebrovascular disease (TIAs and minor stroke) without any 'definable risk factor'. Three of the four patients with myelopathy had a gastrointestinal motility disorder, but evidence for mal-absorption had not been found. Averbuch-Heller *et al.* (1992) argued that CNS events in systemic sclerosis might very well be caused by vasculopathy or by an auto-immune process.

Observations described in case reports lend some support to the view of Averbuch-Heller *et al.* (1992). Brown and Murphy (1985) described a patient with acute transverse myelopathy. The patient, who was a 33-year-old woman who had limited systemic sclerosis for three years without evidence of overlap with another ICTD, experienced an acute onset of sensory disturbances and weakness of the limbs with hyperreflexia, positive Babinski reflexes, and abnormal micturition. Examination of the CSF and myelography were not informative. Transverse myelopathy was diagnosed and was considered vascular in origin. She was treated with corticosteroids and cyclophosphamide and recovered (as far as the myelopathy was concerned) within a matter of months. This was indeed very similar to what was observed in many cases of SLE and Sjögren's syndrome. In addition, there were four patients in the literature with cerebral vasculitis complicating systemic sclerosis (Lee and Haynes, 1967; Estey *et al.*, 1979; Pathak and Gabor, 1991; Ishida *et al.*, 1993). In each case, diagnosis was based on arteriography, and one case was confirmed at post-mortem examination (Lee and Haynes, 1967). Vasculitis is a recognized complication of systemic sclerosis (Oddis *et al.*, 1987; Miller *et al.*, 1997; Dyck *et al.*, 1997). Therefore, we conclude that systemic sclerosis itself causes, in exceptional cases, disorders of the CNS, which at least in some cases are due to vasculitis.

CNS manifestations in systemic sclerosis are so rare that one has never attempted to obtain consensus on treatment. Management is based on experience obtained in related auto-immune diseases (*e.g.* SLE, Sjögren's syndrome).

SYSTEMIC SCLEROSIS ASSOCIATED WITH MULTIPLE SCLEROSIS

There are reports on at least three patients with both multiple sclerosis (MS) and systemic sclerosis (Trostle *et al.*, 1986; Jawad *et al.*, 1997). In each case, MS devel-oped first and was the dominant disorder; skin changes and other evidence of systemic sclerosis followed months or years thereafter. The diagnosis of MS was based on the multiplicity of the lesions and the relapsing and remitting course. One patient had optic neuritis, diplopia, and transverse myelitis; the second had optic neuritis, ataxia, spasticity, and decreased hearing; and the third had optic neuritis and spastic paraplegia. Increased IgG synthesis in the CSF was estab-lished in one case, and in another, abnormal evoked visual responses that are compatible with MS as well as evidence of demyelination at MRI were estab-lished. One of the patients in the series of Hietaharju *et al.* (1993a) had transient signs of optic neuritis. It is very possible that the association of the two diseases is merely coincidental.

TRIGEMINAL NEUROPATHY IN SYSTEMIC SCLEROSIS

Trigeminal neuropathy is also rare in systemic sclerosis, but nevertheless is one of the most frequently occurring neurological manifestations of the disease, and in exceptional cases may even be the first manifestation. Farrell and Medsger (1982) reported that 16 out of 442 consecutively examined and carefully administered patients with systemic sclerosis had trigeminal neuropathy (4%). Among 50 patients, Averbuch-Heller *et al.* (1992) had two with trigeminal neuropathy (4%). Gordon and Silverstein (1970) discovered, however, only one case of facial hypaesthesia in 130 patients, and Lee *et al.* (1984) who followed 125 patients for a mean duration of 31 months diagnosed trigeminal neuropathy once (<1%). The changes developed gradually nearly always and were sensory. With one exception, there was no muscle weakness of trigeminal innervated muscles. All sensory modalities were involved (Teasdall *et al.*, 1980; Lecky *et al.*, 1987). In some patients, the tongue and the inner side of the cheek(s) were also affected, and often taste was impaired. Hypaesthesia was present usually in the territories of the 2 or 3 branches of the nerve, rarely in only one. In some patients, both sides were affected simultaneously or consecutively. Patients complained about numbness, like after dental anaesthesia, and in a variable degree, about paraesthesia, painful itching, electric shock-like experiences when touched at the cheek, an aching or stabbing pain or a lancinating pain several times daily, or a burning sensation. When sensibility was markedly disturbed in the territory of the first branch, the cornea reflex was decreased and the blink reflex could not be elicited. In some cases of trigeminal neuropathy, Teasdall *et al.* (1980) observed impairment of hearing, facial weakness, or hypaesthesia in the glossopharyngeus nerve-innervated territory, but this was never confirmed by other authors. The CSF was mostly normal and had a mildly raised protein content or a slightly increased number of lymphocytes only exceptionally (Lecky *et al.*, 1987). A biopsy of the supraorbital nerve from a patient with severe loss of sensibility showed a marked decrease of the myelinated fibre density compared to an age-matched autopsy control. The endoneurial connective tissue was increased, but the perineurial sheaths and the nerve vasculature were within the normal range (Lecky *et al.*, 1987). Some patients apparently improve somewhat after a variable period.

The combination of trigeminal neuropathy and spinal ganglionopathy has, to the best of our knowledge, not been reported in systemic sclerosis. This is in contrast to primary Sjögren's syndrome and MCTD where patients often show this combination. The cause of trigeminal neuropathy is not definitely known (post-mortem investigations are urgently needed), but the available evidence is in favour of an inflammatory auto-immune disorder of the ganglion Gasseri (see Chapter 2, *Trigeminal Neuropathy*). Ganglion Gasseri lesions are recognized causes of ipsilateral impairment of sensibility and taste (Hughes, 1993).

Management. Attempts to treat patients have not been successful up till now (see also Chapter 2). Corticosteroids have not been effective (Hughes, 1993). There is no reason at all to consider trigeminal neuropathy as an untreatable auto-immune disorder, especially not when the disorder is diagnosed early. Facial hypaesthesia, when not painful, does not seem to disturb patients too much (Hughes, 1993).

OTHER CRANIAL NEUROPATHIES

Impairment of other cranial nerves is very rare and may well be coincidental (Teasdall *et al.*, 1980; Machet *et al.*, 1992). For optic neuritis see the section on systemic sclerosis associated with MS.

SPINAL CALCIFICATIONS

Small, subcutaneus tissue calcifications are frequent in systemic sclerosis, and occur at the fingertips and extensor surfaces of the interphalangeal joints especially (Fam and Prizker, 1992). Less often they appear elsewhere, in the limbs or the face and near large joints or at pressure points. Paraspinal and intraspinal calcifications are also described. These calcified masses may be large and tumour-like. They are centred at synovial articulations (Schweitzer *et al.*, 1991) or intervertebral discs (Walden *et al.*, 1990) and localized in nearby ligaments (Petrocelli *et al.*, 1988). They can occur at the cervical and thoracic level and cause cord compression or radiculopathy (Petrocelli *et al.*, 1988; Pinstein *et al.*, 1989; Walden *et al.*, 1990; Schweitzer *et al.*, 1991; Ward *et al.*, 1997). The underlying bony tissue may show osteolysis or bone erosion. The aetiology of these calcifications is not clear. Evidence for metabolic derangement has so far not been discovered, and authors therefore assume a relation to local soft tissue necrosis (Schweitzer *et al.*, 1991; Walden *et al.*, 1990).

Management. Treatment of symptomatic paraspinal or intraspinal calcifications is surgical to relieve neurological manifestations. An effective medication is not available. However, there are a few interesting case reports on reduction of calcinotic depots by diltiazem (Dolan *et al.*, 1995; Palmieri *et al.*, 1995).

DISTAL AXONAL NEUROPATHY

Meticulous investigation of sensory modalities at the fingers and toes in patients with advanced skin changes and Raynaud's phenomenon reveals, in some cases, cutaneous hypaesthesia, especially of touch sensation (Teasdall *et al.*, 1980; Schady *et al.*, 1991). Electrophysiological studies point to mild, mainly subclinical, distal axonal neuropathy, predominantly at the upper limbs (Mondelli *et al.*, 1985; Hietaharju *et al.*, 1993b; Lori *et al.*, 1996). Possible causes of this distal neuropathy are strangulation of nerve fibres by accumulation of collagen in distal nerve fascicles, ischaemia induced by the Raynaud's phenomenon, and ischaemia due to vasculopathy or vasculitis.

POLYNEUROPATHY AND MONONEURITIS MULTIPLEX

Polyneuropathies and multiple mononeuropathies are described by several authors and occur probably more frequently than explainable by chance. In a retrospective investigation of 130 patients, one patient was reported to have a mixed polyneuropathy (Gordon and Silverstein, 1970). Lee *et al.* (1984) followed 125 patients for a mean duration of 31 months and detected one case of predominantly sensory polyneuropathy and another case of multiple mononeuropathy. Schady *et al.* (1991) found depressed or absent tendon reflexes at the lower limbs in four of 29 patients. Hietaharju *et al.* (1993b) re-examined 32 previously diagnosed patients and discovered one patient with predominantly sensory polyneuropathy. The electrophysio-logical findings by these two latter groups of authors were in support of an axonal disorder. Averbuch-Heller *et al.* (1992), in a retrospective investigation of charts from 50 patients, established that seven patients (an exceptionally high number) had a mild sensomotor polyneuropathy, perhaps in one case related to Sjögren's syndrome. In a case control study of 536 patients with limited sclerosis (CREST syndrome), seven had peripheral neuropathy not related to any other disorder (Dyck *et al.*, 1997). In the control group, only two patients had neuropathy not related to a known disorder, which was significantly less than in the CREST group. Six of the seven peripheral neuropathy cases had predominantly sensory multiple mono-neuropathy, and one patient had sensory painful small fibre neuropathy. There are also case reports on polyneuropathy (DiTrappani *et al.*, 1986; Sukenik *et al.*, 1987; Berth Jones *et al.*, 1990; Herrick *et al.*, 1994) and multiple mononeuropathy (Miller *et al.*, 1997) in systemic sclerosis. Oddis *et al.* (1987) discovered electrophysiological evidence for multiple mononeuropathy in four patients with both CREST syndrome and Sjögren's syndrome who had symptoms of numbess and paraesthesia.

The available evidence points to vasculitis as the cause for the multiple mononeu-ropathies and probably also for the polyneuropathy. The presence of vasculitis was established in the patients reported by Miller *et al.* (1997), Herrick *et al.* (1994), and in the four cases published by Oddis *et al.* (1987). In four sural nerve biopsies stud-ied by Dyck *et al.* (1997), vasculitis was seen in two cases and perivascular mononu-clear cell infiltrations in the two other cases.

Management. If symptoms and signs of polyneuropathy are only mild, one can wait to see how the clinical picture develops while controlling the condition regularly. Progressive and more severe neuropathies with muscle weakness due to vasculitis and obvious mononeuritis multiplex should be treated with immunosuppression as described in the section on vasculitic neuropathy in Chapter 5.

AUTONOMIC DYSFUNCTION

The best evidence for impaired autonomic function in systemic sclerosis stems, at present, from studies of heart rate variability. Ferri *et al.* (1997) compared 24-hour ECG ambulatory recordings of thirty patients with systemic sclerosis, who did not have heart failure, myositis or diabetes mellitus, with a similar number of age and sex matched controls, and established that heart rate was significantly higher and that day and night differences as well as spectral indices of heart rate variability were significantly lower than in controls. This confirms, essentially, the results of other authors, which were obtained with other methods (Dessein *et al.*, 1992; Straub *et al.*, 1996). The exact cause of the autonomic dysfunction has not been elucidated yet. One would expect changes at the limbs if autonomic dysfunction resulted from a disorder of nerve fibres, *e.g.* an autonomic neuropathy comparable to sensomotor polyneuropathy. The most convenient method to establish autonomic dysfunction at the limbs is examination of perspiration. In systemic sclerosis, this is not feasible as the disease causes decrease of dermal appendages, notably sweat glands.

The clinical relevance of the abnormal autonomic tests in systemic sclerosis remains to be demonstrated. Autonomic neuropathy may potentially contribute to the gastrointestinal motility changes in systemic sclerosis. A relation of autonomic neuropathy and cardiovascular mortality is known from studies in diabetics (Ewing *et al.*, 1980). Sudden death, conceivably due to cardiac arrhythmia, occurs in systemic sclerosis (Bulkley *et al.*, 1978; Ferri *et al.*, 1985).

Males with systemic sclerosis may present with complaints about impotence. This abnormality is probably not due to autonomic neuropathy but to small vessel disease and fibrosis of the penile corpora cavernosa (Nowlin *et al.*, 1986; Sukenik *et al.*, 1987).

CARPAL TUNNEL SYNDROME AND OTHER PERIPHERAL NERVE LESIONS

On the basis of case reports, a relation has been suggested between systemic sclerosis and carpal tunnel syndrome (CTS) (Barr and Blair, 1988; Berth Jones *et al.*, 1990; Machet *et al.*, 1992). A few of these patients were male, but the majority were female. The problem is the high percentage of females in the systemic sclerosis population and the high prevalence of CTS in otherwise healthy women (9.2% of women between 25 and 75 years have CTS) (de Krom *et al.*, 1992). An epidemiological investigation that compares findings in systemic sclerosis with age and sex matched controls is necessary to find out whether CTS is indeed more frequent in patients with systemic sclerosis than in controls. Observations on uncontrolled groups of patients are contradictory. In a retrospective study of 130 patients, Gordon and Silverstein (1970) reported no case of CTS. Lee *et al.* (1984) discovered four cases of CTS in 125 patients followed for a mean period of approximately 30 months. Averbuch-Heller *et al.* (1992) discovered one case of CTS in a retrospective investigation of 50 cases, and Hietaharju *et al.* (1993b) who re-examined 32 patients, all previously diagnosed as suffering from systemic sclerosis, found no evidence of CTS. CTS was also not found in a group of 29 extensively examined patients by Schady *et al.* (1991). Gonzales-Alvaro *et al.* (1995) reported on 324 sequentially examined cases of CTS. Two hundred and one fulfilled the inclusion criteria of the study; 12 had rheumatic arthritis and one had systemic sclerosis. Of interest was the observation of inflammatory infiltrates around small vessels in the tissue removed from the carpal tunnel in a case of CTS complicating systemic sclerosis. In a second case, pathological examination revealed only fibrosis (Machet *et al.*, 1992). This short review of the literature shows that, at present, the available data do not justify the conclusion of an increased risk of CTS in patients with systemic sclerosis.

There are communications about other nerve lesions in systemic sclerosis: meralgia paraesthetica (Kaufman and Canoso, 1986), ulnar neuropathy (Averbuch-Heller *et al.*, 1992), brachial plexus neuropathy (Hietaharju *et al.*, 1993b), and phrenicus palsy (Birk and Zeuthen, 1995). No definite causes are revealed in any of these cases.

SYSTEMIC SCLEROSIS AND MYASTHENIA GRAVIS

Association of systemic sclerosis and MG has been described in at least five patients (Mitchell *et al.*, 1975; Bhalla *et al.*, 1993; Arostegui *et al.*, 1995). Both scleroderma and MG may come first with a time interval of months to several years between the two. MG is generalized, not ocular, and seropositive. The combination may be a coincidence or the consequence of an 'auto-immune diathesis' (Bhalla *et al.*, 1993).

MYOPATHY AND MYOSITIS

Muscle force of patients (moving as in armour due to the tightening of the skin with joint contractures) tends to decrease. Serum creatine kinase (CK) in such patients is usually normal or slightly raised, and electromyography may be normal or reveal a varying degree of multiphasic motor-unit potentials (Medsger, 1997; Clements *et al.*, 1978). Perimysial and epimysial connective tissue in muscle biopsies from these patients is estimated to be increased. Inflammatory changes are reported to be absent, though in our experience, an occasional interstitial inflammatory infiltrate or a perivascular infiltrate of mononuclear cells is present. Longitudinal studies reveal that this form of myopathy has a stable course (Medsger, 1997).

Five to ten percent of systemic sclerosis patients eventually present with a more pronounced weakness proximal at the limbs, with some degree of weakness of neck flexors (Hietarinta *et al.* 1996). Such cases are classified either as systemic sclerosis with polymyositis (PM) or as systemic sclerosis in overlap with PM. Laboratory investigations in these patients reveal increased serum CK levels, and at electromyography reveal fibrillation potentials, positive sharp waves, and short duration polyphasic motor-unit potentials. Muscle biopsies show a variable degree of vasculopathy with intimal proliferation, inflammatory changes, and muscle fibre necrosis and regeneration (Ringel *et al.*, 1990). Mild perifascicular atrophy, as in dermatomyositis (DM), is present in some cases (Eduardo and Cavaliere, 1995). The role of antibodies in 'sclero-myositis' is discussed in Chapter 3. Inclusion body myositis (IBM) is occasionally reported in patients with systemic sclerosis (Salama *et al.*, 1980) (see also Chapter 6, *Inclusion Body Myositis*).

Management. Treatment with corticosteroids is effective, as far as return of muscle force is concerned, but continued low-dose medication is usually required. See for a more extensive discussion of PM treatment Chapter 6.

LOCALIZED SCLERODERMA

The term morphea is used when one or more patches of the skin are indurated. These patches can be small (guttata) or somewhat larger (en plaque). When patches become confluent and cover a larger portion of the skin, morphea is considered to be general. Scleroderma is linear when a band-like shape is indurated. In general, localized scleroderma affects not only the skin but also the underlying tissues, including muscle and bone. Local scleroderma may also be confined to tissues under the skin, but this is exceptional (see Table 10.1). In all types, the changes of the skin are qualitatively similar and characterized by thickening and induration with or without hyperpigmentation. In late stages there is atrophy (Seibold, 1997). In childhood, localized scleroderma is much more frequent than systemic sclerosis (Jablonska and Blaszczyk, 1997). In a population-based study in Olmsted County, Rochester, USA, the incidence rate of localized scleroderma per year was 2.7/100 000 (Peterson *et al.*, 1997), and the estimated prevalence at the age of 18 years was 50/100.000. The number of patients identified in this study was 82, and the mean length of follow-up was 9.2 years. In general, females were more frequently affected than males (ratio 2.6:1). For the large majority of patients, the duration of disease activity was 5.5 years or less, which confirms previous communication that the disease was self-limiting. A small number of patients in the Olmsted study had mild arthralgia, synovitis, joint contracture, and CTS, but no increased incidence of oesophagal, cardiac, pulmonary, or renal disorders. Neurological disorders may complicate linear scleroderma (Jablonska and Blaszczyk, 1997).

LINEAR SCLERODERMA, LINEAR SCLERODERMA EN COUP DE SABRE

Linear scleroderma differs from other types of localized scleroderma by a younger mean age at onset (18 years versus 33 for all types of localized scleroderma together) (Falanga *et al.*, 1986), and by presenting preferentially at one of the limbs or on the face ('en coup de sabre') instead of at the trunk. The majority of cases of childhood-onset, localized scleroderma is linear in type (Jablonska and Blaszczyk, 1997). Falanga *et al.* (1986) diagnosed and followed, during a period of 31 years, 52 patients with linear scleroderma. Five of them had scleroderma en coup de sabre in the face (Falanga *et al.*, 1986).

When localized at a limb, linear scleroderma may gradually extend along the whole extremity. The affected limb may remain shorter than the contralateral side when onset of the disorder is in childhood. Linear scleroderma en coup de sabre affects one side of the forehead and the scalp (Fig. 10.3). Some reports mention a

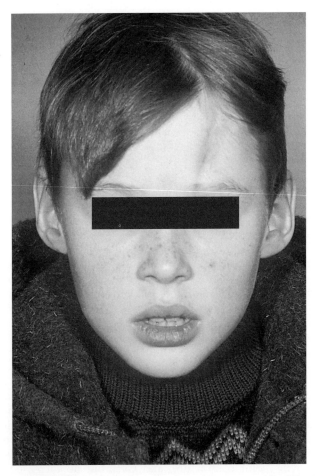

Figure 10.3 Linear scleroderma 'en coup de sabre'. (Courtesy of Dr. Harold Baart de la Faille.)

slight ipsilateral atrophy of the face. Blood eosinophilia, polyclonal hypergamma-globulinaemia, aspecific antibodies against nuclear antigens, and single stranded DNA (ssDNA) are features of linear scleroderma (Seibold, 1997). Biopsies from an early stage of the disorder show muscle atrophy; fibrosis and inflammatory infiltration with lymphocytes in the skin, as in systemic sclerosis, and a localized inflammatory myopathy in the underlying muscle tissue (Miike *et al.*, 1983; Miller III, 1992). Linear scleroderma is considered by most authors as 'immunological' in origin, but the pathogenetic mechanism is still a complete mystery (Pupillo *et al.*, 1996). In some cases, linear scleroderma precedes the onset of SLE (Mackel *et al.*, 1979).

Management. Therapy is topical in mild cases or immunosuppressive when the changes are more severe. Ultraviolet A_1 phototherapy has been attempted (see Lehman, 1996).

Neurology of linear scleroderma
There are several case reports on epilepsy in patients with facial linear scleroderma (Chazen *et al.*, 1962; Dubeau *et al.*, 1988; David *et al.*, 1991; Chung *et al.*, 1995). The case report of Chung *et al.* (1995) is of interest because neuropathological investigation demonstrated that the changes in the brain that caused the seizures were clearly localized and well demarcated beneath the affected part of the skin. The leptomeninx was thickened and opaque, and contained thickened and sclerotic vessels and clusters of such vessels. Gliosis, calcium depositions, and similar abnormal vessels, as in the leptomeninx, were seen in the brain parenchyma. In another case with scleroderma en coup de sabre and seizures, the underlying brain tissue contained scattered microglial nodules and chronic inflammatory changes including 'perivascular infiltrates' (Dubeau *et al.*, 1988). The discrepancies between the neuropathological findings may be due to the different stages of the disease. In each of these cases, the pathological brain tissue was removed and epilepsy improved.

Management. There are no general rules for treating neurological manifestations of localized scleroderma. Treatment of epilepsy is discussed in detail in Chapter 2. Case reports show that abnormal and dysfunctioning brain tissue has been removed in some cases.

PARRY ROMBERG SYNDROME OR HEMIATROPHIA FACEI

The Parry Romberg syndrome (PRS) or hemiatrophia facei is a rare sporadic disorder of unknown origin with onset of clinical changes after birth and usually in the first two decades (Poskanzer, 1975; Gorlin and Sedano, 1977). The disease has a slowly progressive course for two to ten years and plateaus thereafter. The initial changes often concern changes in pigmentation and develop at the lower forehead or below the lower eyelid. PRS differs from linear scleroderma en coup de sabre by extension of atrophy below the eye and the lack of induration of the skin (Lehman, 1992). The changes are not restricted to the skin and involve the underlying tissue including the bone, and in some patients the brain. Ophthalmological abnormalities and neurological manifestations are not rare, but are not present in all cases (see below). Circulating aspecific antibodies against nuclear antigens, RF, and other antibodies are present in a majority of patients, which is comparable to linear scleroderma (Garcia-de-la-Torre *et al.*, 1995). The lack of skin-induration is the reason why most authors do not include the PRS in the scleroderma spectrum but there is no unanimity on this point (see for references Garcia-de-la-Torre *et al.*, 1995). Dupont *et al.* (1997) suggested that the disorder might result from an early malformative process on one side of the rostral neural tube.

Neurological and ophthalmological abnormalities observed in PRS patients are strikingly heterogeneous. They vary from seizures (as the most frequent manifestation) to headache or migraine, cataract, a dilated and fixed pupil, optic atrophy, Horner's syndrome, and hemiparesis (Wolf and Verity, 1974; Gorlin and Sedano, 1977; Lehman, 1992; Fry *et al.*, 1992; Dupont *et al.*, 1997). Results of brain imaging are no less diverse and include no changes at all, cortical thickening or atrophy, ill defined sulci, white matter lesions, vascular malformations and calcifications, and lateral ventricle widening. Brain changes are predominantly localized, frontal and temporal. Facial atrophy is ipsilateral (Pensler *et al.*, 1990; Fry *et al.*, 1992; Terstegge *et al.*, 1994: Dupont *et al.*, 1997).

SUMMARY

Disorders of the CNS and PNS in systemic sclerosis are uncommon. When present, vasculitis should be considered as a possible cause. Trigeminal neuropathy occurs in some cases, and is probably not due to vasculitis but to an inflammatory disorder of the ganglion Gasseri. A striking and unusual complication is spinal calcinosis; it may cause cord compression and radiculopathy. Systemic sclerosis is, in 5–10%, associated with clinically relevant symptoms and signs of myositis. In some cases, linear scleroderma in the face is complicated by seizures due to underlying local brain pathology.

REFERENCES

Arostegui J, Gorodo JM and Azamburn JM (1995) Myasthenia gravis and scleroderma. *J Rheumatol* **22**, 792–793.

Artlett CM, Smith B and Jimenez SA (1998) Identification of fetal DNA and cells in skin lesions from women with systemic sclerosis. *N Engl J Med* **338**, 1186–1191.

Averbuch-Heller L, Steiner I and Ambramsky O (1992) Neurologic manifestations of progressive systemic sclerosis. *Arch Neurol* **49**, 1292–1295.

Barr WG and Blair SJ (1988) Carpal tunnel syndrome as the initial manifestation of scleroderma. *J Hand Surg* **13A**, 366–367.

Berth Jones J, Coales PAA, Graham Brown RAC *et al.* (1990) Neurologic complications in scleroderma: A report of three cases and review of the literature. *Clin Exp Dermatol* **15**, 91–94.

Bhalla R, Swedler WI, Lazazeric MB *et al.* (1993) Myasthenia gravis and scleroderma. *J Rheumatol* **20**, 1409–1410.

Birk MA and Zeuthen EL (1995) Phrenicus palsy in progressive systemic sclerosis. *Brit J Rheumatol* **34**, 684–685.

Brown JJ and Murphy MJ (1985) Transverse myelopathy in progressive systemic sclerosis. *Ann Neurol* **17**, 615.

Bulkley BH, Klacsmann PG and Hutchins GM (1978) Angina pectoris, myocardial infarction and sudden cardiac death with normal coronary arteries: A clinico-pathologic study of 9 patients with progressive systemic sclerosis. *Am Heart J* **95**, 563–569.

Bulpitt KJ, Clements PJ, Lachenbruch PA *et al.* (1993) Early undifferentiated connective tissue disease: III. Outcome and prognostic indicators in early scleroderma (systemic sclerosis). *Ann Int Med* **118**, 602–609.

Carwile Roy E (1997) Pathogenesis of systemic sclerosis (scleroderma). In: Koopman WJ (ed) *Arthritis and Allied Conditions. A Textbook of Rheumatology,* 13th ed, pp 1481–1490. Baltimore: Williams and Wilkins.

Chazen FM, Cook CD and Cohen J (1962) Focal scleroderma – report of 19 cases in children. *J Pediatr* **60**, 385–393.

Chung MH, Sum J, Morrell MJ *et al.* (1995) Intracerebral involvement in scleroderma en coup de sabre: Report of a case with neuropathological findings. *Ann Neurol* **37**, 679–681.

Clements PJ, Furst DE, Campon DS *et al.* (1978) Muscle disease in progressive systemic sclerosis. *Arthritis Rheum* **21**, 62–71.

David J, Wilson J and Woo P (1991) Scleroderma 'en coup de sabre'. *Ann Rheum Dis* **50**, 260–266.

De Krom MCTFM, Knipschild PG, Kester ADM *et al.* (1992) Carpal tunnel syndrome. Prevalence in the general population. *J Clin Epidemiol* **45**, 373–375.

Dessein PH, Joffe BI, Metz RM *et al.* (1992) Autonomic dysfunction in systemic sclerosis: Sympathic overactivity and instability. *Am J Med* **93**, 143–150.

DiTrappani G, Tull A, La Cara A *et al.* (1986) Peripheral neuropathy in the course of systemic sclerosis. *Acta Neuropath (Berl)* **72**, 103–110.

Dolan AL, Kassimos D, Gibson T *et al.* (1995) Diltiazem induces remission of calcinosis in scleroderma. *Brit J Rheumatol* **34**, 576–578.

Dubeau F, Andermann F, Robitaille Y *et al.* (1988) Morphea or focal scleroderma of the brain: Intractable epilepsy and clinicopathologic correlation. (abstract) *Epilepsia* **29**, 712.

Dupont S, Catala M, Hasboun D *et al.* (1997) Progressive facial hemiatrophy and epilepsy: A common underlying dysgenetic mechanism. *Neurology* **48**, 1013–1018.

Dyck PJB, Hunder GG and Dyck PJ (1997) A case-control and nerve biopsy study of CREST multiple mononeuropathy. *Neurology* **49**, 1641–1645.

Eduardo E and Cavaliere MJ (1995) Skeletal muscle pathology in systemic sclerosis. *J Rheumatol* **22**, 2246–2249.

Estey E, Lieberman A, Pinto R *et al.* (1979) Cerebral arteritis in scleroderma. *Stroke* **10**, 595–597.

Ewing DJ, Campbell I, Murray A *et al.* (1980) The natural history of diabetic autonomic neuropathy. *Quart J Med* **193**, 95–108.

Falanga V, Medsger Jr TA, Reichlin M *et al.* (1986) Linear scleroderma. Clinical spectrum, prognosis and laboratory abnormalities. *Ann Int Med* **104**, 849–857.

Fam AG and Prizker KPH (1992) Acute calcific periarthritis in scleroderma. *J Rheumatol* **19**, 1580–1585.

Farmer ER, Goltz RW, Graham GF *et al.* (1996) Guidelines of care for scleroderma and scleroid disorders. *J Am Acad Dermatol* **35**, 609–614.

Farrell DA and Medsger Jr TA (1982) Trigeminal neuropathy in progressive systemic sclerosis. *Am J Med* **73**, 57–62.

Ferri C, Bernini L, Bongiorni MG *et al.* (1985) Noninvasive evaluation of cardiac dysrythmias and their relationship with multisystemic symptoms in progressive systemic sclerosis patients. *Arthritis Rheum* **28**, 1259–1266.

Ferri C, Emdin M, Giuggioli D *et al.* (1997) Autonomic dysfunction in systemic sclerosis: Time and frequency domain 24 hour heart rate variability analysis. *Brit J Rheumatol* **36**, 669–676.

Fry JA, Alvarellos A, Fink CW *et al.* (1992) Intracranial findings in progressive facial hemiatrophia. *J Rheumatol* **19**, 956–958.

Garcia-de-la-Torre I, Castello-Sendra J, Esgleyes-Ribot T *et al.* (1995) Auto-antibodies in Parry-Romberg syndrome: A serologic study of 14 patients. *J Rheumatol* **22**, 73–77.

Gonzales-Alvaro I, Carvajal I, Estevez M *et al.* (1995) Carpal tunnel syndrome as initial manifestation of inflammatory connective tissue diseases. *Ann Rheum Dis* **54**, 782.

Gordon RM and Silverstein A (1970) Neurologic manifestations in progressive sclerosis. *Arch Neurol* **22**, 126–134.

Gorlin RJ and Sedano HO (1977) Progressive hemifacial atrophy (Parry Romberg syndrome). In: Vinken PJ and Bruyn GW (eds) *Handbook of Clinical Neurology,* Vol 43, pp 252–255. Amsterdam: North Holland Publishing Co.

Herrick AL, Oogarah P, Brammah TB *et al.* (1994) Nervous system involvement in association with anticardiolipin antibodies in a patient with systemic sclerosis. *Ann Rheum Dis* **53**, 349–350.

Hietaharju A, Jaaskelainen S, Hietarinta M *et al.* (1993a) Central nervous system involvement and psychiatric manifestations in systemic sclerosis (scleroderma): Clinical and neurophysiological evaluation. *Acta Neurol Scand* **87**, 382–387.

Hietaharju A, Jaaskelainen S, Kalimo H *et al.* (1993b) Peripheral neuromuscular manifestations in systemic sclerosis (scleroderma). *Muscle Nerve* **16**, 1204–1212.

Hietarinta M, Meyer O, Haim T *et al.* (1996) Antinuclear and antinucleolar antibodies in patients with scleroderma-polymyositis overlap syndrome. *Brit J Rheumatol* **35**, 1326–1327.

Hughes RAC (1993) Diseases of the fifth cranial nerve. In: Dyck PJ, Thomas PK, Griffin JW *et al.* (eds) *Peripheral Neuropathy*, 3rd ed, pp 801–817. Philadelphia: WB Saunders.

Ishida K, Kamata T, Tsukagoshi H *et al.* (1993) Progressive systemic sclerosis with CNS vasculitis and cyclosporin A therapy (a letter). *J Neurol Neurosurg Psychiat* **56**, 720.

Jablonska S, Maddison PJ and Blaszczyck M (1995) Scleroderma. In: Kater L and Baart de la Faille H (eds) *Multi-Systemic Auto-Immune Diseases: An Integrated Approach*, pp 207–226. Amsterdam: Elsevier.

Jablonska S and Blaszczyk M (1997) Childhood onset scleroderma from a dermatologist's perspective: Comment on the article by Vancheeswaren *et al. Arthritis Rheum* **40**, 1183–1184.

Jawad SH, Askari A and Ward AB (1997) Case history of a patient with multiple sclerosis and scleroderma. *Brit J Rheumatol* **36**, 502–503.

Kaufman J and Canoso JJ (1986) Progressive systemic sclerosis and meralgia paraesthetica. *Ann Int Med* **105**, 973.

Lecky BRF, Hughes RAC and Murray NMF (1987) Trigeminal neuropathy. *Brain* **110**, 1463–1485.

Lee JE and Haynes JM (1967) Carotid arteritis and cerebral infarction. *Neurology* **17**, 18–22.

Lee P, Bruni J and Sukenik S (1984) Neurologic manifestations in progressive systemic sclerosis. *J Rheumatol* **11**, 480–483.

Lehman TJA (1992) The Parry Romberg syndrome of progressive facial hemiatrophy and linear scleroderma en coup de sabre. Mistaken diagnosis or overlapping conditions. *J Rheumatol* **19**, 844–845.

Lehman TJA (1996) Systemic and localized scleroderma in children. *Curr Opin Rheumatol* **8**, 576–579.

Lori S, Matucci-Cerinic M, Casale R *et al.* (1996) Peripheral nervous system involvement in systemic sclerosis: The median nerve as target structure. *Clin Exp Rheumatol* **14**, 601–605.

Mackel SE, Korin F, Ryan LM *et al.* (1979) Concurrent linear scleroderma and systemic lupus erythematosus: A report of two cases. *J Invest Dermatol* **73**, 368–372.

Machet L, Vaillant L, Machet MC *et al.* (1992) Carpal tunnel syndrome and systemic sclerosis. *Dermatology* **185**, 101–103.

Maddison DJ, Skinner RP, Pereira RS *et al.* (1986) Antinuclear antibodies in the relatives and spouses of patients with systemic sclerosis. *Ann Rheum Dis* **45**, 793–796.

Masi AT, Rodnan GP, Medsger Jr TA *et al.* (1980) Subcommittee for scleroderma criteria of the American Rheumatism Association Diagnostic and Therapeutic Criteria Committee: Preliminary criteria for the classification of systemic sclerosis (scleroderma). *Arthritis Rheum* **23**, 581–590.

Matucci Cerinic M, Generini S, Pignone A *et al.* (1996) The nervous system in systemic sclerosis (scleroderma). Clinical features and pathogenetic mechanisms. *Rheumatic Disease Clinics of North America* **22**, 879–892.

Mayes MD (1997) Epidemiology of systemic sclerosis and related diseases. *Curr Opin Rheumatol* **9**, 557–561.

Medsger Jr TA (1997) Systemic sclerosis (scleroderma): Clinical aspects. In: Koopman WJ (ed) *Arthritis and Allied Conditions. A Textbook of Rheumatology*, 13th ed, pp 1433–1464. Baltimore: Williams and Wilkins.

Miike T, Ohtani Y, Hattori S *et al.* (1983) Childhood-type myositis and linear scleroderma. *Neurology (Cleveland)* **33**, 928–930.

Miller A, Ryan PFJ and Dowling J (1997) Vasculitis and thrombotic thrombocytopenic purpura in a patient with limited scleroderma. *J Rheumatol* **24**, 598–600.

Miller III JJ (1992) The fasciitis-morphea complex in children. *Am J Dis Child* **146**, 733–736.

Mitchell GW, Lichtenfeld PJ and McDonald CJ (1975). Systemic sclerosis and myasthenia. *JAMA* **233**, 531.

Mondelli M, Romano C and Porta P della (1995) Electrophysiological evidence of 'entrapment syndromes' and subclinical peripheral neuropathy in progressive systemic sclerosis (scleroderma). *J Neurol* **242**, 185–194.

Nelson JL (1998) Microchimerism and autoimmune disease. *N Engl J Med* **338**, 1224–1225.

Nowlin NS, Brick JE, Weaver DJ *et al.* (1986) Impotence in scleroderma. *Ann Int Med* **104**, 794–798.

Oddis CV, Eisenbeis CH, Reidbord HE *et al.* (1987) Vasculitis in systemic sclerosis: Association with Sjogren's syndrome and the CREST variant. *J Rheumatol* **14**, 942–948.

Palmieri GMA, Sebes JI, Aelion JA *et al.* (1995) Treatment of calcinosis with diltiazem. *Arthritis Rheum* **38**, 1646–1654.

Pathak R and Gabor AJ (1991) Scleroderma and central nervous system vasculitis. *Stroke* **22**, 410–413.

Pensler JM, Murphy GF and Mulliken JB (1990) Clinical and ultrastructural studies of Romberg's hemifacial atrophy. *Plast Reconstr Surg* **85**, 669–674.

Peterson LS, Nelson AM, Su WPD *et al.* (1997) The epidemiology of morphea (localized scleroderma) in Olmsted County 1960–1993. *J Rheumatol* **24**, 73–80.

Petrocelli AR, Bassett LW, Mirra J *et al.* (1988) Scleroderma: Dystrophic calcification with spinal cord compression. *J Rheumatol* **15**, 1733–1735.

Pinstein ML, Sebes JI, Levanthal M *et al.* (1989) Case report 579: Progressive systemic sclerosis with cervical cord compression syndrome, osteolysis and bilateral facet arthropathy. *Skeletal Radiol* **18**, 603–605.

Poskanzer DC (1975) Progressive hemifacial atrophy (Romberg's disease). In: Vinken PJ and Bruyn GW (eds) *Handbook of Clinical Neurology*, vol 22, pp 546–549. Amsterdam: North Holland Publishing Co.

Pupillo G, Andermann F and Dubeau F (1996) Linear scleroderma and intractable epilepsy: Neuropathologic evidence for a chronic inflammatory process. *Ann Neurol* **39**, 277–278.

Report of a meeting of physicians and scientists (1996) Systemic sclerosis: Current pathogenetic concepts and future prospects for targeted therapy. *Lancet* **347**, 1453–1458.

Rendall JR and McKenzie AW (1974) Familial scleroderma. *Br J Dermatol* **91**, 517–522.

Ringel RA, Brick JE, Gutmann L *et al.* (1990) Muscle involvement in the scleroderma syndrome. *Arch Int Med* **150**, 2550–2552.

Salama J, Tome FMS, Lebon P *et al.* (1980) Myosite a inclusions: etude clinique, morphologique et virologique concernant une nouvelle observation associee a une sclerodermie generalisee et a un syndrome de Klinefelter. *Rev Neurol* **136**, 863–878.

Schady W, Sheard A, Hassell A *et al.* (1991) Peripheral nerve dysfunction in scleroderma. *Quart J Med* **80**, 661–675.

Schweitzer ME, Cervilla V, Manaster BJ *et al.* (1991) Cervical paraspinal calcification in collagen vascular diseases. *Am J Roentgenol* **157**, 523–525.

Seibold JR (1997) Scleroderma. In: Kelley WN, Ruddy S, Harris ED Jr *et al.* (eds). *Textbook of Rheumatology*, 5th ed, pp 1133–1162. Philadelphia: WB Saunders.

Silman A and Newman J (1996) Epidemiology of systemic sclerosis. *Curr Opinion Rheumatol* **8**, 585–589.

Shulman HM and Sullivan KM (1988) Graft-versus host disease: Allo- and autoimmunity after bone marrow transplantation. *Concepts Immunopathol* **6**, 141–165.

Steen VD, Oddis CV, Conte CG *et al.* (1997) Incidence of systemic sclerosis in Allegheney County, Pennsylvania. *Arthritis Rheum* **40**, 441–445.

Stephens C, Briggs DC, Whyte J *et al.* (1995) Familial scleroderma: Evidence for environmental versus genetic trigger. *Br J Rheumatol* **33**, 1131–1135.

Straub RH, Zeuner M, Lock G *et al.* (1996) Autonomic and sensorimotor neuropathy in patients with systemic lupus erythematosus and systemic sclerosis. *J Rheumatol* **23**, 87–92.

Sukenik S, Horowitz J, Buskila J *et al.* (1986) Impotence in systemic sclerosis. *Ann Int Med* **106**, 910–911.

Sukenik S, Abarbanel JM, Buskila D *et al.* (1987) Impotence, carpal tunnel syndrome and peripheral neuropathy as presenting symptoms in progressive systemic sclerosis. *J Rheumatol* **14**, 641–642.

Teasdall R, Frayha RA and Shulman LE (1980) Cranial nerve involvement in systemic sclerosis (scleroderma): A report of 10 cases. *Medicine* **59**, 149–159.

Terstegge K, Kuneth B, Felber S *et al.* (1994) MR of brain involvement in progressive facial hemiatrophy (Romberg disease): Reconstruction of a syndrome. *AJNR* **15**, 145–150.

Trostle D, Helfrich D and Medsger Jr TA (1986) Systemic sclerosis (scleroderma) and multiple sclerosis. *Arthritis Rheum* **29**, 124–127.

Tuffanelli D and Winkelman RK (1961) Systemic scleroderma: A clinical study of 727 cases. *Arch Dermatol* **84**, 359–371.

Tuffanelli DL (1969) Scleroderma, immunologic and genetic disease in three families. *Dermatology* **138**, 93–104.

Van den Hoogen FHJ, Boerbooms AMT, Swaak AJG *et al.* (1996) Comparison of methotrexate with placebo in the treatment of systemic sclerosis: A 24 week randomized double-blind trial, followed by a 24 week observational trial. *Br J Rheum* **35**, 364–372.

Van den Hoogen FHJ (1997) Sclerodermie: diagnostiek en behandeling. In: Breedveld FC (redacteur) *Bindweefsel Ziekten*, pp 41–50. Leiden: Boerhaave Commissie.

Van de Putte LBA, Tyndall A, van den Hoogen FHJ *et al.* (1997) Hematopoietic stem cell transplants for autoimmune disease: Role for EULAR. *J Rheumatol*, Suppl. 48, 98–99.

Walden CA, Gilbert P, Rogers LF *et al.* (1990) Case report 620: Progressive systemic sclerosis with paraspinous and intraspinous calcifications. *Skeletal Radiol* **19**, 377–378.

Ward M, Cure J, Schabel S *et al.* (1997) Symptomatic spinal calcinosis in systemic sclerosis (scleroderma). *Arthritis Rheum* **40**, 1892–1895.

Wolf SM and Verity MA (1974) Neurological complications of progressive focal hemiatrophy. *J Neurol Neurosurg Psychiat* **37**, 997–1004.

11

Sjögren's Syndrome

INTRODUCTION

Sjögren's syndrome (Ss) is considered to be an auto-immune disease and is characterized clinically by keratoconjunctivitis sicca and xerostomia and pathologically by progressive lymphocytic and plasma cell infiltration of the salivary and lacrimal glands (Anaya and Talal, 1997). The manifestations of the disease are usually mild, but the disease carries the risk of developing into malignant lymphoma. A difference is made between primary Ss (pSs), which is not associated with another inflammatory connective tissue disease (ICTD), and secondary Ss (sSs), in which another ICTD (rheumatoid arthritis, systemic lupus erythematosus, systemic sclerosis) is also present. Salivary gland enlargement, predominantly the parotid glands, occurs in two-thirds of pSs patients and varies in frequency in sSs patients (Kruize *et al.*, 1996; Moutsopoulos *et al.*, 1979) (Fig. 11.1). Extraglandular manifestations are present in approximately 30 to 60% of pSs patients (Anaya and Talal, 1997; Moutsopoulos *et al.*, 1980). Manifestations of the peripheral nervous system (PNS) are frequent, and those of the central nervous system (CNS) are disputed.

In this chapter we first present a short general description of the disease and then, in the second part, the psychiatrical and neurological aspects are dealt with. Previous reviews on the neurology of Sjögren's syndrome were published by Alexander in 1986 and Kaplan *et al.* in 1990.

SJÖGREN'S SYNDROME: A SHORT GENERAL DESCRIPTION

EPIDEMIOLOGY

There are several sets of diagnostic criteria for Ss and this greatly impedes comparison of different epidemiological studies. Onset of the disease is mostly in the fourth

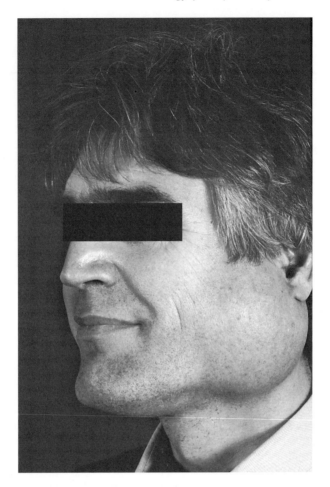

Figure 11.1 Enlargement of the parotid gland in a patient with primary Sjögren's syndrome. (Courtesy of Dr. O. Paul van Bijsterveld.)

or fifth decade, but younger persons and even children may be affected also (Moutsopoulos *et al.*, 1995). Approximately 90% of patients with pSs are female (Kruize *et al.*, 1996). Clinical and serological expression of the disease is similar in children, men, and women (Anaya *et al.*, 1995a and 1995b). According to Swedish authors, the prevalence of pSs in middle aged people is 2.7%, which means that it may be the most common ICTD (Jacobson *et al.*, 1989).

AETIOLOGY

As usual in the ICTDs, the aetiology is unknown. Several factors point to genetic predisposition. The prevalence of pSs, other ICTDs and serological auto-immune changes is higher in family members than in age and sex matched controls (Reveille *et al.*, 1984; Youinou and Pennec, 1987). There is, in addition, an association of pSs with some of the HLA genes (Moutsopoulos *et al.*, 1995). Triggering of Ss by viral or bacterial infections has been suggested but support for this view has not been discovered so far (see Moutsopoulos *et al.*, 1995 and Fox, 1996).

PATHOGENESIS

The two main auto-immune changes that have been recognized in Ss are B-lymphocyte hyperactivity and infiltration of the exocrine glands by lymphocytes and plasma cells. The B-cell hyperactivity is expressed by hypergammaglobulinaemia and the presence of polyclonal and oligoclonal or monoclonal circulating antibodies (Kater and de Wilde, 1992). Auto-antibodies against two ribonucleoprotein antigens (Ro/SS-A and La/SS-B) are frequent in Ss, and are associated, in comparison to Ss without these antibodies, with earlier disease onset, longer disease duration, recurrent enlargement of parotid glands, splenomegaly, lymphadenopathy, and vasculitis (Manoussakis *et al.*, 1986). These auto-antibodies are not disease specific and may be found in other auto-immune diseases as well, especially in SLE. In Ss there are antibodies against cytoskeletal proteins in epithelial and myoepithelial cells of exocrine glands (Saku *et al.*, 1990; Moutsopoulos *et al.*, 1995). These antibodies occur also in RA and are probably secondary in nature.

Monoclonal light chains, or immunoglobulins often behaving as cryoglobulins, have been demonstrated in the serum of approximately 80% of patients with pSs and extraglandular (systemic) manifestations. Analysis has shown that these immunoglobulins are comparable to mixed monoclonal cryoglobulins (type II) containing an IgM/kappa monoclonal RF (see Chapter 5, *Essential Cryoglobulinaemia*). Patients with these immunoglobulins run an increased risk of lymphoid malignancy (Tzioufas *et al.*, 1987; Moutsopoulos *et al.*, 1995).

PATHOLOGY

Mononuclear inflammatory infiltrates consisting mainly of activated B- and T-lymphocytes (mainly CD4+) and plasma cells are present in the major salivary glands, especially around dilated ducts (Moutsopoulos *et al.*, 1993) (Fig. 11.2). This infiltration increases until the glandular parenchyma is almost completely replaced. The minor salivary glands in the oral mucosa show focal lymphocytic adenitis. Two definitions are used to facilitate quantification of inflammation in the minor salivary glands: lymphocytic focus and lymphocytic focus score. A *lymphocytic focus* is an aggregate of at least 50 lymphocytes and histiocytes. These foci are often localized near or around intralobular ducts. The *lymphocytic focus score* is defined as the number of lymphocytic foci per 4 mm^2 salivary gland tissue. A score of more than one is of diagnostic significance. Scores higher than 1 are, however, not only found in Ss, but also in other ICTDs, graft-versus-host disease, HIV infection, primary biliary cirrhosis, MG, and in 5–10% of healthy individuals. The sensitivity and specificity of a lymphocytic score > 1 as criterion for Ss are reported to be 83.5% and 81.8% respectively (Vitali *et al.*, 1993). Specificity and sensitivity increase to more than 95% when the percentage of plasma cells in the infiltrates containing IgA is lower than 70% (de Wilde *et al.*, 1989; Bodeutsch *et al.*, 1992a; Bodeutsch *et al.*, 1992b).

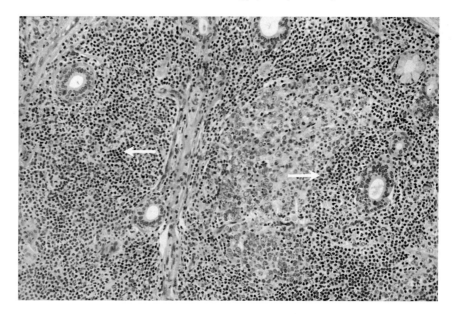

Figure 11.2 Micrograph of sublabial salivary gland in a patient with primary Sjögren's syndrome. The parenchyma of the gland is replaced by confluent lymphocytic foci (arrows). [From Moutsopoulos *et al.* (1995), with permission.]

CLINICAL FEATURES AND DIAGNOSIS

The most common clinical manifestations are dry eyes, dry mouth, fatigue, myalgia, arthralgia and arthritis, Raynaud's phenomenon, exanthema, salivary gland enlargement, vaginal dryness, and neurological and psychiatrical changes. The initial manifestations are insidious and often nonspecific. It may take as long as a decade before the disease becomes clinically manifest (Pavlidis *et al.*, 1982; Markusse, 1992). Keratoconjunctivitis sicca is not specific for Ss and may occur in a large number of other conditions (Anaya and Talal, 1997). The symptoms and signs for keratoconjunctivitis sicca are listed in Table 11.1. Several tests, including Schirmer's test, are used for measuring tear secretion.

Xerostomia is a side effect of many drugs and may be caused by autonomic neuropathy, salivary gland diseases (viral infections, sarcoidosis, chronic graft-versus-host disease), and radiation. Salivary flow rates differ considerably in normal individuals. Table 11.2 lists the symptoms and signs of xerostomia, and Table 11.3 gives the cumulative frequencies of extraglandular manifestations in pSs.

There are at least six frequently used, slightly different sets of classification criteria. Five of them have decreased secretion of lacrimal and/or salivary glands and an increased lymphocytic focus score in a lip biopsy is common (Fox *et al.*, 1986; Homma *et al.*, 1986; Manthorpe *et al.*, 1986; Skopouli *et al.*, 1986; Daniels and Talal, 1987; Vitali *et al.*, 1993; Kater and Provost, 1995). The sets differ in their criteria for decreased secretion, and do not allow classification of possible or probable Ss. At present the European set of criteria receives much support (Table 11.4) (Vitali *et al.*,

Table 11.1 Symptoms and signs of keratoconjunctivitis sicca

Symptoms
   Foreign body sensation
   Burning sensation
   Tiredness with/without difficulty in opening the eyes
   Dry feeling often with inadequate response to physical and/or chemical irritants
   Redness
   Blurred vision
   Itchiness
   Aches
   Soreness
   Photophobia
   Inability to tolerate contact lenses
Signs
   Dilatation of the bulbar conjunctival vessels
   Mild pericorneal injection
   Irregularity of the corneal image
   Discharge
   Dullness of the conjunctiva and/or cornea

From Moutsopoulos *et al.* (1995), with permission.

Table 11.2 Symptoms and signs of xerostomia

Symptoms
   Difficulty in swallowing dry food
   Inability to speak for prolonged periods
   Burning sensation
   Changes in the sense of taste
   Disturbance of nightly sleep by dry mouth
Signs
   Dry, erythematous oral mucosa
   Atrophy of the filiform tongue papillae
   Inability to express saliva from the major salivary glands or only cloudy saliva is
      expressible
   Increased dental caries
   Badly fitting dental prostheses

1993; Anaya and Talal, 1997). A method for measuring disease activity is not available.

THERAPY

As Ss is a chronic incurable disease with a wide clinical spectrum, patients should remain under regular observation to allow for early diagnosis and treatment of significant functional deterioration and signs of complications. Topical therapy is applied for dryness of the eyes, oral cavity, and skin. Dental control every six months is required for prevention and treatment of caries. pSs was previously treated with antimalarials (hydroxychloroquine), but this had no clear clinical effect (Kruize *et al.*, 1993). Severe extraglandular manifestations are treated with corticosteroids and cytostatic agents.

Table 11.3 Cumulative frequencies of extraglandular manifestations in primary Sjögren's syndrome.

Systemic manifestations	Mean (%)	Range
Arthralgia	53	9–94
Arthritis	7	0–17
Myalgias	22	0–54
Myositis	12	0–39
Skin	38	31–45
Vasculitis, cutaneous	8	3–17
Vasculitis, systemic	3	0–13
Raynaud's phenomenon	38	20–81
Pulmonary	20	8–43
Renal	12	0–38
Anaemia	6	2–10
Leukopenia	22	6–42
Lymphadenopathy	20	6–50
Splenomegaly	14	4–23
Malignant lymphoma	6	2–14
CNS disorders	6	0–13
PNS disorders	7	0–15
Gastrointestinal	10	2–24

From Anaya and Talal (1997), with permission.

PROGNOSIS

An epidemiological study of 136 women with Ss revealed that the relative risk for developing malignant non-Hodgkin's lymphoma was about 44 times higher than in the general population. For patients with a history of parotid gland enlargement, splenomegaly and lymphadenopathy were an additional risk (Kassan *et al.*, 1978). A 10-year follow-up of patients with pSs showed that the course of the disease was quite stable and that few patients developed new extraglandular manifestations or auto-immune diseases. Malignant lymphoma occurred in 9% of patients with pSs (Kruize *et al.*, 1996).

NEUROLOGY, PSYCHIATRY, AND MYOLOGY OF SJÖGREN'S SYNDROME

EPIDEMIOLOGY OF CNS DISORDERS IN pSs

The uncertainty about the percentage of patients who remain undiagnosed greatly hampers an accurate estimation of the prevalence of neurological and psychiatrical manifestations. It appears that, for many patients, symptoms of dry eyes and dry mouth are not sufficient reason to consult a physician. Ss is diagnosed only when extraglandular manifestations force the patient to ask for help, if at least the physician is sufficiently alert to ask for Ss symptoms or to perform the required investigations.

Until approximately 1980, there was only little interest in nervous system mani-

Table 11.4 European criteria for Sjögren's syndrome

Criterion	Definition
Ocular symptoms: a positive response to at least one of the three selected questions	Daily, persistent, troublesome dry eyes for more than 3 months Recurrent sensation of sand or gravel in the eyes Tear substitutes more than 3 times a day obligatory
Oral symptoms: a positive response to at least one of the three selected questions	Daily feeling of dry mouth for more than 3 months Recurrently or persistently swollen salivary glands as an adult Frequent drinking of liquids to aid in swallowing dry food
Ocular signs, *i.e.* objective evidence of ocular involvement defined as a positive result in at least one of two tests	Schirmer's I test (<5 mm in 5 min) Rose Bengal score (>4 according to van Bijsterveld's scoring system)
Histopathology: a focus score >1 in a minor salivary gland biopsy (a focus is defined as an agglomerate of at least 50 mononuclear cells around an intralobular duct; the focus score is defined by the number of foci in 4 mm² of glandular tissue)	
Salivary gland involvement: objective evidence of salivary gland involvement defined by a positive result in at least one of these three diagnostic tests	Salivary scintigraphy Parotid sialography (Fig. 11.3) Unstimulated salivary flow 1.5 ml in 15 min)
Auto-antibodies: presence in the serum of at least one of these auto-antibodies	Antibodies to Ro/SS-A or La/SS-B antigens ANA RF

Exclusion criteria: pre-existing lymphoma, acquired immunodeficiency disease (AIDS), sarcoidosis, graft-vs-host disease. Sjögren's syndrome can be diagnosed if any of 4 or more of the 6 criteria are present. This yields a sensitivity of 93% and a specificity of 93%.
From: Vitali *et al.* (1993), with permission.

festations of Ss (Pittsley and Talal, 1980; Alexander *et al.*, 1982a). This changed completely when a series of papers on a gradually expanding number of selected patients with pSs and nervous system disorders were written by Alexander and co-workers at Johns Hopkins in Baltimore (Alexander *et al.*, 1981; Alexander *et al.*, 1982a; Alexander *et al.*, 1986a). These patients were of great interest because of their unexpectedly severe CNS disease and because of a remitting and relapsing course in some of them. The Baltimore group never published a prospective study on the prevalence of nervous system disease in Ss and based their opinion in this regard on retrospective investigations. The figure they supplied came as a surprise: 20% of the patients with pSs in their institute had evidence of CNS involvement (Alexander *et al.*, 1986a). It should be stressed that the authors did not specify whether patients

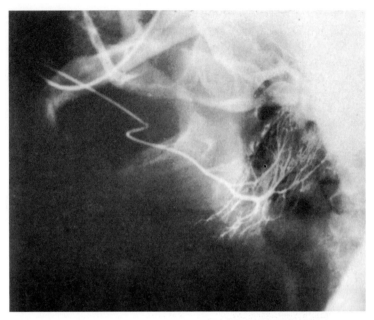

Figure 11.3A. Sialogram in a control subject. The normal salivary duct system of a salivary gland. See Fig. 11.3B.

with headache, migraine, or depression were included in this figure. The group of Andonopoulos in Greece examined 63 consecutive patients with pSs for nervous system disorders (Drosos *et al.*, 1989; Andonopoulos *et al.*, 1990). Headache, migraine, and depression were apparently left out of consideration. Several patients had evidence of peripheral neuropathy. In one patient, pSs was diagnosed when she was admitted for a stroke. In the other 62 patients, evidence of CNS disease was not present. Hietaharju *et al.* (1990) in Finland neurologically re-examined the patients with definite or probable pSs, who in a 10-year period had attended their rheumatology department, and discovered evidence for CNS involvement in eight of 48 cases: cognitive impairment (1), pyramidal tract signs (3), epilepsy (1), monocular papilloedema (1), trigeminal neuropathy (1), trigeminal neuralgia (2) and aseptic meningitis (1). Headache, depression, and migraine were probably not included. In the Netherlands, Markusse *et al.* (1992) studied charts of 450 patients who, in the period from 1975–1990, had been seen in their department and who had been suspected to suffer from pSs. The diagnosis was considered to be definite in 50 cases; these patients were re-examined in 1990. CNS disease was present or had been present in three patients: cerebrovascular 'incident' (1), transverse myelitis (1), and pyramidal tract signs (1). In addition, three patients had migraine and three others

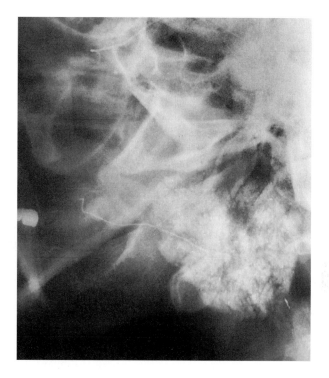

Figure 11.3B. Sialogram in a patient with primary Sjögren's syndrome. Retention of water soluble medium at endpoints of the duct system.

previously experienced depression. Moll *et al.* (1993) (from the same department as Markusse) reported on their findings in 45 consecutive patients with pSs. CNS manifestations were present in four cases: organic brain syndrome (1) (see Chapter 2 for the meaning of this term), transverse myelitis (1), stroke (1) and pyramidal signs (1). In addition, seven patients had migraine and two had depression. It may be concluded that a well-planned prospective study on the prevalence of CNS manifestations in pSs is urgently required. The prevalence figures provided by Alexander *et al.* (1986a) are relatively high. Several factors that have been mentioned as possible explanations for the discrepancy with findings in other centres are: selection bias (Andonopoulos *et al.*, 1990; Moutsopoulos *et al.*, 1993), lack of adherence to strict diagnostic criteria, and the existence of a true pSs-SLE overlap syndrome (Moutsopoulos *et al.*, 1993).

THE RANGE OF CNS MANIFESTATIONS IN pSs

No-one disputes that the range of CNS manifestations in pSs is wide, albeit probably less wide than in SLE (Table 11.5). Large vessel occlusion is probably not

Table 11.5 CNS disorders in SLE and primary Sjögren's syndrome (pSs)

CNS disorders	SLE	pSs	References pSs*
Neuropsychological syndrome	+	+/−	Malinow *et al.*, 1985, Drosos *et al.*, 1989
Headache/migraine	+	+	Pal *et al.*, 1989 Moll *et al.*, 1993
Epilepsy	+	+	Alexander *et al.*, 1982a Bansal *et al.*, 1987
TIAs	+	−	
Stroke	+	+/−	Andonopoulos *et al.*, 1990, Moll *et al.*, 1993
CNS vasculitis	+	+	Sato *et al.*, 1987, Kaltreider and Talal, 1969
Small vessel encephalitis	+	−	
Aseptic meningo-encephalitis	+	+	Alexander and Alexander, 1983, Caselli 1991
Cerebral venous thrombosis	+	+/−	Urban *et al.*, 1994
Hemiplegia, aphasia	+	+	Alexander *et al.*, 1986a, Ohtsuka *et al.*, 1995
Idiopathic intracranial hypertension	+	−	
Acute amnesia	+	−	
Chorea/ballism	+	−	
Parkinsonism	+	+	Visser *et al.*, 1993, Créange *et al.*, 1997
Optic neuropathy	+	+	Harada *et al.*, 1995, Tesar *et al.*, 1992
Inappropriate ADH secretion	+	−	
INO**, nystagmus	+	+	Alexander *et al.*, 1986a, Tesar *et al.*, 1992
Cerebellar ataxia	+	+	Alexander *et al.*, 1986a, Tesar *et al.*, 1992
Cranial neuropathies	+	+	Matsukawa *et al.*, 1995, Tesar *et al.*, 1992
Myelopathy	+	+	Alexander *et al.*, 1982b, Urban *et al.*, 1994
Neuroinfections	+	−	

*References concern only Sjögren's syndrome; **internuclear opthalmoplegia.

a feature of pSs. Small vessel encephalopathy and chorea have not been described so far. Aseptic meningo-encephalitis with perivascular inflammatory cell infiltrations in the meninges and, to a lesser extent, in the superficial layers of the brain seems a more prominent manifestation in pSs than in SLE.

DO CNS SYNDROMES IN pSs MIMICK MULTIPLE SCLEROSIS?

Alexander *et al.* (1986a) put forward that the CNS changes in pSs could mimick MS. They argued that quite a number of neurological changes, more or less characteristic for MS, occurred in a similar fashion in pSs: optic neuropathy, internuclear ophthalmoplegia (INO), and cerebellar ataxia in combination with pyramidal changes. CNS disease in pSs had, in some cases, a remitting and relapsing course, and the CSF of these patients often showed evidence of intrathecal synthesis of IgG with a raised IgG index and one or several oligoclonal bands at agar gel electrophoresis (see this Chapter, *Cerebrospinal Fluid*). In some cases, a mild degree of pleocytosis was also present, exactly as in MS. They suggested that pSs should be included in the differential diagnosis of MS, and that minor salivary gland biopsies should be taken from patients suspected of MS. These patients should also be examined for changes that are frequent in pSs but rare in MS, *i.e.* peripheral neuropathy, myositis, serological abnormalities, and cutaneous vasculitis. A remitting and relapsing course of pSs was subsequently described by other authors also in case reports (Tesar *et al.*, 1992; Caselli *et al.*, 1993; Ohtsuka *et al.*, 1995). These suggestions stimulated clinicians caring for MS patients to examine a number of them for symptoms and signs of Ss. The results were disappointing: only three out of 364 patients with definite or probable MS proved to have pSs, which is well within the range of prevalence figures of pSs in the population (Noseworthy *et al.*, 1989; Montecucco *et al.*, 1989; Metz *et al.*, 1989; Miro *et al.*, 1990; Sandberg-Wollheim *et al.*, 1992). The conclusion may be that there are apparently CNS changes in pSs that mimic MS. The number of such patients is probably very small. There is no increased frequency of pSs in cohorts of patients with MS.

ASEPTIC MENINGO-ENCEPHALITIS IN pSs

Perivascular inflammatory infiltrates in the leptomeninx and subarachnoid space are a well documented feature of Ss. de la Monte *et al.* (1983) described such infiltrates in post-mortem material in nine out of 11 cases of Ss. The infiltrates were not only present in five cases with neurological manifestations (two with pSs and three with sSs), but also in four others that were neurologically asymptomatic. The infiltrates consisted of lymphocytes, plasma cells, and variable numbers of macrophages and polymorphonuclear leucocytes. The inflammation was mild to moderate, or focal. In one case, infiltration of the leptomeninx was associated with a necrotizing vasculitis. In biopsy material of another case, the infiltrates extended into the parenchyma of the brain tissue (Caselli *et al.*, 1991).

The clinical manifestations related to this form of aseptic meningo-encephalitis are variable. In some patients, symptoms are entirely lacking, as already mentioned. Other patients complained about pain in the limbs, back and other body regions (de la Monte *et al.*, 1983; Alexander and Alexander, 1983). Recurrent episodes of fever, headache, meningismus, confusion, and even delirium and dementia were reported (Alexander and Alexander, 1983; Caselli *et al.*, 1991; Caselli *et al.*, 1993). Epilepsy, transient paresis of cranial nerves, and transverse myelitis were also present in some cases. CSF pressure was often raised. Changes in the composition of the CSF were sometimes restricted to the protein content and to evidence of intrathecal synthesis of Ig. In most cases, however, there was a moderate degree of pleocytosis with lymphocytes, plasma cells, polymorphonuclear leucocytes, and macrophages (Alexander and Alexander, 1983; de la Monte *et al.*, 1983). Results of CT scanning and angiography were, as a rule, disappointing. Gadolinium MRI is conceivably the best technique to demonstrate the changes in the blood-brain barrier in the leptomeninx and in the border-zone of the CNS parenchyma (Caselli *et al.*, 1993). However, reports in support of this suggestion are not available yet.

Diagnosis and management. Aseptic meningo-encephalitis should be considered in the differential diagnosis of every patient with Ss and CNS manifestations, whether or not there are any symptoms or signs of meningismus. The main laboratory methods to confirm or rule out the diagnosis are CSF examination and probably gadolinium MRI. Symptoms and signs of aseptic meningo-encephalitis may disappear spontaneously, and have been observed to improve after administration of moderate doses of corticosteroids (Alexander and Alexander, 1983; Caselli *et al.*, 1991; Caselli *et al.*, 1993).

CEREBRAL VENOUS THROMBOSIS IN pSs

There is one case in the literature of a woman with thrombosis of the right transverse and sigmoid sinus as demonstrated by MRI. This syndrome became manifest shortly after she had developed quadriplegia, which was presumably related to a cervical cord lesion (Urban *et al.*, 1994). She satisfied the diagnostic criteria for pSs. She had no ACAs and serum levels of antithrombin III, protein C, and protein S were normal (see Chapter, 7 to compare with venous sinus thrombosis in SLE; see also Chapter, 2). She was anticoagulated first with heparin and thereafter with warfarin. Weakness improved markedly following administration of a moderate dose of prednisone.

CEREBRAL VASCULITIS IN pSs

Vasculitis in the skin is a common finding in Ss. It may be leucocytoclastic (see Chapter 5 to compare with idiopathic cutaneous leucocytoclastic vasculitis) or exclusively mononuclear. The leucocytoclastic type is usually associated with the presence of anti Ro/SS-A and anti La/SS-B antibodies, rheumatoid factor, and ANAs. The mononuclear type of skin vasculitis is mostly seronegative (Molina *et al.*, 1985a). CNS disorders occur in patients with either type of skin vasculitis (Molina *et al.*, 1985b). Vasculitis is probably much less common in the visceral organs than in the skin. To what extent vasculitis plays a role in brain and spinal cord disease is not definitely known. Vasculitis has been documented at autopsy of patients with Sjögren's syndrome as the underlying cause of CNS disease, as appears from a few case reports (Kaltreider and Talal, 1969; Alexander *et al.*, 1982b; Sato *et al.*, 1987). According to Alexander *et al.* (1994), angiography revealed changes in 10–15% of patients with CNS disease. In some selected cases (18!), stenosis and dilatation or occlusion of predominantly small cerebral blood vessels were seen, which was compatible with vasculitis (Alexander *et al.*, 1994). Five of these 18 patients had multiple aneurysms of small blood vessels.

PSYCHIATRIC MANIFESTATIONS IN pSs

Cognitive impairment and psychiatrical manifestations are to be expected in patients with brain disease. This holds also for Ss. However, studies to document neuro-psychiatrical changes in Ss are few. Malinow *et al.* (1985) from Johns Hopkins in Baltimore performed psychiatrical examination in 40 patients. Ss was diagnosed in the large majority of these patients, following referral to Johns Hopkins for other reasons. Many patients had extraglandular manifestations, but none met criteria for other ICTDs. Sixteen patients had CNS disease. Psychiatrical evaluation disclosed that 25 patients (60%) had psychiatrical disturbances. Cognition was examined with a limited test battery in 16 patients. Attention and concentration were considered insufficient in seven patients, for reasons not specified. Control groups were not included, which limits the value of this study. Drosos *et al.* (1989) performed a psychiatrical investigation in 31 pSs patients and compared the results with those in 33 healthy women and in 41 women with malignancies. The investigation revealed some differences with the control groups (a significantly higher level of introverted hostility and higher scores on paranoid ideation, somatization, and obsessive compulsiveness), which were explained as expressions of coping difficulties with a chronic, incurable, and progressive disease.

Depression is one of the disorders mentioned in reviews of neuropsychiatrical aspects of pSs (Alexander *et al.*, 1986a; Markusse *et al.*, 1992; Moll *et al.*, 1993) and is described in case histories (Caselli *et al.*, 1993; Créange *et al.*, 1997).

Diagnosis and management. See section on depression in Chapter 7.

HEADACHE AND MIGRAINE IN pSs

There is some evidence for a higher prevalence of migraine in pSs than in controls. In an investigation by Pal *et al.* (1989), 16 of 35 patients with pSs suffered from migraine, according to data obtained from a questionnaire, compared with three of 26 controls (11%). Moll *et al.* (1993) reported that seven of 45 consecutive patients with pSs in their department (15%) had migraine. Headache is one of the complaints of patients with aseptic meningo-encephalitis; the CSF pressure in these patients is often raised (see this Chapter, *Aseptic Meningo-Encephalitis*) (Roos, 1997).

Diagnosis and Management. See section on headache in Chapter 7.

EPILEPSY

Partial epilepsy and secondary generalized epilepsy may occur in patients with Ss, as appears from studies of groups of patients with Ss and from reviews (Alexander *et al.*, 1982b; Alexander and Alexander, 1983; Hietaharju *et al.*, 1990a; Alexander *et al.*, 1994). A single case of epilepsia partialis continua has been described (Bansal *et al.*, 1987).

Diagnosis and management. See section on epilepsy in Chapter 2.

FOCAL CEREBRAL DISORDERS IN pSs

Hemiparesis, hemidysaesthesia, aphasia, internuclear ophthalmoplegia, and ataxia have been reported by several authors in selected patients (Alexander *et al.*, 1982a; Alexander *et al.*, 1986a; Kontttinen *et al.*, 1987; Alexander *et al.*, 1988; Wise and Agudelo, 1988; Ohtsuka *et al.*, 1995). Onset and course of these disorders are, in most articles, not described in detail and the age of the patients is not always given, which is a pity since Ss often affects old people with an increased risk of cerebrovascular disorders. Focal cerebral changes in pSs occur either subacutely or gradually. They are often transient or react favourably to therapy with corticosteroids mostly. Findings at CT scans and MRI are compatible with infarcts or inflammatory lesions (Wise and Agudelo, 1988; Alexander *et al.*, 1988; Alexander *et al.*, 1994; Ohtsuka *et al.*, 1995). Focal cerebral disorders were not observed in retrospective or prospective investigations (Andonoupolos *et al.*, 1990; Hietaharju *et al.*, 1990; Markusse *et al.*, 1992; Moll *et al.*, 1993, Kruize *et al.*, 1996). Stroke has been reported in 2 cases however (Andonopoulos *et al.*, 1990; Moll *et al.*, 1993).

PARKINSONISM IN pSs

There have been two case reports on parkinsonism in patients with pSs. One concerned a 55-year-old woman with left sided hemiparkinsonism who at MRI showed linear lesions with increased signal intensity on T2-weighted images in the contralateral striatum (Visser *et al.*, 1993). The CSF was not examined. The second report was about a 44-year-old woman with a progressive Parkinson syndrome, normal CSF, and at MRI two symmetrical high-intensity signals on T2-weighted images in the posterior parts of the globus pallidus (Créange *et al.*, 1997). The lesions in the basal ganglia were considered as possibly related to inflammatory changes and did not resemble infarcts. In both studies, a relation of the clinical features with the MRI lesions seemed likely. Such lesions are not seen in idiopathic Parkinson disease.

Management. The first patient did not respond to a moderate dose of corticosteroids. The second patient improved slightly after a high dose of intravenous (IV) methyl-prednisolone (1 g daily for 3 days) and a five day course of IVIG (20 g daily). This second patient did not respond to repeat courses of IVIG, a moderate daily dose of prednisone, intravenous cyclophosphamide, and L-DOPA.

OPTIC NEUROPATHY IN pSs

Transient monocular visual loss was first described by Alexander *et al.* (1982a and 1986a). In 1986 an article appeared in the Japanese literature on optic neuritis in Ss (Shimode *et al.*, 1986). Since then, at least seven other reports were published. The descriptions were remarkable because of the variable course of the disease and the complexity of the associated CNS manifestations (Wise and Agudelo, 1988; Tesar *et al.*, 1992; Harada *et al.*, 1995). There was not sufficient evidence for MS or SLE in any of these patients. In six of seven cases, both eyes were affected, either one after the other or both eyes simultaneously. In some cases, visual loss came about suddenly, suggesting a vascular cause, and was preceded or accompanied by orbital or retro-orbital pain. Two patients discovered loss of vision in one eye in the morning on awakening. In several instances, episodes of blurred vision or visual loss were remitting and relapsing. Ophthalmological investigation revealed optic disc oedema in one or both eyes of four patients, and in later stages there was optic nerve atrophy. Myelopathy was associated with optic neuropathy in two patients. There were signs of brainstem and possible basal ganglia involvement in one, and pyra-midal signs with multiple cranial neuropathies in another case as well. One other patient had intermittent paraesthesiae on one side of the body for several years.

Diagnosis and management. Routine neurological and ophthalmological investiga-tions in addition to MRI of the optic nerves and the chiasm are required. CSF exam-ination is advisable to demonstrate or rule out aseptic meningitis. In case histories published so far, loss of vision seemed to respond favourably to IV methylpred-nisolone 1 g/day for 3 days or to IV pulse-dose of cyclophosphamide, in some instances. Spontaneous improvement was observed as well (see Chapter 2 *Optic Neuritis*, diagnosis and treatment).

CRANIAL NEUROPATHY IN pSs

Sensory trigeminal neuropathy is relatively frequent among the cranial neuro-pathies in Ss (Kaltreider and Talal, 1969; Grant *et al.*, 1997). It causes a disturbance of sensation in the second or third division of the trigeminal nerve or in all three terri-tories (Hughes, 1993). It may remain unilateral but often it becomes bilateral. Motor functions are nearly always preserved. Taste may be impaired also. In many patients, onset is subacute and may be followed by a slowly progressive course. Trigeminal neuropathy in pSs often forms part of a larger neurological syndrome with symptoms and signs of sensory neuronopathy at one or several limbs and the trunk (Sobue *et al.*, 1993) (see this Chapter, *Sensory Neuronopathy*). In a minority of the patients, trigeminal neuropathy is transient, but in most cases it is permanent. According to the experience of Hughes (1993), patients are usually not distressed too much by facial numbness. Electrophysiological investigations (Förster *et al.*, 1996), MRI (Förster *et al.*, 1996; Rorick *et al.*, 1996), and histological studies (Hughes, 1993) all point to an inflammatory disorder of the ganglion Gasseri and the preganglionic part of the Vth nerve (see Chapter 2). Trigeminal neuralgia has also been reported in patients with pSs (Hietaharju *et al.*, 1990), and may be due to a lesion in the root entry zone of the trigeminal nerve in the pons (Hughes, 1993).

Other cranial nerves that are occasionally affected in Ss are the nn VI, III, VII, VIII, IV and IX in that order of frequency (Attwood and Poser, 1961; Alexander and Alexander, 1983; Alexander *et al.*, 1986a; Tesar *et al.*, 1992; Moll *et al.*, 1993; Matsukawa *et al.*, 1995; Grant *et al.*, 1997). For unknown reasons, the three lowest cranial nerves are only very rarely involved, exactly as in SLE. Multiple and recurrent cranial neuropathies have been reported as well (Attwood and Poser, 1961; Alexander and Alexander, 1983; Vincent *et al.*, 1985; Pou Serradel and Vinas Gaya, 1993). The cause of the cranial neuropathies is obscure in most cases. In a few patients, a relation with aseptic meningitis was likely (Alexander and Alexander, 1983).

Management. Trigeminal neuropathy is resistant to common forms of therapy with corticosteroids or cytostatic agents. The question is, however, whether rapid interventions shortly after onset with IV methylprednisolone or IV pulse-dose cyclophosphamide will also be ineffective. For obscure reasons, other cranial neuropathies (except optic neuropathy) are mostly transient (Alexander *et al.*, 1983; Tesar *et al.*, 1992; Matsukawa *et al.*, 1995).

TRANSVERSE MYELITIS OR MYELOPATHY IN pSs

Spinal cord lesions in pSs are mentioned in overviews of selected cases (Alexander *et al.*, 1986a; Moll *et al.*, 1993), and are described in case reports (Alexander *et al.*, 1982b; Konttinen *et al.*, 1987; Urban *et al.*, 1994; Harada *et al.*, 1995). The clinical features, course of the disease, and the outcome all resemble transverse myelitis in SLE (see Chapters 2 and 7, sections on *Transverse Myelitis*). The pathogenesis is usually presumed to be vasculitis or vasculopathy and is even less well understood than in SLE. A patient described by Konttinen *et al.* (1987) is of interest because of the association of transverse myelitis and aseptic meningitis. Another patient with transverse myelitis and aseptic meningitis is mentioned by Alexander and Alexander, (1983).

Diagnosis and management. Diagnosis is based primarily on neurological examination and may be confirmed by MRI. There are case reports of favourable results using early and vigorous immunosuppression with intravenous corticosteroid or cyclophosphamide pulse therapy for transverse myelitis in SLE (Baca *et al.*, 1996; Harisdangkui *et al.*, 1995) (see Chapters 2 and 7, sections on *Transverse Myelitis*).

EPIDEMIOLOGY OF PERIPHERAL NERVE LESIONS IN pSs

The generally held opinion is that peripheral nerve disorders are more common than CNS disorders. In 43 consecutive cases of pSs without other relevant diseases (*e.g.* diabetes mellitus), 11 had evidence of polyneuropathy (Moll *et al.*, 1993). In a retrospective investigation of 48 cases, 10 had peripheral nerve disorders (entrapment neuropathy and radiculopathy not included) (Hietaharju *et al.*, 1990). In yet another series of 46 consecutive patients, 10 had peripheral neuropathy (Gemignani *et al.*, 1994). Peripheral nerve disorders in pSs are strikingly heterogeneous (Kaplan *et al.*, 1990). There are sensory and sensori-motor neuropathies, sensory neurono-pathies (or polygangliopathies), chronic inflammatory demyelinating polyneuro-pathies (CIDP), autonomic neuropathies, multiple mononeuropathy, and cranial neuropathies. The last mentioned type has already been discussed in the foregoing. Entrapment neuropathies, more specifically carpal tunnel syndrome (CTS), are mentioned in several reviews on neurological disorders in Ss. Ss is, however, a disease of predominantly middle aged women and the prevalence of CTS among women at this age is high (9.2%) (de Krom *et al.*, 1992). In our view, CTS is not very likely to be related to Ss and will therefore not be discussed.

SENSORY AND SENSOMOTOR AXONAL POLYNEUROPATHIES IN pSs

Sensory or sensomotor polyneuropathy is the most frequent form of polyneuro-pathy in Ss, and is the presenting feature in some cases (Grant *et al.*, 1997; Mellgren *et al.*, 1989). The main clinical characteristics of this neuropathy are sensory distur-bances of vital (small sensory nerve fibres) and gnostic (large sensory nerve fibres) qualities in a symmetrical distribution. The changes are predominantly distal and affect the lower limbs more than the upper limbs. Some degree of motor involve-ment (weakness) is present in a minority of the patients. In occasional patients, sen-sory loss concerns predominantly small sensory nerve fibre qualities (Grant *et al.*, 1997). Signs of autonomic changes are not rare (see below). The CSF is normal or shows a slight rise of protein content and a minor degree of pleocytosis very occa-sionally (Grant *et al.*, 1997; Mellgren *et al.*, 1989). This neuropathy is axonal in origin, as demonstrated by electrophysiological and histological examinations (Gemignani *et al.*, 1994; Grant *et al.*, 1997). The pathogenetic mechanism is obscure. Sural nerve biopsies often reveal small or moderate perivascular mononuclear cell infiltrates in the epineurium (Kaltreider and Talal, 1969; Mellgren *et al.*, 1989; Gemignani *et al.*, 1994; Grant *et al.*, 1997). There is no evidence at present for the assumption that these predominantly sensory polyneuropathies are all due to ischaemia, induced by necrotizing vasculitis (see, however, this Chapter, *Mononeuritis Multiplex*).

Van Dijk *et al.* (1997) discovered three cases (all female) of pSs in a group of 49 patients with chronic idiopathic axonal polyneuropathy (CIAP), which was proba-bly slightly more than might be expected on the basis of prevalence figures of Ss in the population (Jacobson *et al.*, 1989). The authors suggested that in all women with CIAP a full workup for Ss should be performed. In males with CIAP, this is advisable only when ocular or oral sicca symptoms are present.

Management. Intervention studies on effects of therapy have not been performed. We refrain from immunosuppressive therapy as long as symptoms are mild. In more severe and progressive cases, we prescribe corticosteroids or corticosteroids in combination with a cytostatic agent like for instance azathioprine (see Chapter 4 for dosages and side effects).

MONONEURITIS MULTIPLEX IN pSs

Mononeuritis multiplex in pSs has been demonstrated convincingly in case reports (Kaltreider and Talal, 1969; Pou Serradell and Vinas Gaya, 1993), but is probably rare.

Three of 53 patients with sicca complex and peripheral neuropathy had mononeuritis multiplex (Grant *et al.*, 1997). Sural nerve biopsies from these three patients revealed necrotizing arteritis in one case and probable necrotizing arteritis in another. Kaltreider and Talal (1969) established peripheral neuropathy in nine out of 109 cases of Ss, and diagnosed mononeuritis multiplex in one case. Gemignani *et al.* (1994) discovered peripheral neuropathy in 10 of 46 consecutive patients with pSs; one had multiple mononeuropathy. The observation of vasculitis-induced multiple neuropathy in pSs makes it likely that at least some of the cases of predominantly sensory polyneuropathy are also due to vasculitis. Sufficient data on effects of therapy are not available.

SENSORY NEURONOPATHY IN pSs

Sensory neuronopathy or ganglionitis is an inflammatory disorder of the dorsal root ganglia and probably often the autonomic ganglia (see Chapter 2, *Sensory Neuronopathy*) (Malinow *et al.*, 1986; Font *et al.*, 1990; Griffin *et al.*, 1990; Kaplan and Schaumburg, 1991; Sobue *et al.*, 1993). Sensory neuronopathy in pSs differs from sensory polyneuropathy by (1) a more rapid onset in most cases, (2) asymmetry at least at onset, (3) pseudoathetosis and other signs of severe disturbance of gnostic sensation, and (4) somewhat more prominent autonomic dysfunction, comprising Adie's pupils, widespread anhidrosis, cardiac arrhythmia and abnormal responses to Valsalva test (Griffin *et al.*, 1990; Sobue *et al.*, 1993, Kumazawa *et al.*, 1993, Grant *et al.*, 1997). The protein content of the CSF may be slightly raised and the cell content is usually normal. Sensory neuronopathy in pSs differs clinically from the idiopathic and carcinomatous sensory neuronopathies by being more frequent in women and by more prominent autonomic manifestations. A relation with a specific antibody has not been detected. Biopsies from dorsal root ganglia (Malinow *et al.*, 1986; Griffin *et al.*, 1990) show degeneration and loss of sensory neurones and mononuclear cell infiltrates throughout the ganglia and around nerve cell bodies and blood vessels. The inflammatory cells are mainly CD8+ T-cells (T-cells in the salivary glands are predominantly CD4+ cells!). The sural nerve in this disorder shows characteristic changes if it is in an affected part of the body. In the acute stage, there is Wallerian degeneration; in late stages, the predominant abnormality is loss of large sensory nerve fibres. There is little evidence of regeneration. In some cases, perivascular mononuclear cell infiltrates are present in the epineurium. Griffin *et al.* (1990) stress that they have not observed necrotizing vasculitis in any of the 12 sural nerve biopsies they have examined.

Management. There are no publications on intervention studies. Treatment with corticosteroids or by immunosuppression is reputedly unsuccessful. In view of the neuronal (axonal) degeneration in this condition, the chances of a beneficial effect of treatment are likely to decrease the longer the condition exists. Attempts to influence the course of the disorder should therefore concentrate on early diagnosis. Intravenous methylprednisolone, cyclophosphamide or intravenous immunoglobulin infusions offer the best chance on a rapid beneficial effect.

AUTONOMIC NEUROPATHY IN pSs

Autonomic dysfunction is only rarely symptomatic. In a retrospective study of 53 patients with sicca complex and peripheral neuropathy (of whom 21 had been screened for autonomic dysfunction), only one patient was discovered with symptoms due to autonomic dysfunction. Symptomatic sudomotor dysfunction seems to be the most frequent abnormality (Grant *et al.*, 1997). Adie's pupils have also been reported.

CHRONIC INFLAMMATORY DEMYELINATING POLYNEUROPATHY (CIDP) IN pSs

At least five patients have been reported with CIDP associated to pSs (Gross, 1987, 1 case; Léger *et al.*, 1991, 1 case; Pou Serradell and Vinas Gaya, 1993, 1 case; Grant *et al.*, 1997, 2 cases). Associations of two immune-mediated conditions are not likely to be fortuitous. Genetic predisposition to auto-immune reactions may be a (or the) reason for such combinations.

EPIDEMIOLOGY AND CLINICAL FEATURES OF POLYMYOSITIS IN pSs

According to some authors, up to one third of the patients with pSs complain about myalgia. Clinical evidence of muscle disease is usually lacking (Martinez-Lavin *et al.*, 1979). Muscle biopsies from asymptomatic cases of pSs often reveal inflammatory, predominantly perivascular, infiltrates of mononuclear cells (Vrethem *et al.*, 1990). Clinical symptoms and signs of polymositis (PM) with weakness of proximal limb muscles are, however, rare (Gran and Myclebust, 1992; Kraus *et al.*, 1994). Weakness (when present) is localized predominantly proximal at the lower limbs and is not associated with skin abnormalities, as it is in dermatomysitis (DM). Biopsies from these cases show inflammatory mononuclear infiltrates and degeneration and regeneration of muscle fibres. Skin purpura, compatible with skin vasculitis, is present occasionally. PM in pSs has no specific features, either clinically, pathologically, or serologically.

Management. A beneficial effect of corticosteroid treatment on symptoms of PM has been reported (see Chapter 6, *Treatment of Dermatomyositis and Polymyositis*).

CEREBROSPINAL FLUID IN pSs

The CSF in patients with active CNS disease is, in most cases, abnormal and provides evidence for an immunologically-mediated process. This conclusion is based on findings by Alexander *et al.* (1986b) in a group of 50 patients, 30 of whom had active CNS disease. These 30 patients had an elevated IgG index, one or more oligoclonal bands at agargel electrophoresis, or both. Similar discrete bands at agargel electrophoresis were not present in serum. An elevated IgG index, oligoclonal bands, or both were present in only seven of 20 patients without active CNS disease. Fifty percent of the patients with active CNS disease had a slight increase of white blood cells in the CSF; cytological investigation revealed the presence of lymphocytes, plasma cells, and other mononuclear cells in 60%. These findings all support intrathecal synthesis of IgG.

AUTO–ANTIBODIES IN PATIENTS WITH pSs AND NERVOUS SYSTEM DISEASE

Why do a minority of patients with pSs develop nervous system manifestations? One possible mechanism might involve auto-antibodies. Moll *et al.* (1993) discovered antineuronal auto-antibodies more frequently in patients with pSs and nervous system disease than in pSs patients without nervous system disease. Antineuronal antibodies were not present in sera of control groups. Anti-Ro/SS-A antibodies were found by the same authors in 63% of patients with nervous system involvement and in an almost similar percentage (71%) of other patients with pSs. Alexander *et al.* (1994) examined the relation between anti-Ro/SS-A antibodies in pSs with CNS disease. It appeared that in patients with established, active CNS disease, anti-Ro/SS-A antibodies occurred more frequently than in pSs patients without CNS disease. Significant CNS disease was, however, also present in some seronegative patients.

IMAGING OF THE CENTRAL NERVOUS SYSTEM

MRI of 16 patients with CNS disease showed many more lesions than MRI in 22 patients without signs of CNS disease (Alexander *et al.*, 1988). Most of these lesions were small distinct areas of increased signal intensity on T2-weighted images. These small lesions were seen more often in the subcortical white matter than in the grey matter. Larger focal areas of increased signal intensity in T2-weighted images that were consistent with oedema, demyelination, or infarcts were present also. CT scanning revealed the presence of infarcts in some cases. Vascular changes of small intracerebral vessels that were consistent with, but did not prove, vasculitis were seen at angiography (Alexander *et al.*, 1994).

PATHOGENETIC MECHANISMS

There is some, still very weak evidence for a role of antibodies in the nervous system disorders in pSs (see this Chapter, *Antibodies*). Studies on the pathology of CNS changes in pSs are few (Kaltreider and Talal, 1969; Alexander *et al.*, 1982b; de la Monte *et al.*, 1983; Caselli *et al.*, 1991). Mononuclear inflammatory cell infiltrates and vasculitis are observed. At present, it is not known to what extent each of these changes is responsible for the clinical signs. Mononuclear inflammatory cell infiltrates are seen also in the PNS and in the musculature. Vasculitis seems exceptional. Axonal (neuronal) degeneration is more frequent in the PNS than demyelination.

CONCLUSIONS

CNS changes occur occasionally in pSs, as authors from several centres have reported, and are very heterogeneous. In many ways, these changes are similar to those in SLE. The changes are likely due to auto-immune processes. pSs should be included in the differential diagnosis of patients with unexplained CNS disease. PNS manifestations are also heterogeneous and occur in a sizable minority of pSs patients. They may be the presenting feature of pSs. Our present knowledge on nervous system manifestations in pSs is still very incomplete, especially concerning effects of therapy and outcome. A clinical syndrome of PM in pSs is rare.

REFERENCES

Alexander EL (1986) Central nervous system (CNS) manifestations of primary Sjögren's syndrome: An overview. *Scand J Rheumatol* **61** (suppl), 161–165.

Alexander EL and Alexander GE (1983) Aseptic meningoencephalitis in primary Sjögren's syndrome. *Neurology* **33**, 593–598.

Alexander GE, Stevens MB, Provost TT *et al* (1981) Sjögren syndrome: Central nervous system manifestations. *Neurology* **31**, 1391–1396.

Alexander EL, Provost TT, Stevens MB *et al* (1982a) Neurologic complications of primary Sjögren's syndrome. *Medicine* **61**, 247–257.

Alexander EH, Craft C, Dorsch C *et al* (1982b) Necrotising arteritis and spinal subarachnoid hemorrhage in Sjögren syndrome. *Ann Neurol* **11**, 632–635.

Alexander EL, Malinow K, Lejewski JE *et al* (1986a) Primary Sjögren's syndrome with central nervous system disease mimicking multiple sclerosis. *Ann Int Med* **104**, 323–330.

Alexander EL, Lijeski JE, Jerdan MS *et al* (1986b) Evidence of an immunopathogenetic basis for central nervous system disease in primary Sjögren's syndrome. *Arthritis Rheum* **29**, 1223–1231.

Alexander EL, Beall SS, Gordon B *et al* (1988) Magnetic resonance imaging of cerebral lesions in patients with Sjögren syndrome. *Ann Int Med* **108**, 815–823.

Alexander EL, Ranzenbach MR, Kumar AJ *et al* (1994) Anti-Ro (SS-A) autoantibodies in central nervous system disease associated with Sjögren's syndrome (CNS-SS): Clinical, neuroimaging, and angiographic correlates. *Neurology* **44**, 899–908.

Anaya JM and Talal N (1997) Sjögren's syndrome and connective tissue diseases associated with other immunologic disorders. In: Koopman WJ (ed) *Arthritis and Allied Conditions. A Textbook of Rheumatology*, vol 2, 13th ed, pp 1561–1580. Baltimore: Williams and Wilkins.

Anaya JM, Ogawa N and Talal N (1995a) Sjögren's syndrome in childhood. *J Rheumatol* **22**, 1152–1158.

Anaya JM, Liu GT, D'Souza E *et al* (1995b) Sjögren's syndrome in men. *Ann Rheum Dis* **54**, 748–751.

Andonoupolos AP, Lagos G, Drosos AA *et al* (1990) The spectrum of neurological involvement in Sjögren's syndrome. *Brit J Rheumatol* **29**, 21–23.

Attwood W and Poser C (1961) Neurologic complications of Sjögren's syndrome. *Neurology (Minneap)* **11**, 1034–1041.

Baca V, Sanchez-Vaca G, Martinez I *et al* (1996) Successful treatment of transverse myelitis in a child with lupus erythematosus. *Neuropaediatrics* **27**, 42–44.

Bansal SK, Sawhney IMS and Chopra JS (1987) Epilepsia partialis continua in Sjögren's syndrome. *Epilepsia* **28**, 362–363.

Bodeutsch C, De Wilde PCM, Kater L *et al* (1992a) Quantitative immunohistologic criteria are superior to the lymphocytic focus score criterion for the diagnosis of Sjögren's syndrome. *Arthritis Rheum* **35**, 1075–1087.

Bodeutsch C, De Wilde PCM, Kater L *et al* (1992b) Quantitative immunohistologic study of lip biopsies. Evaluation of diagnostic and prognostic value in Sjögren's syndrome. *Path Res Pract* **188**, 599–602.

Caselli RJ, Scheithauer BW, Bowles CA *et al* (1991) The treatable dementia of Sjögren's syndrome. *Ann Neurol* **30**, 98–101.

Caselli RJ, Scheithauer BW, O'Duffy JD *et al* (1993) Chronic inflammatory meningoencephalitis should not be mistaken for Alzheimer's disease. *Mayo Clin Proc* **68**, 846–853.

Créange A, Brugières P, Voisin M-C *et al* (1997) Primary Sjögren's syndrome presenting as progressive Parkinsonian syndrome. *Mov Disord* **12**, 121–123.

Daniels TE and Talal N (1987) Diagnosis and differential diagnosis of Sjögren's syndrome. In: Talal N, Moutsopoulos HM and Kassan SS (eds) *Sjögren's Syndrome. Clinical and Immunological Aspects*, pp 193–199. Berlin: Springer.

de Krom MCTFM, Knipschild PG, Kester ADM *et al* (1992) Carpal tunnel syndrome. Prevalence in the general population. *J Clin Epidemiol* **45**, 373–375.

de la Monte SM, Hutchins GM and Gupta PK (1983) Polymorphous meningitis with atypical mononuclear cells in Sjögren's syndrome. *Ann Neurol* **14**, 455–461.

de Wilde PCM, Kater L, Baak JPA *et al* (1989) A new and highly sensitive immunohistologic diagnostic criterion for Sjögren's syndrome. *Arthritis Rheum* **32**, 1214–1220.

Drosos AA, Andonopoulos AP, Lagos *et al* (1989) Neuropsychiatric abnormalities in primary Sjögren's syndrome. *Clin Exp Rheum* **7**, 207–209.

Font J, Valls J, Cervera R, *et al* (1990) Pure sensory neuropathy in patients with primary Sjögren's syndrome: Clinical, immunological, and electromyographic findings. *Ann Rheum Dis* **49**, 775–778.

Förster C, Brandt MD, Meink HM *et al* (1996) Trigeminal sensory neuropathy in connective tissue disease; Evidence for the site of the lesion. *Neurology* **46**, 270–271.

Fox RI (1996) Clinical features, pathogenesis, and treatment of Sjögren's syndrome. *Curr Opin Rheumatol* **8**, 438–445.

Fox RI, Robinson C, Curd J *et al* (1986) Sjögren's syndrome. Proposed criteria for classification. *Arthritis Rheum* **29**, 577–585.

Gemignani F, Marbini A, Pavesi G *et al* (1994) Peripheral neuropathy associated with primary Sjögren's syndrome. *J Neurol Neurosurg Psychiat* **57**, 983–986.

Gran JT and Myclebust G (1992) The concomitant occurrence of Sjögren's syndrome and polymyositis. *Scand J Rheumatol* **21**, 150–154.

Grant IA, Hunder GG, Homburger HA *et al* (1997) Peripheral neuropathy associated with sicca complex. *Neurology* **48**, 855–862.

Griffin JW, Cornblath DR, Alexander MD *et al* (1990) Ataxic sensory neuropathy and dorsal root ganglionitis associated with Sjögren's syndrome. *Ann Neurol* **27**, 304–315.

Gross M (1987) Chronic relapsing inflammatory polyneuropathy complicating sicca syndrome. *J Neurol Neurosurg Psychiat* **50**, 939–940.

Harada T, Ohashi T, Miyagishi R *et al* (1995) Optic neuropathy and acute transverse myelopathy in primary Sjögren's syndrome. *Jpn J Ophthalmol* **39**, 162–165.

Harisdangkui V, Doorenbos D and Subramony SH (1995) Lupus transverse myelopathy: Better outcome with early recognition and aggressive high dose intravenous corticosteroid pulse treatment. *J Neurol* **242**, 326–331.

Hietaharju A, Yli-Kerttula U, Häkkinen V *et al* (1990) Nervous system manifestation in Sjögren's syndrome. *Acta Neurol Scand* **81**, 144–152.

Homma M, Tojo T and Akizuki M (1986) Criteria for Sjögren's syndrome in Japan. *Scand J Rheumatol* **61**(Suppl), 26–27.

Hughes RAC (1993) Diseases of the fifth cranial nerve. In: Dyck PJ, Thomas PK, Griffin JW *et al* (eds) *Peripheral Neuropathy*, vol 2, 3rd ed, pp 801–817. Philadelphia: WB Saunders.

Jacobson LTH, Axell TE, Hansen BU *et al* (1989) An epidemiological study in Swedish adults with special reference to primary Sjögren's syndrome. *J Autoimmunity* **2**, 521–527.

Kaltreider HB and Talal N (1969) The neuropathy of Sjögren's syndrome. Trigeminal nerve involvement. *Ann Int Med* **70**, 751–762.

Kaplan JG, Rosenberg R, Reinitz E *et al* (1990) Invited review: Peripheral neuropathy in Sjögren's syndrome. *Muscle Nerve* **13**, 570–579.

Kaplan JG and Schaumburg HH (1991) Predominantly unilateral sensory neuronopathy in Sjögren's syndrome. *Neurology* **41**, 948–949.

Kassan SS, Thomas TL, Moutsopoulos HM *et al* (1978) Increased risk of lymphoma in Sjögren's syndrome. *Ann Intern Med* **43**, 50–65.

Kater L and de Wilde PCM (1992) New developments in Sjögren's syndrome. *Curr Opin Rheumatol* **4**, 657–665.

Kater L and Provost TT (1995) Classification criteria, disease activity criteria and chronicity criteria. In: Kater L and Baart de la Faille H (eds) *Multi-Systemic Auto-Immune Diseases: An Integrated Approach*, pp 43–59. Amsterdam: Elsevier.

Konttinen YT, Kinnunen E, Bonsdorff von M *et al* (1987) Acute transverse myelopathy successfully treated with plasmapheresis and prednisone in a patient with primary Sjögren's syndrome. *Arthritis Rheum* **30**, 339–344.

Kraus A, Cifuentes M, Villa AR *et al* (1994) Myositis in primary Sjögren's syndrome. Report of 3 cases. *J Rheumatol* **21**, 649–653.

Kruize AA, Hené RJ, Kallenberg CGM *et al* (1993) Hydroxychloroquine treatment for primary Sjögren's syndrome: A two year, double blind crossover trial. *Ann Rheum Dis* **52**, 360–364.

Kruize AA, Hené RJ, van der Heide A *et al* (1996) Long-term follow up of patients with Sjögren's syndrome. *Arthritis Rheum* **39**, 297–303.

Kumazawa K, Sobue G, Yamamoto K *et al* (1993) Segmental anhidrosis in the spinal dermatomes in Sjögren's syndrome-associated neuropathy. *Neurology* **43**, 1820–1823.

Léger JM, Bouche P, Wechsler B *et al* (1991) Peripheral neuropathy in primary Sjögren syndrome: A prospective and retrospective study. *Neurology* **41**(Suppl), 132.

Malinow KL, Molina R, Gordon B *et al* (1985) Neuropsychiatric dysfunction in primary Sjögren's syndrome. *Ann Int Med* **103**, 344–349.

Malinow K, Yannakakis GD, Glusman SM *et al* (1986) Subacute sensory neuronopathy secondary to dorsal root ganglionitis in primary Sjögren's syndrome. *Ann Neurol* **20**, 535–537.

Manoussakis MN, Tzioufas AG, Pange PJE *et al* (1986) Serological profiles in subgroups of patients with Sjögren's syndrome. *Scand J Rheumatol* **61**(Suppl), 89–92.

Manthorpe R, Oxholm P, Prause JU *et al* (1986) The Copenhagen criteria for Sjögren's syndrome. *Scand J Rheumatol* **61** (Suppl), 19–21.

Markusse HM (1992) *Primary Sjögren's syndrome in rheumatology. Clinical and diagnostic aspects.* PhD Thesis. University of Leiden.

Markusse HM, Oudkerk M, Vroom TM *et al* (1992) Primary Sjögren's syndrome: Clinical spectrum and mode of presentation based on an analysis of 50 patients selected from a department of rheumatology. *Neth J Med* **40**, 125–134.

Martinez-Lavin M, Vaughan JH and Tan EM (1979) Autoantibodies and the spectrum of Sjögren's syndrome. *Ann Int Med* **91**, 185–190.

Matsukawa Y, Nishinarita S, Horie T *et al* (1995) Abducens and trochlear palsies in a patient with Sjögren's syndrome. *Brit J Rheumatol* **34**, 484–485.

Mellgren SI, Conn DL, Stevens C *et al* (1989) Peripheral neuropathy in primary Sjögren's syndrome. *Neurology* **39**, 390–394.

Metz LM, Seland TP and Fritzler MJ (1989) An analysis of the frequency of Sjögren's syndrome in a population of multiple sclerosis patients. *J Clin Lab Immunol* **30**, 121–125.

Miro J, Pena-Sagredo JL, Berciano J *et al* (1990) Prevalence of primary Sjögren's syndrome in patients with multiple sclerosis. *Ann Neurol* **27**, 582–584.

Molina R, Provost TT and Alexander EL (1985a) Two types of inflammatory vascular disease in Sjögren's syndrome. *Arthritis Rheum* **28**, 1251–1258.

Molina R, Provost TT and Alexander EL (1985b) Peripheral inflammatory vascular disease in Sjögren's syndrome. Association with nervous system complications. *Arthritis Rheum* **28**, 1341–1347.

Moll JWB, Markusse HM, Pijnenburg JJJM *et al* (1993) Antineuronal antibodies in patients with neurologic complications of primary Sjögren's syndrome. *Neurology* **43**, 2574–2581.

Montecucco C, Franciotta DM, Caporali R *et al* (1989) Sicca syndrome and anti-SSA/Ro antibodies in patients with suspected or definite multiple sclerosis. *Scand J Rheumatol* **18**, 407–412.

Moutsopoulos HM, Sarmas JH and Talal N (1993) Is central nervous system involvement a systemic manifestation of primary Sjögren's syndrome. *Rheum Dis Clin North Amer* **19**, 909–912.

Moutsopoulos HM, Velthuis PJ, de Wilde PCM *et al* (1995) Sjögren's syndrome. In: Kater L and Baart de la Faille H (eds) *Multisystemic Auto-Immune Disease*, pp 173–205. Amsterdam: Elsevier.

Moutsopoulos HM, Chused TM, Mann DL *et al* (1980) Sjögren's syndrome (sicca syndrome): Current issues. *Ann Int Med* **92**, 212–226.

Moutsopoulos HM, Webber BL, Vlagopoulos TP *et al* (1979) Differences in the clinical manifestations of the sicca syndrome in the presence and absence of rheumatoid arthritis. *Am J Med* **66**, 733–736.

Noseworthy JH, Bass BH, Vandervoort MK *et al* (1989) The prevalence of primary Sjögren's syndrome in a multiple sclerosis population. *Ann Neurol* **25**, 95–98.

Ohtsuka T, Saito Y, Hasegawa M *et al* (1995) Central nervous system disease in a child with primary Sjögren's syndrome. *J Pediatr* **127**, 961–963.

Pal B, Gibson C, Passmore J *et al* (1989) A study of headaches and migraine in Sjögren's syndrome and other rheumatic disorders. *Ann Rheum Dis* **48**, 312–316.

Pavlidis NA, Karsh J and Moutsopoulos HM (1982) The clinical picture of primary Sjögren's syndrome. A retrospective study. *J Rheumatol* **9**, 685–690.

Pittsley RA and Talal N (1980) Neuromuscular complications of Sjögren's syndrome. In: Vinken PJ and Bruyn GW (eds) *Handbook of Clinical Neurology*, vol 39, pp 419–433. Amsterdam: North-Holland Publishing Co.

Pou Serradell A and Vinas Gaya J (1993) Trois cas de neuropathies périphériques rares associées au syndromes de Gougerot-Sjögren's primitif. *Rev Neurol* **149**, 481–484.

Reveille JD, Wilson RW, Provost TT *et al* (1984) Primary Sjögren's syndrome and other autoimmune diseases in families. Prevalence and immunogenetic studies in 6 kindreds. *Ann Int Med* **101**, 748–756.

Roos KL (1997) Viral meningitis and aseptic meningitis. In: Roos KL (ed) *Central Nervous System Infectious Diseases and Therapy*, pp 127–139. New York: Marcel Dekker.

Rorick MB, Chandar K and Colombi BJ (1996) Inflammatory trigeminal sensory neuropathy mimicking trigeminal neurinoma. *Neurology* **46**, 1455–1457.

Saku T, Shibata Y, Cheng J et al (1990) Autoantibodies to keratin in Sjögren's syndrome. *J Oral Pathol Med* **19**, 45–48.

Sandberg-Wollheim M, Axell T, Hansen BU et al (1992) Primary Sjögren's syndrome in patients with multiple sclerosis. *Neurology* **42**, 845–847.

Sato K, Miyasaka N, Nishioka K et al (1987) Primary Sjögren's syndrome associated with systemic vasculitis. *Arthritis Rheum* **30**, 717–718.

Shimode K, Kobayashi S, Kitani M et al (1986) Optic neuritis in primary Sjögren's syndrome. *Rinsho Shinkeigaku* **26**, 433–436.

Skopouli FN, Drosos AA, Papaioannou T et al (1986) Preliminary diagnostic criteria for Sjögren's syndrome. *Scand J Rheumatol* **61** (Suppl), 26–27.

Sobue G, Yasuda T, Kachi T et al (1993) Chronic progressive sensory ataxic neuropathy: Clinicopathological features of idiopathic and Sjögren's syndrome-associated cases. *J Neurol* **240**, 1–7.

Tesar JT, McMillan V, Molina R et al (1992) Optic neuropathy and central nervous system disease associated with primary Sjögren's syndrome. *Am J Med* **92**, 686–692.

Tzioufas AG, Moutsopoulos Hm and Talal N (1987) Lymphoid malignancy and monoclonal proteins. In: Talal N, Moutsopoulos HM and Kassan SS (eds) *Sjögren's Syndrome. Clinical and Immunological Aspects*, pp 129–136. Berlin: Springer.

Urban E, Jabbari B and Robles H (1994) Concurrent cerebral venous sinus thombosis and myelo-radiculopathy in Sjögren's syndrome. *Neurology* **44**, 554–556.

van Dijk GW, Notermans NC, Kater L et al (1997) Sjögren's syndrome in patients with chronic idiopathic axonal polyneuropathy. *J Neurol Neurosurg Psychiat* **63**, 376–378.

Vincent D, Lozon P, Awada A et al (1985) Paralysies multiples et récidivantes des nerf craniën. Syndromes de Gougerot-Sjögren. *Rev Neurol (Paris)* **141**, 318–321.

Visser LH, Koudstaal PJ and van de Merwe JP (1993) Hemiparkinsonism in a patient with primary Sjögren's syndrome. A case report and a review of the literature. *Clin Neurol Neurosurg* **95**, 141–145.

Vitali C, Bombardieri S, Moutsopoulos HM et al (1993) Preliminary criteria for the classification of Sjögren's syndrome. Results of a prospective concerted action supported by the European Community. *Arthritis Rheum* **36**, 340–347.

Vrethem M, Lindvall VM, Holmgren H et al (1990) Neuropathy and myopathy in primary Sjögren's syndrome; neurophysiological, immunological and muscle biopsy results. *Acta Neurol Scand* **82**, 126–131.

Wise CM and Agudelo CA (1988) Optic neuropathy as an initial manifestation of Sjögren's syndrome. *J Rheumatol* **15**, 799–802.

Youinou P and Pennec Y (1987) Immunopathological features of primary Sjögren's syndrome. *Clin Exp Rheumatol* **5**, 173–194.

12

Relapsing Polychondritis, Polymyalgia Rheumatica, Undifferentiated Connective Tissue Disease, Overlap Syndromes and Mixed Connective Tissue Disease

INTRODUCTION

This chapter is devoted to five disorders. The first two are entities on their own and the last three are mutually related. The first disorder is relapsing polychondritis, which is an auto-immune disease primarily of cartilagenous tissues. Next, follows polymyalgia rheumatica, which is not a muscle disease as the name erroneously suggests but a disorder of bursae, synoviae, and tendons. The chapter closes with descriptions of mixed connective tissue disease (MCTD), overlap syndromes, and undifferentiated connective tissue disease (UCTD), which are a group of disorders related to each other and to several other inflammatory connective tissue diseases (ICTDs).

RELAPSING POLYCHONDRITIS

Relapsing polychondritis is a rare and remarkable disease of unknown aetiology that is characterized by episodes of inflammation of cartilagenous structures and tissues rich in glycosaminoglycans (see Maddison, 1998). Figures on incidence and prevalence are not available. A series of patients with relapsing polychondritis diagnosed in the Mayo Clinics and published retrospectively is approximately 50% longer than a comparable series of patients with Churg-Strauss vasculitis from the same centre (Michet *et al.*, 1986) (see also Chap. 5). Relapsing polychondritis may affect subjects of all races and individuals older than 30 years in particular. It is considered to be an immunological disorder because of its relapsing and remitting course, its association with other auto-immune diseases in approximately 30% of patients (rheumatoid arthritis, systemic lupus erythematosus, Sjögren's syndrome, thyroiditis, ulcerative colitis and others), and because of the presence of antibodies against type II collagen in 50% and of ANCA and ANA in 24% and 20% respectively (McAdam *et al.*, 1976). Circulating immune complexes are demonstrable in most patients. The description of a neonate who was born from a mother with relapsing polychondritis and who had features of the disease that recovered spontaneously is also in favour of an auto-immune origin (see Maddison, 1998). At microscopy, biopsies from inflamed pinnae show infiltrates composed of neutrophils, lymphocytes, macrophages, and plasma cells.

CLINICAL CHARACTERISTICS

The organs involved in this disorder are manifold as shown in Box 12.1. Vessel occlusion is uncommon, even in patients with anticardiolipin antibodies (ACAs) (present in eight of 21 patients) (Zeuner *et al.*, 1998). There is an association of relapsing polychondritis with myelodysplastic processes (see Case Records of the Massachusetts General Hospital, case 38, 1997).

Box 12.1 Organs involved in relapsing polychondritis

1. Episodes of inflammation of cartilagenous portion of one or both ears (Fig. 12.1). This is the most frequent sign of the disease and often the presenting sign. It is present in 80–90% of patients.
2. Episodes of inflammation of cartilagenous portion of the nose resulting, in some cases, in a saddle nose. Less frequent than number 1, but still present overall in approximately 50%. In a minority of patients it is a presenting sign.
3. Inflammation and breakdown of laryngeal and tracheal cartilage. Approximately similar in frequency as number 2.
4. Arthralgia and mostly nonerosive arthritis of large and small joints. Approximately similar in frequency as numbers 2 and 3.
5. Inflammation of the eyes causing episcleritis, cornea thinning, uveitis, retinal vasculitis, optic neuritis, orbital inflammation, inflammation of orbital muscles, and papilloedema. Approximately similar in frequency as numbers 2, 3, and 4, but is less often the presenting sign.
6. Involvement of the inner ear with cochlear and vestibular dysfunction. Develops in 25–45% of patients, but usually not from onset.
7. A wide range of non-specific skin changes with leucocytoclastic vasculitis. Develops in 1/3rd of patients. Usually not present from onset.
8. Renal manifestations with necrotizing glomerulonephritis. Develops in 10–20% of patients.
9. Heart involvement with aortic insufficiency either from dilatation of the aortic root or valvular destruction. Also present are pericarditis, myocarditis, heart block, and aorta aneurysm. Develops in approximately 10%.
10. Vasculitis involving large and medium-sized vessels. In approximately 5–10%.
11. Seldom CNS involvement.

Data from Michet *et al.* (1986) and Maddison (1998).

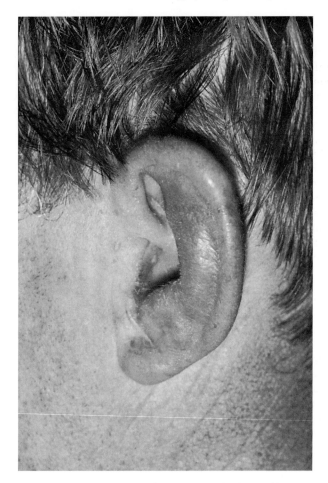

Figure 12.1 Relapsing polychondritis. Inflammation of left ear. (Courtesy of Prof. Wim A. van Vloten.)

DIAGNOSIS, COURSE AND TREATMENT

McAdam *et al.* (1976) proposed that the presence of three or more of the following would be diagnostic for the disease: recurrent chondritis of both ears; non-erosive polyarthritis; chondritis of the nasal cartilage; ocular inflammation including conjunctivitis, keratitis, scleritis, episcleritis, uveitis; involvement of laryngeal and tracheal cartilage; and cochlear and vestibular involvement. Michet *et al.* (1986) used the follow-up data from 112 patients, all diagnosed in the Mayo Clinics, to define the natural history and outcome of the disease. The probabilities of survival five and 10 years after diagnosis were 74 and 55%. Maddison (1998) suggested that the actual figures might be much more favourable, because mild cases of relapsing polychondritis were likely to go unrecognized.

Effects of treatment are not easy to establish because of the relapsing nature of the disease. Mild symptoms are often treated empirically with non-steroidal anti-inflammatory drugs (NSAIDs), and more severe manifestations are treated with oral prednisone. The prednisone-effect varies for different manifestations. General features of inflammation often respond quickly, but hearing loss is mostly definite. Prospective intervention studies have not been performed.

NEUROLOGICAL ASPECTS OF RELAPSING POLYCHONDRITIS

In handbooks, neurological manifestations of relapsing polychondritis are stated to be rare (Maddison, 1998; Zeuner *et al.* 1997). In part, this view is based on the retrospective analysis done in the Mayo Clinics by Michet *et al.* (1986): neurological manifestations in the 112 patients diagnosed are not described, and among 41 causes of death only one, an intracranial abscess, is obviously neurological.

In a literature search by Sundaram and Rajput (1983), reports were found on 10 patients (mean age 44, range 20–58 years) with neurological abnormalities. These abnormalities concerned optic neuritis and extra-ocular palsies in six cases; aphasia and hemiparesis in two; seizures and mental disorders that were not due to other concomitant disorders in one; and deafness in three. Two of the deaf patients had gait ataxia and VIIth nerve palsy. Since 1983, at least 15 other cases with neurological symptoms have been reported (Sundaram and Rajput, 1983; Willis *et al.*, 1984; Hull and Morgan, 1984; Brod and Boose, 1988; Hashimoto *et al.*, 1988; Stewart *et al.*, 1988; Wasserfallen and Schaller, 1992; Hanslik *et al.*, 1994; Berg *et al.*, 1996; Ragnaud *et al.*, 1996; Watanabe *et al.*, 1997; Othmani *et al.*, 1997). Data on 10 of these cases are given in Table 12.1. From the descriptions, it appears that in most patients onset of neurological abnormalities is acute with fever, signs of relapsing polychondritis, and a raised erythrocyte sedimentation rate (ESR). Nearly all patients have evidence of aseptic meningitis, often with mental abnormalities indicating implication of cortical structures. Several patients have hearing loss, mostly in combination with cerebellar ataxia, facial palsy, or nystagmus, which is apparently due to involvement of infratentorial structures. Few patients have bilateral pyramidal abnormalities due either to brainstem or spinal cord disorders. Neuro-imaging has not been done in all cases. MRI has shown, in one case, meningeal enhancement that is compatible with inflammatory changes of the meninges and hydrocephalus and, in another case, multiple small lesions predominantly in the white matter that are perhaps due to vasculitis. In one case, a brain and meningeal biopsy has revealed meningeal infiltration by lymphocytes, and an autopsy investigation has provided evidence of small and medium vessel vasculitis in the brain in one other case.

Management of neurological manifestations. The rarity of neurological manifestations in a disease that itself is also rare has precluded a systematic therapeutic approach. Aseptic meningitis is treated with oral corticosteroids and antituberculous medication. When evidence of meningeal inflammation is lacking, only corticosteroids are given. Organic brain syndrome and delirium are treated as described in Chapter 7.

POLYMYALGIA RHEUMATICA (PMR)

In contrast to what the name suggests, this disease is not due to myopathy or myositis but to inflammatory changes of synovia, tendon sheaths, and bursae (Salvarini *et*

Table 12.1 Summary of clinical data from 10 patients with relapsing polychondritis

Authors	Gender and age	Clinical features	Laboratory
Berg et al., 1996	Male, 60 yrs	Headache, hearing loss, ataxia, decreased short term memory	CSF: pleocytosis (200 WBC/mm³). Protein content raised (1.4/g/l). Gadolinium MRI: meningeal enhancement, hydrocephalus
Ragnaud et al., 1996	Male, 70 yrs	Bilateral hearing loss, meningitis, 6 episodes	CSF: pleocytosis and raised protein content
Hanslik et al., 1994	Female, 70 yrs	Headache, confusion, memory disturbance	CSF: slight pleocytosis and protein increase. MRI T2-Wi, multiple bilateral: white matter hypersignals
Wasserfallen and Schaller, 1992	Female, 73 yrs	Right-sided ptosis, R.* facial palsy, R. hearing loss, conjunctivitis, uveitis	CSF: 950 WBC/mm³, mostly PMN; protein 1 g/l.
Brod and Boose, 1988	Female, 30 yrs	Headache, hearing loss, dizziness, unsteady, wide-based gait	CSF: pleocytosis
Brod and Boose, 1988	Male, 75 yrs	Headache, mental changes, hearing loss, horizontal nystagmus, bilateral hyperreflexia and Babinski's	Biopsy meninges and brain: lymphocytic infiltration of meninges
Brod and Boose, 1988	Female, 60 yrs	Hearing loss	CSF: pleocytosis
Stewart et al., 1988	Male, 52 yrs	Headache, delirium, cognitive impairment, seizures, papilloedema, Babinski's	Autopsy: giant cell arteritis of the aorta abdominalis, brain necrotizing vasculitis of medium and small-sized vessels
Hull and Morgan, 1984	Male, 51 yrs	Confusion, cognitive impairment, cerebellar ataxia, hearing loss, facial weakness, horizontal nystagmus	CT scan: cerebral and cerebellar atrophy, old infarct occipital lobe
Sundaram and Rajput, 1983	Female, 58 yrs	Organic brain syndrome with visual hallucinations, rotatory and vertical nystagmus, right-sided facial palsy, hearing loss left, cerebellar ataxia	CT scan: transient low density in midbrain. CSF: normal

*R.= right-sided.

al., 1997a). It is a relatively common clinical syndrome that develops more often in females than males (ratio 2:1) and nearly always in subjects above the age of 50, similar to giant cell arteritis to which it is often associated. The inflammation does not only involve structures proximal in the limbs but, in a minority of patients, it is also distal, *e.g.* the synovia of the knees, wrists, and metacarpophalangeal joints. Distal inflammations are usually not severe and are self-limiting. Synovial biopsies reveal that the inflammatory infiltrates consist predominantly of CD68+ macrophages, more T-cells of CD4+ type than CD8+ type, a predominance of memory T-cells, and expression of HLA class-II antigens on synovial and inflammatory cells but not on endothelial cells (Meliconi *et al.*, 1996). How this inflammation arises is unknown. As in so many of the other ICTDs, theories on the aetiology concentrate on hereditary predisposition and on the role of an environmental factor, perhaps a viral infection. The high incidence of PMR among Scandinavians and Scandinavian descendants and the much lower incidence among those from the Mediterranean is interpreted as pointing to a genetic factor. In most patients with PMR, no other illness is found. When an associated process can be identified, giant cell arteritis (GCA) is by far the most common. Biopsy studies of the temporal artery in population-based studies reveal an incidence of GCA in patients with PMR of approximately 12% (see Salvarini *et al.*, 1997b, and Chapter 5, *Giant Cell Arteritis*).

CLINICAL AND LABORATORY FINDINGS

The hallmarks of the clinical picture are persistent pain or discomfort, with stiffness after a period of rest or in the morning for several hours, that is localized in the shoulders, the upper part of the upper limbs, and less often the neck and the pelvic girdle. These symptoms are, as a rule, bilateral though onset may be unilateral. A large minority of patients complain at onset about fatigue, weight loss, and lack of appetite. They may also have fever. The stiffness may impede movements to such a degree that patients feel forced to stay in bed. The clinical examination reveals little that is abnormal, except for the abnormal movement pattern. A minority of the patients (19 patients from a community-based cohort of 245) shows distal limb swelling with pitting oedema either in the upper, lower, or upper and lower limbs. Only one limb may be involved; however, usually multiple limbs are affected (Salvarini *et al.*, 1996a). Some patients have symptoms of carpal tunnel syndrome (CTS), perhaps as a consequence of wrist tenosynovitis (Salvarini *et al.*, 1996a; Herrera *et al.*, 1997).

Until not very long ago, PMR would not have been diagnosed definitely if the ESR was not markedly raised (above 40 mm/hour). Now, however, it appears that in up to 10 to 20% of patients with the typical clinical features of PMR, the ESR is normal. When it is normal, C reactive protein is often normal as well (Helfgott and Kieval, 1996; Ortiz and Tugwell, 1996; Salvarini *et al.*, 1996b). The typical clinical features are more important for the diagnosis than the laboratory findings!

Management. Randomized, placebo-controlled studies of different forms of treatment have not been performed. When symptoms are mild and do not cause changes in the patterns of living, one may start therapy by trying NSAIDs. A favourable response should be obtained within 2–4 weeks. When the effect of this approach is insufficient or when symptoms clearly derange the living pattern, low-dose corticosteroid medication is preferred. Salvarini *et al.* (1997b) advise to commence with

12.5 mg prednisone, once daily. In most cases this is sufficient. Occasionally, a higher dose is necessary to suppress symptoms fully. The effect of corticosteroids is, however, usually very striking, and some authors consider this response even as a criterion for the diagnosis (Healy, 1984). The duration of treatment has not been decided. Salvarini *et al.* (1997b) reduces the dose after one month when the response has been rapid and ESR is normal or has normalized. Decrease of the daily dose below 10 mg is done in steps of 1 mg per 2–4 weeks. In the first two years after onset of the disease, relapses are common and are independent of the corticosteroid reduction programme (Salvarini *et al.*, 1987). Side effects of corticosteroids are not to be underestimated, even when corticosteroid doses are low (see Chapter 4, *Corticosteroids*). At onset of therapy, the bone mineral density should be measured and when it is too low or appears to decrease at repeat measurement, measures should be taken to protect the bone tissue (see Table 4.4).

MCTD, OVERLAP SYNDROMES AND UCTD

It is estimated that in at least 25% of patients with features of ICTDs, the syndromes cannot be classified into one of the entities described so far (Calvo-Alen *et al.*, 1996). Three labels are available for these remaining disorders: (1) Mixed connective tissue disease has clinical characteristics of several other ICTDs and is associated with a specific serological feature that is decisive for the diagnosis; (2) the term overlap syndrome is used for conditions that comply to the criteria of two or more ICTDs; and (3) the term undifferentiated connective tissue disease is used when symptoms and signs are not sufficiently evolved for a definite diagnosis.

MIXED CONNECTIVE TISSUE DISEASE (MCTD)

MCTD was initially described as an ICTD with clinical features of SLE, sclero-derma, and polymyositis. Its characteristics were suggested to be absence of cerebral manifestations, renal disease, and vasculitis; a relatively benign course; good response to corticosteroids; a high titre of an anti-nuclear antibody (ANA), with a speckled pattern on indirect immunofluorescence; and a haemagglutina-tion reaction to a RNAse-sensitive component of a buffered saline-extracted nuclear antigen. The haemagglutination reaction appeared to be due to the pres-ence of an antibody against a subfraction of nuclear ribonuclear protein (U1RNP). The proposed clinical and laboratory features are summarized in Box 12.2. The syndrome, as delineated here, is reported to occur at any age, predomi-nantly from the 2nd to the 4th decade, but also in children, though this is less frequent than SLE and myositis. The large majority of affected persons is female (see Reichlin, 1997; Soriano and McHugh, 1998). The aetiology is not known; there are, however, speculations about a hereditary predisposition and a role of environmental factors, *e.g.* toxins like vinyl chloride. The pathology is insuffi-ciently studied. In handbook reviews, however, it is stated that a proliferative angiopathy of small and large arteries with narrowing of lumina is the most prominent histological feature. The pathology would resemble the angiopathy of scleroderma, though the associated perivascular fibrosis would be much less than in systemic sclerosis.

Box 12.2 Originally proposed clinical and laboratory core features of MCTD

1. Presence of Raynaud's phenomenon, arthralgia and arthritis, puffy hands, abnormal oesophageal motility, myositis and lymphadenopathy.
2. Absence of cerebral and renal disease and of vasculitis.
3. Favourable response to corticosteroid treatment.
4. Benign prognosis.
5. High titre of antibody against U1RNP.

From Maddison and Jablonska (1995), with permission.

Since the initial description, doubt on the existence of this syndrome has arisen and steadily increased for the following reasons:

1. The spectrum of clinical features is much wider than initially suggested. Arthritis is sometimes erosive and deforming and may be associated with the presence of multiple subcutaneous (rheumatic) nodules near tendons in hands and forearms. SLE or dermatomyositis-like skin changes may occur. Some patients develop serositis, mostly pericarditis, and some have verrucous thickenings of anterior valvular leaflets. Patients may have pulmonary hypertension, and many have evidence of interstitial pulmonary fibrosis.
2. The clinical features may gradually evolve to systemic sclerosis or SLE.
3. The prognosis is less benign than initially conceived. Fatal cases due to renal vascular disease (as in sclerodermia), cardiac failure, and progressive vasculopathy have been reported (Mier *et al.*, 1996). CNS manifestations are indeed rare, but are not absent (see below), and the association of MCTD with vasculitis has been documented (Black and Isenberg, 1992).
4. Antibodies against U1RNP may disappear during the course of MCTD. Approximately 50% of patients with antibodies against U1RNP have no features of MCTD.
5. In studies of series of patients with overlap syndromes that are defined by clinical criteria, differences between patients with and without anti-U1RNP are not obvious.

Some authors feel, therefore, that MCTD is just a form of UCTD or is not different from other overlap syndromes (Leroy *et al.*, 1980).

Diagnosis and management. Though the concept of MCTD is contested, several sets of classification criteria have been proposed. The simplest of these is presented in Table 12.2.

Intervention studies in MCTD have not been performed and therefore therapy is entirely determined by the experience of experts and by what has become customary. NSAIDs and anti-malarials are used for mild conditions and corticosteroids and cytostatic agents for more severe manifestations, as specified in Chapter 4 on guidelines for immunotherapy.

Neurological manifestations in MCTD
Subclinical myositis is frequent and suggested to be present in up to 2/3rd of all these patients. The percentage of patients with weakness due to myositis is much lower (Table 12.3). Second in frequency in MCTD is trigeminal neuropathy, which

Table 12.2 Classification criteria for mixed connective tissue disease proposed by Alarcon-Segovia *et al.*, 1987

Serological criterion	Clinical criteria
Positive anti-U1RNP at a haemagglutination titre of 1:1600 or higher	Oedema of the hands
	Raynaud's phenomenon (2 or 3 colour phase)
	Acrosclerosis
	Synovitis
	Myositis (laboratory or biopsy proven)

Requirements for diagnosis: 1. serological, 2. at least 3 clinical criteria, 3. the association of oedema of the hands, Raynaud's phenomenon, and acrosclerosis requires at least 1 of the other two criteria. From Kater and Provost (1995), with permission.

Table 12.3 Neurological and myological manifestations in MCTD

Estimated incidence	Manifestations	References
Relatively high	Clinical evidence of myositis (10–25%)	Maddison and Jablonska, 1995; Mier *et al.*, 1996; Soriano and McHugh, 1998.
	Trigeminal neuropathy (up to 10%)	Bennet and O'Connell, 1980; Lazaro *et al.*, 1989; Hagen *et al.*, 1990; Hughes, 1993
	Peripheral neuropathy (up to 10%)	Bennet and O'Connell, 1980; Olney, 1992; Katada *et al.*, 1997
Low	Psychosis	Bennet and O'Connell, 1980; Alarcon *et al.*, 1991
	Seizures	Bennet and O'Connell, 1980; Alarcon *et al.*, 1991
	Aseptic/pachymeningitis	Bennet and O'Connell, 1980; Singsen *et al.*, 1977; Fujimoto *et al.*, 1993
	Transverse myelitis or myelopathy	Weiss *et al.*, 1978; Pedersen *et al.*, 1987; Lazaro *et al.*, 1989
Single case reports, e.g.:	Intracerebral haemorrhage	Graf *et al.*, 1993
	Large vessel occlusion	Graf *et al.*, 1993
	Optic neuropathy	Gressel and Tomsak, 1983
	Atlanto-axial subluxation	Stuart and Maddison, 1991; Pirainen, 1990

is estimated to occur in up to 10% of patients. Some patients present with symptoms of aseptic meningitis and develop other features of MCTD subsequently. Other brain and spinal cord manifestations are all rare (Maddison and Jablonska, 1995). An axonal form of polyneuropathy is, however, not very exceptional, and acute radiculopolyneuropathy and mononeuritis multiplex have been reported also (Katada *et al.*, 1997; Lazaro *et al.*, 1989). There are also single case reports on combinations of MCTD with focal myositis, pravastatin-induced rhabdomyolysis, choreoathetosis, cerebellar syndrome, white matter lesions, large vessel occlusion, and other abnormalities (McKenna *et al.*, 1986; Schneider, 1991; Graf *et al.*, 1993; Hino *et al.*, 1996; Rivest *et al.*, 1996; (see also Table 12.1)).

In recent publications, attention is drawn to the rarity of clotting events and other manifestations of Hughes' (antiphospholipid) syndrome, despite the fact that ACAs occur more frequently in patients with MCTD than in controls. Two possible explanations have been put forward: ACAs in MCTD are usually not directed to phospholipid binding β_2 glycoproteins, and ACA titres in MCTD are relatively low in contrast to ACAs in SLE and Hughes' syndrome (Komatireddy *et al.*, 1997; Mendonca *et al.*, 1998).

Management of neurological complications. The neurological manifestations of MCTD occur in a similar fashion to those in SLE and require a similar treatment. For more extensive descriptions of these manifestations, see Chapters 2 and 7; for their management see Chapters 4 and 7. Therapy of myositis is described in Chapter 6.

OVERLAP SYNDROMES

Patients with overlap syndromes comply to the criteria for two or more ICTDs, *e.g.* rheumatoid arthritis and SLE (Brand *et al.*, 1992) or SLE and Sjögren's syndrome (see Chapter 11). They may reveal the neurological manifestations that are associated with each of these diseases. The combination of scleroderma and myositis is not uncommon (Venables, 1996). Occasional patients show combinations of RA, Sjögren's syndrome, SLE, and scleroderma, with or without myositis.

Scleromyositis
Myositis or dermatomyositis (DM) in patients with scleroderma does, according to Maddison and Jablonska (1995), often (in ± 50% of adults) not give rise to elevated levels of serum CK activity. Visceral involvement is reported to be less frequent and less severe than in other patients with scleroderma. The course of scleromyositis is variable and often benign, even with regression of myositis symptoms. Patients with anti-PM/Scl antibodies have either scleroderma or scleroderma and polymyositis. The antibody is directed against a nucleolar protein complex of 11–16 polypeptides of unknown function.

UNDIFFERENTIATED CONNECTIVE TISSUE DISEASE (UCTD)

UCTD is defined as a condition with clinical manifestations suggestive of connective tissue disease in association with the presence of at least one non-organ specific auto-antibody (ANA, anti-dsDNA, or anti-extractable nuclear antigen antibodies). The literature on UCTD has recently been summarized by Mosca *et al.* (1998). Onset of symptoms may occur in any decade, and the large majority of patients are female. The most frequent clinical manifestations are presented in Box 12.3.

Neuropsychiatrical abnormalities comprise seizures, personality changes, psychosis, cranial nerve palsy, and peripheral neuropathies. These abnormalities commonly remain in the background and are present, at least in the first year of the disease, in no more than approximately 15% of patients (Alarcon *et al.*, 1991). In 10–15% of patients, the disease progresses within 1–8 years to SLE. In the majority, the disease remains unclassifiable, and exhibits a relatively mild and stable course

Box 12.3 Clinical and serological features of UCTD

---

1. Clinical features: arthralgia, Raynaud's phenomenon, arthritis, leukopenia, sicca symptoms, alopecia, photosensitivity
2. Specific antinuclear antibodies are present in the majority: anti-Ro/SS-A, anti-RNP, anti-Sm (rarely)
3. Undefined antinuclear antibodies are found in a minority

---

with little change in the antibody profile (Mosca *et al.*, 1998; Calvo-Alen *et al.*, 1996; Ganczarczyk *et al.*, 1989; Greer and Pannush, 1989). Treatment remains often limited to NSAIDs, antimalarials, or low-dose steroids.

REFERENCES

Alarcon GS, Williams GV, Singer JZ *et al* (1991) Early undifferentiated connective tissue diseases. I Early clinical manifestations in a large cohort of patients with undifferentiated tissue diseases compared with cohorts of well established connective tissue disease. *J Rheumatol* **18**, 1332–1339.

Bennett RM and O'Connell DJ (1980) Mixed connective tissue disease: A clinicopathologic study of 20 cases. *Sem Arthritis Rheum* **10**, 25–51.

Berg AM, Kasznica J, Hopkins P *et al* (1996) Relapsing polychondritis and aseptic meningitis. *J Rheumatol* **23**, 567–569.

Black C and Isenberg DA (1992) Mixed connective tissue disease – goodbye to all that. *Br J Rheumatol* **31**, 695–700.

Brand CA, Rowley MJ, Tait BD *et al* (1992) Co-existent rheumatoid arthritis and systemic lupus erythematosus: Clinical, serological and phenotypic features. *Ann Rheum Dis* **51**, 173–176.

Brod S and Boose J (1988) Idiopathic CSF phagocytosis in relapsing polychondritis. *Neurology* **38**, 322–323.

Calvo-Alen J, Alarcon GS, Burgard SL *et al* (1996) Systemic lupus erythematosus: Predictors of its occurrence among a cohort of patients with early undifferentiated connective tissue disease: Multivariate analyses and identification of risk factors. *J Rheumatol* **23**, 469–475.

Ganczarczyk L, Urowitz MB and Gladman DD (1989) 'Latent lupus'. *J Rheumatol* **16**, 475–478.

Case records of the Massachusetts General Hospital. Weekly clinicopathological exercises. Case 38 (1997) Inflammation of the ears, anemia and fever 21 years after treatment for Hodgkin's disease. *N Engl J Med* **337**, 1753–1760.

Graf WD, Milstein JM and Sherry DD (1993) Stroke and mixed connective tissue disease. *J Child Neurol* **8**, 256–259.

Greer JM and Panush RS (1989) Incomplete lupus. *Arch Intern Med* **149**, 2473–2481.

Gressel MG and Tomsak RL (1983) Recurrent bilateral optic neuropathy in mixed connective tissue disease. *J Clin Neuro-Ophthalmology* **3**, 101–104.

Fujimoto M, Kira J, Murai H *et al* (1993) Hypertrophic cranial pachymeningitis associated with mixed connective tissue disease: A comparison with idiopathic and infectious pachymeningitis. *Intern Med* **32**, 510–512.

Hagen NA, Stevens JC and Michet CJ (1990) Trigeminal sensory neuropathy associated with connective tissue diseases. *Neurology* **40**, 891–896.

Hanslik T, Wechsler B, Piette J-C *et al* (1994) Central nervous system involvement in relapsing polychondritis. *Clin Exp Rheumatology* **12**, 539–541.

Hashimoto K, Masahari S and Sakuta M (1988) A case of relapsing polychondritis with neurological symptoms and abnormal CSF findings. *Clin Neurol* **28**, 1004–1007.

Healy LA (1984) Long-term follow-up of polymyalgia rheumatica: Evidence for synovitis. *Sem Arthritis Rheum* **13**, 322–328.

Helfgott SM and Kieval RI (1996) Polymyalgia rheumatica in patients with a normal erythrocyte sedimentation rate. *Arthritis Rheum* **39**, 304–307.

Herrera B, Sanmarti R, Ponce A *et al* (1997) Carpal tunnel syndrome heralding polymyalgia rheumatica. *Scand J Rheumatol* **26**, 222–224.

Hino I, Akama H, Furuya T *et al* (1996) Pravastatin-induced rhabdomyolysis in a patient with mixed connective tissue disease. *Arthritis Rheum* **39**, 1259–1260.

Hughes RAC (1993) Diseases of the fifth cranial nerve. In: Dyck PJ, Thomas PK, Griffin JW *et al* (eds), *Peripheral Neuropathy*, 3rd ed, pp 801–817. Philadelphia: WB Saunders.

Hull RG and Morgan SH (1984) The nervous system and relapsing polychondritis. *Neurology* **34**, 557.

Katada E, Ojika K, Uemura M *et al* (1997) Mixed connective tissue disease associated with acute polyradiculoneuropathy. *Intern Med* **36**, 118–124.

Kater L and Provost TT (1995) Classification criteria, disease activity criteria and chronicity criteria. In: Kater L and Baart de la Faille H (eds) *Multi-Systemic Auto-Immune Diseases: An Integrated Approach*, pp 43–59. Amsterdam: Elsevier.

Komatireddy GR, Wang GS, Sharp GC *et al* (1997) Antiphospholipid antibodies among anti-U1-70 kDa autoantibody positive patients with mixed connective tissue disease. *J Rheumatol* **24**, 319–322.

Lazaro MA, Maldonado Cocco JA, Catoggio LJ *et al* (1989) Clinical and serologic characteristics of patients with overlap syndrome: Is mixed connective tissue disease a distinct clinical entity? *Medicine* **68**, 58–65.

Leroy EC, Maricq HR and Kahalch MB (1980) Undifferentiated connective tissue syndromes. *Arthritis Rheum* **23**, 341–343.

Maddison PJ (1998) Diseases of bone, cartilage and synovium. In: Maddison PJ, Isenberg DA, Woo P *et al* (eds) *Oxford Textbook of Rheumatology*, 2nd ed, pp 1624–1629. Oxford: Oxford University Press.

Maddison PJ and Jablonska S (1995) Overlap syndromes. In: Kater L and Baart de la Faille H (eds) *Multi-Systemic Autoimmune Diseases*, pp 227–240. Amsterdam: Elsevier.

McAdam LP, O'Hanlan MA, Bluestone R *et al* (1976) Relapsing polychondritis: Prospective study of 23 patients and a review of the literature. *Medicine (Baltimore)* **55**, 193–215.

McKenna F, Eccles J and Neumann VC (1986) Neuropsychiatric disorders in mixed connective tissue disease. *Br J Rheumatol* **25**, 225–226.

Meliconi R, Pulsatelli L, Uguccioni M *et al* (1996) Leucocyte infiltration in synovial tissue from the shoulder of patients with polymyalgia rheumatica. Quantitative analysis and influence of corticosteroid treatment. *Arthritis Rheum* **39**, 1199–1207.

Mendonca LL, Amengual O, Atsumi O *et al* (1998) Most anticardiolipin antibodies in mixed connective tissue disease are beta 2-glycoprotein independent (letter). *J Rheumatol* **25**, 189–190.

Mier R, Ansell B, Hall MA *et al* (1996) Long term follow-up of children with mixed connective tissue disease. *Lupus* **5**, 221–226.

Michet CJ, McKenna CH, Harvindrer S *et al* (1986) Relapsing polychondritis. Survival and predictive role of early disease manifestations. *Ann Int Medicine* **104**, 74–78.

Mosca M, Tavoni A, Neri R *et al* (1998) Undifferentiated connective tissue diseases: The clinical and serological profiles of 91 patients followed for at least 1 year. *Lupus* **7**, 95–100.

Olney RK (1992) AAEM Minimonograph #38: Neuropathies in connective tissue disease. *Muscle Nerve* **15**, 985–988.

Ortiz Z and Tugwell P (1996) Raised ESR in polymyalgia rheumatica no longer a sine qua non? *Lancet* **348**, 4–5.

Othmani S, Bahri N, Louzir B *et al* (1997) Complications neurologique de la polychondrite atrophiante. *Ann Med Interne Paris* **148**, 509–511.

Pedersen C, Bonen H and Boesen F (1987) Transverse myelitis in mixed connective tissue disease. *Arthritis Rheum* **20**, 985–988.

Pirainen HI (1990) Patients with arthritis and anti-U1RNP antibodies: A 10-year follow-up. *Br J Rheumatology* **29**, 345–348.

Ragnaud JM, Tahbar A, Morlat P *et al* (1996) Recurrent aseptic purulent meningitis in a patient with relapsing polychondritis. *Clin Infect* **22**, 374–375.

Reichlin M (1997) Undifferentiated connective tissue diseases, overlap syndromes and mixed connective tissue diseases. In: Koopman WJ (ed) *Arthritis and Allied Conditions. A Textbook of Rheumatology*, 13th ed, pp 1309–1318. Baltimore: Williams and Wilkins.

Rivest C, Miller FW, Love LA *et al* (1996) Focal myositis presenting as pseudothrombophlebitis of the neck in a patient with mixed connective tissue disease. *Arthritis Rheum* **39**, 1254–1258.

Salvarini C, Macchioni PL, Tartoni PL *et al* (1987) Polymyalgia rheumatica and giant cell arteritis: A 5-year epidemiologic and clinical study in Reggio Emilia, Italy. *Clin Exp Rheumatol* **5**, 205–215.

Salvarini C, Gabriel S, Hunder GG (1996a) Distal extremity swelling with pitting edema in polymyalgia rheumatica. Report of nineteen cases. *Arthritis Rheum* **39**, 73–80.

Salvarini C, Boiardi L, Macchioni L *et al* (1996b) Polymyalgia rheumatica. Letter. *Lancet* **348**, 550–551.

Salvarini C, Macchioni P and Boiardi L (1997a) Polymyalgia rheumatica. Seminar. *Lancet* **350**, 43–47.

Salvarini C, Cantini F, Olivieri I *et al* (1997b) Proximal bursitis in active polymyalgia rheumatica. *Ann Intern Med* **127**, 27–31.

Schneider F (1991) Progressive multifocale leukencephalopathie als ursache neurologischer symptomatik bei Sharp-syndrom. *Z Rheumatol* **50**, 222–224.

Singsen BH, Kornreich HK and Koster-King K (1977) Mixed connective tissue disease in children. *Arthritis Rheum* **20**, 355–360.

Soriano ER and McHugh NJ (1998) Overlap syndromes in adults and children. In: Maddison PJ, Isenberg DA, Woo P *et al* (eds) *Oxford Textbook of Rheumatology*, 2nd edn, pp 1413–1432. Oxford: Oxford University Press.

Stewart SS, Ashizawa T, Dudley JAW *et al* (1988) Cerebral vasculitis in relapsing polychondritis. *Neurology* **38**, 150–152.

Stuart RA and Maddison PJ (1991) Atlantoaxial subluxation in a patient with mixed connective tissue disease. *J Rheumatol* **18**, 1617–1620.

Sundaram MBM and Rajput AH (1983) Nervous system complications of relapsing polychondritis. *Neurology* **33**, 513–515.

Taborcias D, Rubiales A, Altadill A et al (1996) Policondritis recidivante y meningoencephalitis. *Med Clin Barc* **107**, 597–598.

Venables PJ (1996) Polymyositis-associated overlap syndromes (editorial). *Br J Rheumatol* **35**, 305–306.

Wasserfallen JB and Schaller MD (1992) Unusual rhombencephalitis in relapsing polychondritis. *Ann Rheum Dis* **51**, 1184.

Watanabe T, Yasuda Y, Tanaka H *et al* (1997) Relapsing polychondritis with mental disorders: A case report. *Rinsho-Shinkeigaku* **37**, 243–248.

Weiss TD, Nelson JS, Woolsey RM *et al* (1978) Transverse myelitis in mixed connective tissue disease. *Arthritis Rheum* **21**, 982–986.

Willis J, Atack EA and Kraag G (1984) Relapsing polychondritis with multifocal neurological abnormalities. *Can J Neurol Sci* **11**, 402–404.

Zeuner M, Straub RH, Rauh G *et al* (1997) Relapsing polychondritis: clinical and immunogenetic analysis of 62 patients. *J Rheumatol* **24**, 96–101.

Zeuner M, Straub RH, Schlosser U *et al* (1998) Anti-phospholipid-antibodies in patients with relapsing polychondritis. *Lupus* **7**, 12–14.

Index

Note: Page numbers in *italics* refer to Figures; those in **bold** refer to Tables